ESSENTIALS OF
CLINICAL ONCOLOGY

ESSENTIALS OF CLINICAL ONCOLOGY

SECOND EDITION

AMIL SHAH, MDCM FRCPC FACP

Medical Oncologist, British Columbia Cancer Agency
Clinical Professor of Medicine
University of British Columbia
Vancouver, Canada

Somerset Publishing
Vancouver, Canada

Published in Canada in 2008
Somerset Publishing
1691 Somerset Crescent
Vancouver, BC
Canada V6M 1S3

The contents in this book are believed to be true and accurate at the date of publication, and the author or publisher accepts no legal responsibility or liability for any errors or omissions. The reader is requested to review and evaluate the information provided in the package insert or instructions for each drug before administering any of the drugs recommended in this book.

Canadian Library Cataloguing-in-Publication Data

A catalogue record for this book is available from the Canadian Library
ISBN 9780973579703

Medical Illustrators: Jane Rowlands and Ken Smith
Cover Design: Adam Tanner
Typesetting/Book Design: Adam Tanner and Eye Candy Creative

For ordering and customer service, contact Somerset Publishing at somersetpublishing@shaw.ca or by Fax 604.877.0585

1 2 3 4 5 6 7 8 9 10

Printed in Canada

PREFACE

Essentials of Clinical Oncology is a concise book written primarily for the undergraduate medical student, who needs a synopsis of the material included in the large, standard textbooks of oncology. It also has obvious usefulness for the postgraduate physician who is looking for an initial survey of the subject, and for the family doctor or generalist, who needs a brief and easily located summary of present oncology practice. In addition, it is hoped that this overview of oncology will be a good source of information for other health care professionals.

The emphasis is on the principles of clinical oncology practice with inclusion of the recent advances in the field as well as the theoretical concepts of obvious merit. The book is divided into three sections. The first section introduces the science that forms the basis of modern treatment; the second deals with the general approach to diagnosis and management; and the third reviews the clinical details and management of the common cancers.

I thank Drs. Kaushik Bhagat and Dorothy Harrison for the radiological images. I am also grateful to Drs. David Owen and John Hay for their input in the chapters on cancer pathology and treatment.

Vancouver, Canada
June 2008

TABLE OF CONTENTS

Chapter 1

CANCER EPIDEMIOLOGY

KEY POINTS

- Cancer is a major health problem globally
- In North America, four cancers – lung, breast, prostate and colorectal cancers – account for almost 50% of all cancer cases
- Lung cancer is the leading cause of cancer deaths in both men and women
- Lifestyles, personal habits and environmental exposure account for the majority of cancers, and some of these, especially cigarette smoking, are avoidable
- Screening for early cancer can reduce deaths from cervical, breast and colorectal cancers
- Chemoprevention by natural or synthetic compounds is promising for some cancers

THE CANCER BURDEN

Cancer is a major health problem worldwide. The distribution of the different types of cancer varies from one region to the next, but the burden in both developed and developing countries is high. To some extent, this is due to the relatively advanced age to which people now live, since cancer is more common in older persons. The median age at diagnosis of cancer is 67 years; Table 1.1 shows the age distribution at diagnosis.

Table 1.1 Age distribution of cancer

Age group	Percent of cancer
<20	1.1
20-34	2.7
35-44	5.9
45-54	13.6
55-64	20.9
65-74	25.8
75-84	22.6
>85	7.4

Tables 1.2 and 1.3 (pages 2 and 3) show the incidence and mortality rates of the major cancers in Canada (2007) and the United States (2007). The estimated number of new cases of cancer in 2007 in Canada is 159,900, and the number of deaths is 72,700; in the US, the number of new cases is 1,444,920, and the number of deaths is 559,650.

Four types of cancer account for at least 50% of new cancer cases: breast, lung and colorectal cancers in women, and prostate, lung and colorectal cancers in men. Table 1.4 shows the risk of developing one of these cancers over a lifetime. Lung cancer is the leading cause of cancer deaths in both men and women, accounting for over one-quarter of cancer deaths.

Table 1.4 Estimates of lifetime risk of cancers

Site	Risk	
	Men	Women
Lung	1 in 12	1 in 16
Breast	1 in 1200	1 in 9
Prostate	1 in 8	-
Colorectum	1 in 14	1 in 16

TRENDS IN INCIDENCE AND MORTALITY

Among men, the cancer incidence rose in the early 1990s because of the sharp increase in the incidence of prostate cancer, but has since been slowly decreasing. Cancer mortality for all cancers reached a peak in 1988, and has declined by 4% since then due primarily to a decrease in mortality rates for lung, colorectal and certain other cancers. Among women, since

1989, the cancer incidence has risen slightly, but has been declining since 2001. Overall, cancer mortality has declined about 3% since 1990. If lung cancer is excluded, the cancer mortality rates for women have fallen by 20% since 1978.

Lung cancer

Following a steady increase in incidence and mortality rates for several decades, the number of new lung cancer cases in men has been declining since the mid-1980s, and death rates have dropped since 1994. On the contrary, the incidence and mortality rates from lung cancer in women have increased in the past three decades, reflecting an increase in smoking among women since the 1940s. However, due to the decline in smoking rates among women, the number of new lung cancer cases may be levelling off.

Table 1.2 Estimated new cases and deaths in Canada 2007

	New Cases			Deaths		
	M	F	Total	M	F	Total
All cancers	**82700**	**77200**	**159900**	**38400**	**34300**	**72700**
Lung	12400	10900	23300	11000	8900	19900
Breast	170	22300	22470	50	5300	5350
Prostate	22300	0	22300	4300	0	4300
Colorectum	11400	9400	20800	4700	4000	8700
Non-Hodgkin's lymphoma	3700	3100	6800	1700	1400	3100
Bladder	5000	1700	6700	1250	520	1770
Kidney	3000	1800	4800	1000	620	1620
Melanoma	2500	2100	4600	560	340	900
Leukemia	2500	1750	4200	1400	980	2400
Uterus	0	4100	4100	0	740	740
Thyroid	790	2900	3700	65	110	175
Pancreas	1750	1850	3600	1750	1850	3600
Oral	2100	1050	3150	740	360	1100
Stomach	1850	1000	2850	1150	730	1880
Brain	1450	1150	2600	980	740	1720
Ovary	0	2400	2400	0	1700	1700
Multiple myeloma	1100	900	2000	530	470	1000
Esophagus	1150	410	1560	1300	430	1730
Liver	1050	310	1360	510	150	660
Cervix	0	1350	1350	0	390	390
Larynx	950	220	1170	420	90	510
Hodgkin's lymphoma	480	400	880	65	50	115
Testis	830	0	830	30	0	30
Other sites	6300	6000	12300	4900	4400	9300

(Excludes basal and squamous cell skin cancers and in situ carcinomas)
Source: National Cancer Institute of Canada Cancer Statistics 2007 http://www.cancer.ca

Breast cancer

Over the past three decades, breast cancer incidence showed a small but steady increase, but has levelled off since 1999. Much of this may be attributable to the introduction of screening mammography. Mortality rates have declined steadily since 1986, likely due to earlier diagnosis through screening and improved treatment.

Prostate cancer

Prostate cancer incidence showed a rapid increase for several years due to early detection of cases by Prostate Specific Antigen (PSA) measurements, but the incidence has declined since the mid-1990s. Mortality rates have also peaked between 1991 and 1995, and have since declined.

Table 1.3 Estimated new cases and deaths in US in 2007

	New Cases			Deaths		
	M	F	Total	M	F	Total
All cancers	**766860**	**678060**	**1444920**	**289550**	**270100**	**559650**
Prostate	218890	0	218890	27050	0	27050
Lung	114760	98620	213380	89510	70880	160390
Breast	2030	178480	180510	450	40460	40910
Colorectum	79130	74630	153760	26000	26180	52180
Bladder	50040	17120	67160	9630	4120	13750
Non-Hodgkin's lymphoma	34200	28990	63190	9600	9060	18660
Melanoma	33910	26030	59940	5220	2890	8110
Kidney	31590	19600	51190	8080	4810	12890
Leukemia	24800	19440	44240	12320	9470	21790
Uterus	0	39080	39080	0	7400	7400
Pancreas	18830	18340	37170	16840	16530	33370
Oral	24180	10180	34360	5180	2370	7550
Thyroid	8070	25480	33550	650	880	1530
Ovary	0	22430	22430	0	15280	15280
Stomach	13000	8260	21260	6610	4600	11210
Brain	11170	9330	20500	7150	5590	12740
Multiple myeloma	10960	8940	19900	5550	5240	10790
Liver	13650	5510	19160	11280	5500	16780
Esophagus	12130	3430	15560	10900	3040	13940
Larynx	8960	2340	11300	2900	760	3660
Cervix	0	11150	11150	0	3670	3670
Hodgkin's lymphoma	4470	3720	8190	770	300	1070
Testis	7920	0	7920	380	0	380
Other sites	44170	46960	91130	38660	31070	69730

(Excludes basal and squamous cell skin cancers and in situ carcinomas)
Source: American Cancer Society http://www.cancer.org/docroot/STT/stt_0.asp

Colorectal cancer

Colorectal cancer is the third most common cancer in men and women and the second leading cause of all cancer deaths. The incidence rates have been stable between 1994 and 2003. There is a decrease in mortality rates in both sexes, probably due to earlier diagnosis and better treatment.

Non-Hodgkin's lymphomas

Non-Hodgkin's lymphomas are the fifth most common cancer for both men and women. The incidence rates increased by 50% between 1978 and the late 1990s, but have since stabilized. Mortality rates have shown a similar trend, although there is a significant decline in men since 1999.

Other cancers

Five other cancers that have increased in incidence in the past few decades are kidney cancer, skin melanoma, thyroid cancer, liver cancer and testicular cancer. Although some of these increases could be due to better diagnosis and reporting, a real increase in incidence is probable. There has been a significant decrease in gastric cancer since the early 1900s, but recently cancer of the gastro-esophageal junction has been increasing sharply. In addition, incidence rates of larynx cancer and cervical cancer are declining. The mortality rates for Hodgkin's lymphoma have declined since 1970, whereas the incidence remains stable. Despite a small increase in incidence of testicular cancer, mortality rates have decline since 1994.

CANCER RISK FACTORS

A risk factor is an aspect of personal behavior or lifestyle, an environmental exposure, or an inborn or inherited characteristic, which is known to be associated with a particular cancer type. Risk factors can be identified through various methods.

• Descriptive/ecological study

This is an uncontrolled study based on the experience of individual physicians, hospitals and registries, in which the units of analysis are populations or groups of people, rather than individuals. An example is the study of association between median income and cancer mortality rates in administrative jurisdictions, such as provinces or states or counties.

• Case-control study

Case-control study refers to a retrospective, observational study of persons with the disease (cases) and a suitable control group of persons without the disease, in which the past history of exposure to the suspected risk factor is compared between "cases" and "controls."

• Cohort study

A cohort study is a prospective, observational study in which large numbers of persons, initially without disease, are followed over a long period of time with comparison of incidence rates of disease in groups that differ in exposure levels to the factor of interest.

• Intervention study

Interventional study involves an intentional change in some aspect of the status of the subjects, e.g. introduction of a preventive or therapeutic regimen, such as in a randomized, controlled trial.

In order to establish causation, several criteria must be satisfied. First, there must be a good level of evidence that the suspected risk factor is the cause of the disease. The different types of studies provide an indication of the level of evidence; from weakest to strongest, they are: descriptive studies, case-control studies, cohort studies and intervention studies. Second, there must be a recognized association between the disease occurrence and the risk factor; the strength of this association is defined as relative risk. Third, a consistency of association between the disease and risk factor must be observed. Fourth, a dose-response relationship must be documented; different levels of exposure to the risk factor result in proportional risks of cancer development. Fifth, a temporal relationship between exposure and cancer formation is required. Finally, there must be a biologically plausible mechanism to explain the association of the suspected risk factor and the disease.

A number of risk factors are implicated in the formation of the common cancers. They are broadly divided into environmental factors and genetic factors. While a large majority of cancers are due to environmental causes, and in theory, therefore, avoidable, these are not always clearly identified for the common cancers. For example, they can include a wide range of dietary, social and cultural habits, and this makes it difficult to recommend specific preventive strategies. Table 1.5 lists the recognized environmental risk factors.

Table 1.5 Risk estimates for the main causes of cancer mortality

Risk Factor	Estimate (%)
Tobacco	30
Diet	35
Infective processes	10
Reproductive & sexual behavior	7
Occupation	4
Geophysical factors	3
Alcohol	3

Source: Doll R, Peto R. The causes of cancer. Oxford University Press, Oxford, England, 1981.

CANCER CONTROL

Although cancer risk factors are not all specifically defined, some are clearly related to cancer and avoidance of these can reduce the cancer incidence. This is primary prevention. A cogent example is the risk of lung cancer from tobacco smoking. When a clear causative factor is not identifiable, the cancer mortality can be reduced by finding the disease at an early, potentially curable stage. This is secondary prevention or screening. A new area of active investigation is the suppression or reversal of carcinogenesis by specific compounds; this is chemoprevention.

PRIMARY PREVENTION

Tobacco

Tobacco smoking is the largest, single avoidable cause of cancer in North America as well as the rest of the world. It is estimated that 30% of cancers are caused by tobacco smoking. In addition to lung cancer, carcinogens in tobacco smoke have been linked to cancers of the oral cavity, larynx, esophagus, pancreas, bladder and kidney. Recently, the importance of second-hand or environmental tobacco smoke exposure as a cause of cancer has been recognized, and an increasing number of lung cancers are due to passive inhalation of cigarette smoke.

Diet and nutritional factors

Interest in the role of diet and nutritional factors as the cause of cancer arose from international comparisons of estimated national per capita food consumption with cancer death rates. As the epidemiological methodology improved, certain correlations emerged.

- A diet high in fat as well as red meat is associated with increased rates of breast,

colorectal, uterine, renal and, probably, prostate cancer
- High consumption of fruits and vegetables is associated with reduced rates of cancers of lung, oral cavity, larynx, esophagus, bladder and stomach
- Obesity with an increased body mass index is associated with an increased risk for cancers of the breast, colon, uterus, esophagus and kidney

In addition, certain carcinogens are now recognized in food; some are a natural part of the foodstuffs, while others are produced by cooking or through microbial contamination. For example, N-nitroso compounds are found in salted, smoked or pickled meat and have been implicated in stomach cancer. Also, alfatoxins, produced by Aspergillus molds on the surface of corn or ground nuts, can lead to the development of hepatocellular carcinoma.

Infections

A number of infections are implicated in the formation of some cancers.
- Human papillomavirus (HPV) with cervical and other anogenital cancers as well as oropharyngeal cancers
- Hepatitis B (HBV) and C (HCV) with hepatocellular carcinoma
- Human T-cell lymphotropic virus (HTLV-I) with adult T-cell leukemia
- Human herpesvirus 8 (HHV-8) with Kaposi's sarcoma and primary effusion lymphoma
- Epstein-Barr virus (EBV) with Burkitt's lymphoma, B-cell lymphomas, mixed cellularity Hodgkin's lymphoma, nasopharyngeal cancers and some gastric cancers
- *Helicobacter pylori* with gastric cancer and MALToma
- *Schistosoma* with bladder cancer
- *Opisthorchis* with cholangiocarcinoma
- *Clonorchis* with cholangiocarcinoma

In addition, some infections contribute indirectly to oncogenesis. For example, the human immunodeficiency virus (HIV) induces immunosuppression, which results in the emergence of other virus-related malignancies.

Some of these cancers, such as hepatocellular, cervical and stomach cancers, are major health problems in less developed countries, and successful eradication or control of the infections associated with them can have a significant impact in reducing their incidence. For example, in Taiwan, universal vaccination against hepatitis B in infants, who contract the virus from their mothers, was introduced in the 1980s. This has brought about a drastic reduction of persistent HBV infection with a consequent marked decline in the incidence of hepatocellular cancer among children. Similarly, vaccination against HPV 16 and 18 have shown promising results in prevention of persistent HPV infection and early precursors lesions of cervical cancer.

Hormonal and reproductive factors

Hormonal and reproductive factors influence the development of cancers of breast, uterus and ovary. Breast cancer risk is increased in women who are nulliparous and in those with late age of menopause. Oral contraceptive use and postmenopausal estrogen replacement therapy are associated with a small increase in the risk of breast cancer. Uterine cancer risk is increased in women who use oral contraceptive or estrogen replacement therapy containing unopposed estrogens; however, use of the combination of estrogen and progesterone reduces the risk. Ovarian cancer risk is increased among women with low parity, but is decreased in women who use oral contraceptives.

Sexual behavior

Certain risk factors for uterine cervical cancer are associated with sexual behavior. Early age of first sexual activity and multiple sexual partners, especially with men who themselves had multiple partners, increase the risk. This may be related to the transmission of the human papillomavirus (HPV). Presence of HPV appears to be necessary for development of both squamous cell and adenocarcinoma of the cervix. HPV-16 accounts for 50% of cervical cancers, and HPV-18 accounts for an additional 15-20% of cases.

Sunlight exposure

Cancers of the skin are caused by excessive sun exposure. Malignant melanoma of the skin has increased sharply in many developed countries, likely due to intense, intermittent recreational sun exposure from sunbathing or outdoor sports. Individuals at higher risk have multiple nevi, fair hair color and show a tendency for sunburn without tanning.

Occupational exposures

Several risk factors and chemicals have been identified in the workplace that may incite cancer formation. Chief among these are ionizing radiation and asbestos.

Alcohol

Alcohol has been implicated in cancers of the oral cavity, pharynx, larynx and esophagus. By itself, alcohol is a weak carcinogen, but it exerts a synergistic effect in combination with tobacco smoke. Alcoholic cirrhosis increases the risk for hepatocellular cancer.

SECONDARY PREVENTION

Cancer can be detected at an early stage through a screening test. Screening is the search for disease in asymptomatic persons. An asymptomatic person is someone who does not have symptoms or who does not recognize the symptoms as being related to disease. The World Health Organization criteria for a successful screening program include:

- The disease being screened for should be a common and important health problem
- There must be an effective treatment for patients suffering from localized disease
- There must be an identifiable latent or early asymptomatic stage of the disease
- The natural history of the disease, including the progression from the latent phase to clinical disease, must be sufficiently known
- The technique to be used for screening must be effective and acceptable to the general population being screened
- The expense of screening must be acceptable

Breast cancer

Between the ages of 20 and 39 years, women should undergo clinical breast examination every three years, and annually after age 40 years. Annual screening by mammography can reduce mortality by 25-40% in women between 40 and 79 years of age. The results for screening women under 50 years of age are somewhat controversial. The controversy arises, in part, from the decreased sensitivity of mammography in dense breasts in younger women. Nonetheless, regular screening is recommended for women over 40 years.

Colorectal cancer

There are several options for colorectal cancer screening and the choice depends on individual risks and preference. Screening should begin at age 50 years for average risk persons. At present, the strongest evidence points to the use of guaiac-based fecal occult blood testing (FOBT) as a screening test for colorectal cancer. Annual FOBT significantly reduces mortality rates from colorectal cancer by 33%; biennial FOBT screening produces a smaller reduction in mortality rates, about 15-18%. The high false positive rates for FOBT have led to a debate about the optimal method of colorectal cancer screening. A newer fecal immunochemical test (FIT) has the potential advantage to increase the specificity of testing, since it detects only human hemoglobin and not food sources of blood. In addition, because blood from the upper gastrointestinal tract is digested before it reaches the colon, bleeding at this site is not picked up by FIT. Sigmoidoscopy, with or without annual FOBT, every 5 years or colonoscopy every 10 years are other options for screening. One clear advantage of endoscopic screening is the potential to remove the precursor polyps, which over time could also reduce the incidence of the cancer.

Cervical cancer

Screening for cervical cancer by examination of a cervical smear, called the Papanicolaou or Pap smear, reduces mortality from cervical cancer. For the conventional Pap smear, sensitivity is 30-87% and specificity is 86-100% for detection of cervical cancer and its precursors (cervical intraepithelial neoplasia). Cervical cancer is associated with human papillomavirus (HPV) infection, and detecting HPV is a potential screening tool. Because of the high sensitivity of HPV testing, a negative HPV test could allow a significant reduction in cervical screening frequency. Clinical trials are in progress to establish what role HPV testing may have as a primary screening tool in combination with cytology screening for women over 30 years of age.

The recent introduction of the HPV vaccine for adolescent women is anticipated to have a significant impact on their risk for cervical abnormalities. Information is not yet available on whether the approach to cervical cancer screening should be modified in women who have received an HPV vaccine. Until data are available, standard screening recommendations should be observed.

Prostate cancer

The use of PSA as a screening test for prostate cancer is being debated. The reason for the controversy is that the PSA test does not yet meet the generally accepted criteria for a screening test in that no scientifically valid study has shown a benefit in terms of men's survival rate. However, the PSA test is the best way to detect prostate cancer at an early stage of the disease, when there is a good chance of cure. Large-scale studies are underway to determine whether PSA testing can decrease prostate cancer mortality. Until the data from these are available, it is appropriate that men should be informed about the benefits and limitations of PSA testing for early detection of prostate cancer. A reasonable approach if a man chooses to have a PSA test is for it to be done annually for 2-3 years, and if normal and stable, it may then be done every 2-3 years.

Lung cancer

Screening for lung cancer by sputum cytology and/or chest x-ray has not been shown to be beneficial. With newer technology for lung imaging, such as low-dose helical CT scans, or detection of early neoplastic cells by molecular markers in the sputum, there is a resurgence of interest in lung cancer screening, but the data are preliminary. The US Preventive Services Task Force (USPSTF) concluded that current evidence was insufficient to recommend for, or against, screening for lung cancer.

Gastric cancer

Because of the high incidence of gastric cancer in regions such as eastern Asia and western South America, nationwide screening programs to detect gastric cancer have been implemented in countries such as Japan, Venezuela and Chile, and have led to some improvements in mortality associated with gastric cancer. In North America, the incidence of stomach cancer is much lower, and population screening is not recommended.

Ovarian cancer

Screening trials for ovarian cancer with tumor markers (CA125) and ultrasonography are in progress to determine whether either approach reduces mortality from ovarian cancer. Until the results of these studies are available, there is a consensus that women at average risk for ovarian cancer should not undergo screening by either method.

Endometrial cancer

There is insufficient evidence for routine screening for endometrial cancer in women at average risk or at somewhat increased risk because of use of unopposed estrogen therapy, tamoxifen therapy for cancer, late menopause, nulliparity, infertility or other risk factors.

Other cancers

Screening tests for oral cancer, nasopharyngeal cancer and neuroblastoma are undergoing evaluation.

The recommendations for early detection of cancer from the American Cancer Society are prudent guidelines for cancer screening in average-risk individuals (Table 1.6).

CHEMOPREVENTION

A new area of research is the use of natural or synthetic compounds to reverse or suppress carcinogenesis in the early or pre-malignant stage and, thus, prevent the development of invasive cancer. The basis of this is the multi-step process of cancer development, during which progression from the pre-malignant state to the fully malignant state can be arrested or even reversed pharmacologically. Chemoprevention can be considered in two categories: primary chemoprevention is directed at individuals with *de novo* pre-malignant lesions, while secondary chemoprevention is directed at cancer patients, who have undergone potentially curative therapy, to prevent recurrent disease. A wide range of compounds are undergoing testing for their chemopreventive properties.

Retinoids

Retinoids are vitamin A and its natural and synthetic analogues. They promote orderly growth and differentiation of epithelial cells, and in pharmacological doses they may reverse pre-malignant lesions. Preliminary data suggest that they may prevent the development of cancer in certain sites, such as the oral cavity, and reduce the occurrence of second primary cancers in individuals with a prior history of head and neck cancers. Retinoids may prevent skin cancer in certain high-risk persons, such as immunosuppressed patients or those with xeroderma pigmentosum.

On the contrary, retinoids, as well as alpha tocopherol or beta carotene, are not beneficial for primary or secondary chemoprevention of lung cancer in smokers and former smokers.

Aspirin and non-steroidal anti-inflammatory drugs (NSAIDS)

Regular use of aspirin or NSAIDs may reduce

Table 1.6 American Cancer Society recommendations for early detection of cancer in average-risk, asymptomatic persons

Cancer Site	Population	Test or Procedure	Frequency
Breast	Women age >20 years	Breast self-exam (BSE)	Beginning in their early 20s, women should be told about the benefits and limitations of BSE. The importance of prompt reporting of any new breast symptoms to a health professional should be emphasized. Women who choose to do BSE should receive instruction and have their technique reviewed on the occasion of a periodic health examination. It is acceptable for women to choose not to do BSE or to do BSE irregularly
		Clinical breast exam (CBE)	For women in their 20s and 30s, it is recommended that CBE be part of a periodic health examination, preferably at least every 3 years. Asymptomatic women aged >40 years should continue to receive CBE as part of a periodic health examination, preferably annually
		Mammography	Begin annual mammography at age 40 years
Colorectum	Men/women age >50 years	Fecal occult blood test (FOBT) or fecal immunochemical test (FIT)	Annual, starting at age 50 years
		or Flexible sigmoidoscopy	Every 5 years, starting at age 50 years
		or FOBT or FIT and flexible sigmoidoscopy	Annual FOBT or FIT and flexible sigmoidoscopy every 5 years, starting at age 50 years
		or Colonoscopy	Every 10 years, starting at age 50 years
		or Double-contrast barium enema	Every 5 years, starting at age 50 years
Prostate	Men age >50 years	Digital rectal exam (DRE) and Prostate Specific antigen (PSA)	PSA and DRE should be offered annually, starting at age 50 years for men who have a life expectancy of at least 10 years
Cervix	Women age >18 years	Papanicolaou (Pap) smear	Cervical cancer screening should begin approximately 3 years after a woman begins having vaginal intercourse, but no later than 21 years of age. Screening should be done every year with conventional Pap tests or every 2 years using liquid-based Pap tests. At or after age 30, women who have had 3 normal test results in a row may get screened every 2-3 years with cervical cytology (conventional or liquid-based Pap tests) alone, or every 3 years with a human papillomavirus DNA test plus cervical cytology. Women >70 years who have had 3 or more normal Pap tests and no abnormal Pap tests in the last 10 years and women who have had a total hysterectomy may choose to stop cervical cancer screening
Cancer-related	Men/women age >20 years		On the occasion of a periodic health examination, the cancer-related check-up should include examination for cancers of the thyroid, testicles, ovaries, lymph nodes, oral cavity, and skin, as well as health counselling about tobacco, sun exposure, diet and nutrition, risk factors, sexual practices, and environmental and occupational exposures

Source: Smith RA. Cancer Screening in the United States, 2007. CA Cancer J Clin. 2007;57:90-104

the risk of colon cancer and the precursor adenomatous polyps by 20-40% in average risk individuals. The benefit is observed in those who use these agents for a long time (>10 years) and in adequate doses (usually 4-6 tablets of aspirin per week). The NSAID Sulindac can reverse or prevent new polyp formation in individuals with familial adenomatous polyposis, a rare genetic condition in which affected persons form numerous colorectal polyps by age 20.

There is a small risk for hemorrhagic stroke and gastrointestinal bleeding with aspirin and increased cardiovascular risk with NSAIDs. Therefore, routine use of these drugs for chemoprevention in healthy people at average risk for colorectal cancer cannot be made until the results of ongoing prospective studies are available. Similarly, further studies are needed to understand the net benefits and risks in high-risk groups, such as those with familial adenomatous polyposis and hereditary nonpolyposis colorectal cancer or a personal history of colorectal cancer of adenoma.

Calcium

Calcium may prevent formation of colon cancer by binding to carcinogenic substances, such as fatty acids or bile acids. In addition, oral calcium reduces the proliferative rates of colonic mucosal cells. Multiple observational studies have demonstrated that higher calcium intake (either dietary or supplements) reduces the risk of colorectal cancer. There may be a minimum level of calcium intake, around 700 mg/day. However, the results of clinical trials are inconsistent and firm recommendations for the use of calcium as a chemopreventive agent must await further clinical trials. In contrast, other studies suggest that high calcium intake (>2000 mg/d) may increase the risk of prostate cancer and may be associated with advanced

and metastatic prostate cancer. It is speculated that high calcium levels may down-regulate the active form of vitamin D, thus interfering with vitamin D's proposed inhibition of tumor growth and metastasis.

Selenium

Selenium is an essential trace element with antioxidant properties. Deficiency of selenium has been correlated with cancers of the breast, colon, prostate, lung and bladder in several epidemiological studies, but the evidence for its chemopreventive potential is preliminary.

Lycopene

Lycopene is a carotenoid with antioxidative properties found in certain foods, such as tomatoes and strawberries. Preliminary studies suggest that lycopene may reduce prostate cancer risk.

Finasteride

Finasteride is a 5α-reductase inhibitor that inhibits the conversion of testosterone to its active metabolite, dihydrotestosterone. It is used in the treatment of benign prostatic hypertrophy and may be a potential chemopreventive agent for prostate cancer. A large, randomized study, the Prostate Cancer Prevention Trial (PCPT), demonstrated that finasteride produced a 25% reduction in the 7-year prevalence of prostate cancer in men over age 55 years with normal digital rectal examination and initial PSA <3 ng/mL. However, finasteride was associated with a slightly higher occurrence of prostate cancers with poor prognostic features. Several observations from the PCPT study data suggested that the increase in high-grade disease may have been due to detection bias rather than a change in the biology of the disease. Nonetheless, the routine prescription of finasteride as a chemopreventive agent for prostate cancer is not presently recommended. In contrast, finasteride is a useful drug for treatment of men with benign prostatic hypertrophy.

Tamoxifen and raloxifene

Tamoxifen acts as an anti-estrogenic agent in breast tissues. In postmenopausal women with previous breast cancer, treatment with tamoxifen can reduce the risk of development of a second primary breast cancer. In a large chemopreventive study, conducted by the US National Surgical Adjuvant Breast Project, tamoxifen decreased the likelihood of cancer development in women at high risk of breast cancer. Because tamoxifen causes a small increase in uterine cancer due to its pro-estrogenic action on uterine tissues, raloxifene, which lacks uterine pro-estrogenic activity, may be a better choice and studies of its efficacy are underway. The USPSTF concluded that, at present, there is fair evidence that treatment with tamoxifen can significantly reduce the risk for breast cancer in women at high risk for breast cancer and that the likelihood of benefit increases as the risk for breast cancer increases.

There is also consistent but less strong evidence for the benefit of raloxifene. While the balance of benefits and harms may be favorable for some high-risk women, neither tamoxifen nor raloxifene is recommended for women at low or average risk for breast cancer.

GENERAL RECOMMENDATIONS FOR CANCER PREVENTION

Many cancers are preventable. Basic lifestyle changes can have a significant impact on the rates of cancer. It is noteworthy that these recommendations are also applicable to other chronic diseases (cardiovascular disease, stroke and diabetes). General lifestyle recommendations include:

- Avoid tobacco
- Be physically active
- Maintain a healthy weight
- Eat a diet rich in fruits, vegetables, and whole grains, and low in saturated/trans fat
- Limit alcohol
- Protect against sexually transmitted infections
- Avoid excess sun
- Get regular screening

Chapter 2

CANCER GENETICS

KEY POINTS

- In normal cells, the cell cycle is tightly regulated and various checkpoints exist to ensure that the process is carried out accurately
- Cancer is a genetic disease caused by mutations in genes that control or regulate cell proliferation, cell differentiation and cell death
- Two classes of cancer genes have been identified: oncogenes and tumor suppressor genes
- Several genes become mutated and act in concert in the formation of a cancer
- Distinct heritable forms of cancer due to specific mutations have been identified

CELL CYCLE CONTROL

The adult human body comprises about 10^{15} cells. All of these arise from a single pluripotent cell, the zygote. Once full growth is achieved, a steady state is reached, and rates of cell birth and cell death are equal. It is important to realize that cells are continuously being produced to replace old or dying cells. Each day, about 10^{12} cells die and must be replaced to ensure homeostasis. Maintenance of cellular constancy is, therefore, a dynamic process and complex mechanisms are in place to achieve this.

Proliferating cells go through a series of phases during the cell cycle (Figure 2.1). Prior to cell division, the cellular DNA is replicated during the synthetic or S phase to produce an accurate copy of itself. This is followed by the mitotic or M phase, during which the proper distribution of chromosomes to the daughter cells takes place. Between the S and M phases are two other phases, called G or growth phases. G1 precedes S, and G2 precedes M. The boundaries between G1 and S, and G2 and M

are quality control checkpoints.

Cells cannot cross these checkpoints until certain conditions are met. During G1, typically the longest portion of the cell cycle, the cell is preparing for DNA replication, requiring a large pool of enzymes for nucleotide biosynthesis. Although entry into the S phase from the G1-S checkpoint requires coordination of multiple signals from the external environment, a key prerequisite is that cells repair any acquired DNA mutations before they can proceed from the G1 to S phase. The M phase is set in motion during G2. The chromosomes condense in preparation for distribution to the new daughter cells, and the proteins responsible for the physical division of the cell, e.g. those that form the mitotic spindle, are synthesized. To traverse the G2-M checkpoint, the proper conditions for chromosome segregation at mitosis must be in place.

Progression of the cell through the cell cycle is tightly regulated and is under the supervision of two classes of proteins: cyclins and cyclin-dependent kinases (CDKs). Cells have a family of ten CDKs that catalyze different cell cycle transitions. CDKs are activated by a family of cyclins, labelled as cyclins A to H. Different cyclins bind and activate different CDKs, and the activated cyclin-CDK complexes, in turn, phosphorylate various target proteins to control events in the cell cycle. Each member of the cyclin family is expressed briefly with peaks at a different phase in the cell cycle in the following sequence: cyclin D in early G1, E at the G1-S boundary, A during the S phase, and B at the G2-M boundary. Once a specific cyclin is produced, it activates its partner CDK, and following this activation, it is degraded

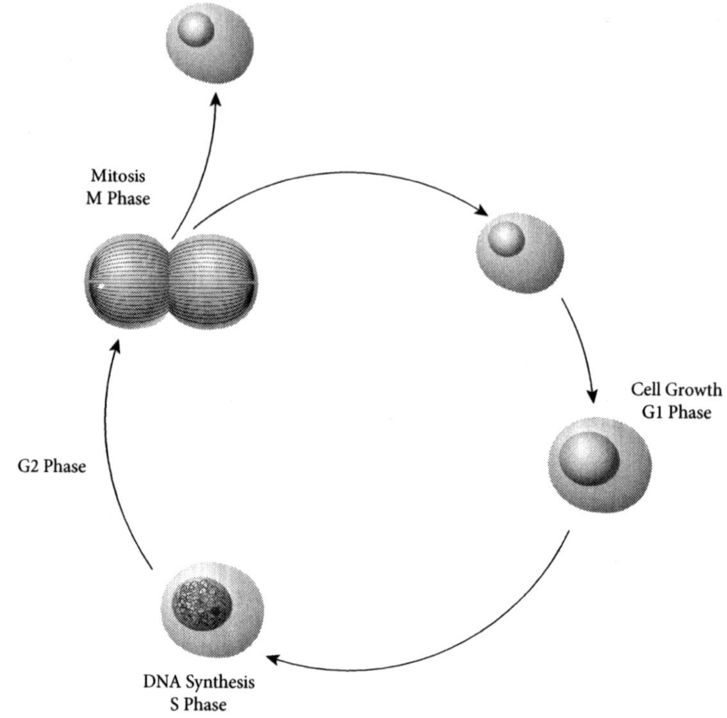

Figure 2.1 Phases of the cell cycle

Mitosis
M Phase

Cell Growth
G1 Phase

G2 Phase

DNA Synthesis
S Phase

rapidly by the ubiquitin proteasomal pathway. This ensures that specific CDKs are active only at specific times during the cell cycle. In addition to activation by cyclins, CDKs are also regulated by CDK inhibitory (CKI) proteins. There are two families of CKIs (kinase inhibitory proteins and inhibitors of CDK4), and over-expression of either causes arrest of the cell in G1.

Normal cells use the cell cycle checkpoints as fail-safe mechanisms to avoid the accumulation of genetic errors during cell division. Cells whose DNA does not pass these quality control checkpoints are diverted into programmed cell death or apoptotic pathways. This ensures that cells with major genetic defects commit suicide and are discarded. Apoptosis is a normal physiological process. It is critically important during embryogenesis, such as the apoptotic loss of cells in the web spaces between fingers and toes during the formation of the hands and feet. Apoptosis proceeds through a series of steps: there is nuclear condensation, cell membrane blebbing, and digestion of the DNA by an endonuclease into small fragments. DNA damage in a cell activates apoptosis and this represents a major protective mechanism against cancer. When this mechanism fails, mutations accumulate and these are passed on to the daughter cells, setting the stage for more mutations and abnormal cell growth.

The cell cycle is deregulated in cancer cells because of increased cyclin expression and inactivation of the CDK inhibitors. Importantly, cancer cells are able to bypass the cell cycle checkpoints even though their DNA is damaged, and this leads to an accumulation of mutations.

GENERAL CLASSES OF CANCER GENES

Cancer results from mutations in the genes that control cell proliferation, differentiation and death. Two classes of genes are intricately involved in these cellular processes: oncogenes and tumor suppressor genes.

ONCOGENES

Oncogenes are abnormally activated versions of normal genes, called proto-oncogenes, which are responsible for normal cell growth and proliferation. Normally, proto-oncogenes become activated in an orderly manner throughout life. They are operational during embryogenesis, growth and tissue repair. Once they have executed their function, however, they are turned off, and they are normally silent. When oncogenes are over-expressed, amplified or mutated, they cause cancer. Oncogenes act in a dominant fashion over the proto-oncogene, and abnormal expression of one copy is sufficient to cause its activation. Oncogenes are labelled by a three-letter code that is often derived from their source of discovery. For example, the first oncogene to be described was detected in chicken sarcoma and is designated src oncogene.

Mechanisms of oncogene activation

Oncogene activation can occur by a number of mechanisms.

- *Point mutation*

A point mutation in the gene leads to a protein product with an altered amino acid sequence. If this change occurs at a critical site, the protein's function can be severely altered. The ras oncogene, for example, becomes activated by a single point mutation, which causes a change in the amino acid sequence in the ras protein.

- *Gene amplification*

Gene amplification leads to multiple copies of the gene with consequent overproduction of its protein. In about 20% of breast cancer, the HER-2 gene is amplified with multiple copies in the breast cancer cells.

- *Chromosomal rearrangement or translocation*

Chromosomal rearrangement or translocation can bring a normally "silent" gene to a transcriptionally active area of another chromosome, causing it to be inadvertently activated. In Burkitt's lymphoma, a high-grade malignancy of B-lymphocytes, the intact myc gene is moved to an immunoglobulin (IG) locus. The strong transcriptional activity of the IG locus in antibody-producing Burkitt's lymphoma cells drives the inappropriate transcription of the myc gene.

A second way in which translocation can deregulate a gene is the formation of a chimeric gene. For example, in chronic myelogenous leukemia, a small portion of the long arms of chromosomes 9 and 22 are exchanged, giving rise to the Philadelphia chromosome. At the molecular level, this translocation t(9:22)(q34;q11) results in the abl proto-oncogene on chromosome 9 being placed next to the bcr (breakpoint cluster region) gene on chromosome 22. This leads to a novel bcr-abl fusion protein, which is more enzymatically potent than the abl protein.

- *Proviral insertion*

The genetic material of animal retroviruses can be inserted into the host genome. If this is near to a cellular proto-oncogene, the strong transcriptional promoters and enhancers of the retrovirus can lead to the proto-oncogene being transcribed inappropriately. While this mechanism is responsible for cancers in animals, it is uncertain if it plays a direct role in human cancers.

Function of oncogenic proteins

The oncogenic proteins form a diverse family that are responsible for the conveying or transduction of signals from the outside of the cell to the nucleus. The ability of cells to receive and respond to external signals is critical for the maintenance of the integrity of an organism. There is an elaborate network of highly regulated circuits, and it is estimated that more than 20% of the coding genes, or 6000 genes, are involved. The signal network is triggered by an external stimulus at the cell surface, followed by the activation of linked cytoplasmic and

nuclear biochemical cascades The transmission of the signal is mediated by proteins, called kinases, which transfer phosphate groups from ATP to the side chains of proteins that contain tyrosine, serine and threonine. This process of phosphorylation activates the protein.

The signal transduction pathways control cellular events, such as cell proliferation, differentiation and cell death. There are four levels at which the oncogenic proteins operate: as extracellular growth factors, cell surface receptors, intracellular messengers and nuclear transcription activators. Another function of oncogenic proteins is anti-apoptosis. Figure 2.2 is a schematic representation of a signal transduction pathway that exists in cells.

- *Extracellular growth factors*

In multi-cellular organisms, cell proliferation

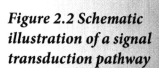

Figure 2.2 Schematic illustration of a signal transduction pathway

Epidermal growth factor binds to its receptor, leading to a cascade of events with eventual activation of DNA transcription

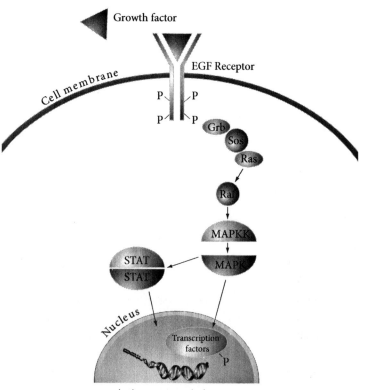

is regulated by secreted proteins, called growth factors or cytokines. If present in abnormal amounts, they provoke excessive cell proliferation by stimulating certain biochemical changes, such as increased tyrosine phosphorylation and altered lipid metabolism, in the cell. Most growth factors are small polypeptide chains. An example is the platelet-derived growth factor or PDGF, which is the protein product of the sis oncogene.

• *Growth factor receptors*

Several oncogenes code for proteins that are surface receptors which span the cell membrane. A common property of the trans-membrane receptors is their ability to phosphorylate themselves as well as other cytoplasmic proteins at tyrosine residues in the presence of their respective growth factors. They are referred to

as receptor protein tyrosine kinases or RPTKs, and a number of RPTK families have been identified. An example is the epidermal growth factor receptor (EGFR) family that comprises four members: EGFR, HER-2, ERBB-3 and ERBB-4

Binding of a growth factor to its receptor results in the pairing of the receptor with another, a process called dimerization (Figure 2.3). Dimerization leads to conformational changes in the receptors that allow each receptor to phosphorylate the other at tyrosine residues. This, in turn, opens up new binding sites in its cytoplasmic portion. As a result, new docking sites are created for other downstream signalling molecules. A cascade of events is set in motion that ultimately activates DNA replication and transcription.

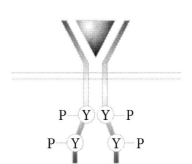

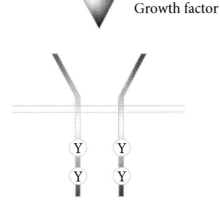

Figure 2.3 Growth factor receptor dimerization and activation

In some cancers, the receptor protein may be altered through a mutation that causes it to exist in an "activated" state even in the absence of any growth factor. Alternatively, the receptors may be present in increased amounts. In either case, the result is the inappropriate activation of cellular pathways that lead to abnormal cell proliferation.

For example the HER-2 protein is over-expressed in approximately 20% of breast cancers due to multiple gene duplication in the chromosome (gene amplification). The overabundance of HER-2 protein on the cell surface leads to a perturbation of signal transduction, tricking the cell into rapid growth.

• Intracellular cytoplasmic messengers

Signalling downstream from the surface receptors is accomplished through the interactions of cytoplasmic proteins. They transmit signals from the cell surface through the cytoplasm to the nucleus. Several unique and overlapping signal transduction pathways can be activated in the process. The pathways that are downstream from the ras protein are a good example of aberrant signal transduction. Ras phosphorylates Raf-1 kinase, which, in turn, phosphorylates MEK1 that then activates ERK1 and ERK2. Mutation or over-expression of the ras protein is present in up to 30% of cancers. Mutation of the ras protein causes it to be trapped in an "activated" state, and it is in the "on" position continuously. The result is the abnormal transmission of growth signals to the cell nucleus.

• *DNA transcription factors*

The transcription of genes is regulated by several transcription factors, which can activate or repress gene expression by binding to specific regions in DNA. The proteins of several oncogenes are localized in the nucleus and play a key role in oncogenesis.

• *Anti-apoptotic proteins*

Apoptosis is controlled by a regulatory network of signalling pathways. An example is the B-cell lymphoma gene-2 (bcl-2 oncogene), which is over-expressed in some cancers. BCL-2 belongs to a family of proteins that includes other pro-survival proteins, such as Bcl-XL and Mcl-1, and pro-apoptotic proteins, such as Bax and Bid. The ratio of members of these two groups determines how the cell responds to growth signals. BCL-2 is over-expressed in leukemias and lymphomas and some other cancers like breast, colon, lung and skin cancers.

The intercellular and intracellular signalling network is complex. For each group of growth factors and receptors, there may be distinct or shared signalling pathways. As a result, there is considerable "cross-talk" between the pathways, emphasizing the elasticity of the system and its consequent vulnerability to perturbations.

TUMOR SUPPRESSOR GENES

Tumor suppressor genes normally suppress cell growth. Unlike oncogenes that act in a dominant manner, it is the loss of function of tumor suppressor genes that leads to uncontrolled cell proliferation. Thus, in cancer cells, expression of tumor suppressor genes is turned off. Another important requirement is that both alleles of the gene must be inactivated to promote the formation of a cancer, and loss of a single allele is, by itself, insufficient.

The genetic material in all cells is made up of equal contribution from the maternal and paternal chromosomes. Small DNA sequence differences, referred to as polymorphism, exist between the pairs of chromosomes. This is termed heterozygosity, and it is of little or no significance, accounting for traits like skin or hair color. In cancers, one allele of a tumor suppressor gene may be mutated, and its normal counterpart is replaced by a defective one, resulting in the absence of polymorphism, termed loss of heterozygosity or LOH (Figure 2.4).

Functions of tumor suppressor genes

More than 20 tumor suppressor genes have been identified. They can be broadly subdivided into two groups: gatekeepers and caretakers. Some tumor suppressor genes belong to both groups. Normally, gatekeeper genes counteract cell proliferation and promote cell death. Mutations of these genes facilitate tumor growth and are

Figure 2.4 Mechanisms of loss of heterozygosity

A mutated gene is present in one chromosome (light grey region). Loss of heterozygosity occurs when the second allele is lost by large deletion, recombination or non-dysjunction and duplication of the remaining copy

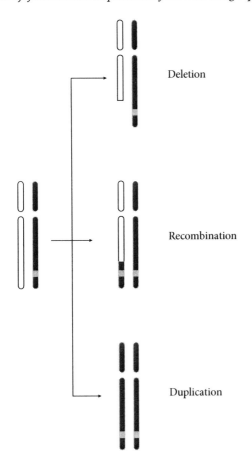

Deletion

Recombination

Duplication

frequently found in both hereditary and sporadic cancers. Caretaker genes are responsible for maintaining genomic stability. It is essential for normal cells to protect and maintain the integrity of its genome, the repository of their genetic information.

Mutations in genes responsible for maintaining genomic stability are important for neoplastic transformation. The formation of a cancer requires several, sequential mutations

to accumulate in a cell. The rate of spontaneous mutation is 10^{-5}-10^{-6}. The probability for two random mutations occurring in a single cell is 10^{-10}-10^{-12}; for three mutations, it is 10^{-15}-10^{-18}. Seen from this perspective, cancer development would be an improbable event; hence, the acquisition of genomic instability appears to be a key prerequisite. Inborn genetic defects in caretaker genes are also frequently associated with inherited cancers.

A number tumor suppressor genes serve as checkpoint controls at different phases of the cell cycle, and they block progression of the cell to the next phase until DNA damage is repaired. Their inactivation contributes to the formation of a cancer by allowing accumulation of DNA changes that would normally have resulted in cell cycle arrest and DNA repair, or cell death. For example, the p53 gene operates between G1 and S; the ATM gene between S and G2; and the RAD and MEC genes between G2 and M. Other cell cycle pathways (MAD, BUB) check for proper attachment of chromosomes to the mitotic spindle, and they delay mitosis if this has not taken place correctly. Mutations in these genes increase the frequency of non-disjunction. Other checkpoint pathways monitor cell growth, cytokinesis and centrosome duplication, and they prevent cell cycle progression if these events are executed incorrectly.

Mechanisms of tumor suppressor inactivation

There are several ways by which tumor suppressor genes can be inactivated.

- *Point mutation or small deletion*

Point mutations or small deletions are commonly found in cancers. In the APC gene, which is mutated in familial adenomatous polyposis, point mutations lead to truncation of the APC protein. The APC gene is also mutated in the sporadic form of colorectal cancer. Likewise, point mutations in the BRCA genes in hereditary breast cancer produce a similar outcome with truncation of their proteins and consequent loss of their function.

- *Large chromosomal deletion or loss*

Large chromosomal deletion or loss of chromosomes can occasionally result in the loss of tumor suppressor genes.

- *Replacement of the normal allele*

Replacement of the normal allele with an abnormal allele may occur through gene conversion or sister chromatid exchange.

- *Gene silencing*

The promoter regions of genes can be silenced through hypermethylation. Frequently, the gene of one or another parent is hypermethylated so that one parental allele – the unmethylated allele – is expressed. In some cancers, the normal allele of a tumor suppressor gene can be inactivated by acquired methylation. For example, von Hippel-Landau disease (hemangioblastoma of the central nervous system and retina, renal cancer and pheochromocytoma) is due to alteration of the VHL tumor suppressor gene. One mechanism of its inactivation is hypermethylation of the normally unmethylated promoter region of VHL. This effectively silences the gene.

Examples of tumor suppressor genes

Rb tumor suppressor gene

A classic tumor suppressor gene is the retinoblastoma gene (rb gene), which plays a key role in cell cycle regulation. It was first described in retinoblastoma, a rare childhood cancer. There are two forms of the disease: an inherited form and a sporadic form. Children with the inherited form develop bilateral cancers at an earlier age

compared with those with the sporadic form. This observation led Knudson to predict that two rate-limiting genetic events or "hits" are required for the cancer to develop. Children with the inherited form of retinoblastoma inherit the first hit from a parent, and only one additional genetic event is, therefore, necessary for the cancer to develop. On the other hand, children with the sporadic form have to acquire both hits after birth, and they are, therefore, unlikely to have bilateral cancers, and they develop the cancer at an older age. This hypothesis can now be understood by the inactivation of both alleles of the rb gene. Children with the inherited form of retinoblastoma are born with one mutated rb gene and the other gene is inactivated by chromosomal deletion or rearrangement after birth. In contrast, children with the sporadic form are born with two functional rb genes, both of which become inactivated after birth. Although first described in a rare childhood cancer, inactivation of the rb gene is now identified in a variety of cancers.

p53 tumor suppressor gene

Another example of tumor suppressor genes is the p53 gene, which is implicated in many types of cancer. The p53 gene codes for a protein that functions as a checkpoint control within the cell cycle and prevents cells with DNA damage from proceeding from G1 to S. The normal p53 protein halts progress through the cell cycle until the DNA has been repaired. Loss of p53 in cancer cells allows cells with damaged DNA to proceed through mitosis and further propagate the mutations. The p53 protein not only inhibits cell cycle progression, but it is critical for the apoptotic pathway for cells with damaged DNA. From this, it is evident that cells with p53 mutations replicate despite DNA damage. Many of these replicating cells will not survive because of the grossly deranged genome, but a small number do survive and set in motion the development of a cancer.

Mismatch repair genes

During DNA replication, billions of nucleotides must be matched correctly. Occasional errors can occur, particularly in sections of the DNA with simple tandem repeats, called microsatellites. These are runs of approximately 4-40 repeated mononucleotides (e.g. TTTT) or dinucleotides (e.g. CACACA), which occur at multiple sites within the genome. Microsatellites are prone to copying errors because the polymerase enzyme that copies the DNA molecule may slip the occasional nucleotide. Normally, repair enzymes, coded by mismatch repair genes or MMR genes, scan the new DNA strand and repair the mistake by replacing the whole segment by matching it to the template strand. Some cancers have a tendency for microsatellite instability due to mutations in the MMR genes. The consequence of this is the accumulation of multiple mutations involving different genes. Mutations in any of six MMR genes are associated with hereditary nonpolyposis colon cancer (HNPCC) syndrome. Individuals with this disorder have a predilection to develop colon cancer as well as a variety of other cancers, such as ovarian and uterine cancers.

DEREGULATION OF THE CELL CYCLE IN CANCER

The cell cycle is deregulated in cancer. This is the result of up-regulation of cyclins or inactivation of CDK inhibitors. In addition, oncogenes and tumor suppressor genes are defective: oncogenes accelerate cell proliferation during G1; tumor suppressor genes malfunction as stop signals at the critical junctions in the cell cycle, and DNA mistakes are not repaired before the chromosomes condense in G2 for mitosis (Figure 2.5).

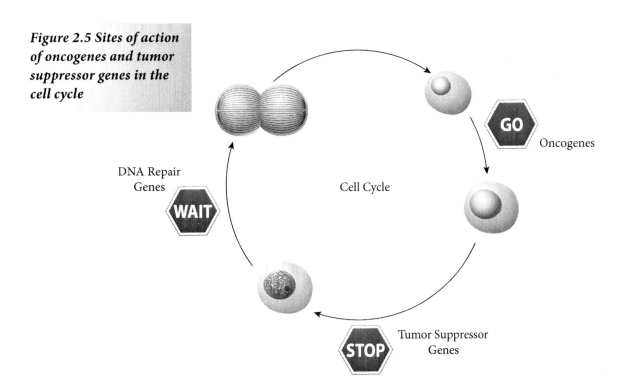

Figure 2.5 Sites of action of oncogenes and tumor suppressor genes in the cell cycle

DNA Repair Genes

WAIT

Cell Cycle

GO

Oncogenes

STOP

Tumor Suppressor Genes

These disrupted mechanisms overlap with dire consequences. As an example, following DNA damage, p53 brings about the arrest of the cell in G1 phase, allowing DNA repair before it enters S phase. p53 induces p21 protein, which blocks specific cyclin-CDK complexes that are important for proper G1-S cell cycle transition (Figure 2.6). These cyclin-CDK complexes normally phosphorylate the rb protein, and this allows the cell to progress past G1. A mutation in the p53 or p21 gene abolishes the inhibitory effect on the specific CDKs, allowing them to phosphorylate rb, which, in turn, removes rb block on cellular proliferation. Mutations of the rb gene can produce a similar outcome by directly subverting its control of events in the cell cycle.

Figure 2.6 Tumor suppressor genes and the cell cycle (see text)

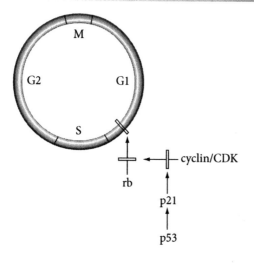

HEREDITARY CANCER SYNDROMES

Cancer is now recognized to be a genetic disease in the sense that it is caused by gene mutations. The majority of cancers are due to acquired gene mutations, i.e. somatic mutations. This should be distinguished from germ-line mutations that are passed from parent to offspring. A small proportion of the common cancers, about 5%, occur in individuals with a known germ-line mutation. The presence of a germ-line mutation should be suspected in the following situations:

- Presence of multiple cases of cancer in several related individuals
- Occurrence of multiple cancers in the same individual; for example, several colon cancers, or bilateral breast cancers, or breast and ovarian cancers
- Young age of onset of cancer
- Familial clustering of cancers that are normally rare in the general population

Many hereditary cancers are due to inheritance of mutated tumor suppressor genes. In these cases, one mutated allele is inherited, and the other allele becomes altered after birth (Knudson's two-hit hypothesis). In rare cases, such as multiple endocrine neoplasia type 2 (MEN-II) or familial papillary renal cancer, mutations in dominant oncogenes are responsible for the cancer syndrome. Table 2.1 lists some of the common hereditary cancer syndromes.

The two most common hereditary cancer syndromes are hereditary breast/ovarian cancer syndrome and hereditary nonpolyposis colon cancer syndrome.

Hereditary breast and ovarian cancer syndrome

Inheritance of mutated BRCA genes predisposes individuals to the development of breast and ovarian cancers. These genes are involved in DNA repair mechanisms. A single copy of BRCA-1 or BRCA-2 is sufficient for normal development, but inheritance of one copy of the mutated gene increases the susceptibility to loss of the other copy and the early development of breast or ovarian cancer.

Table 2.1 Common hereditary cancer syndromes

Cancer syndrome	Gene mutations
Breast/ovarian cancer	BRCA1, BRCA2
Hereditary nonpolyposis colon cancer	MSH2, MLH1, PMS1, PMS2, MSH6, MLH3
Familial adenomatous polyposis coli	APC
Multiple neuroendocrine tumor type I	MEN1
Multiple neuroendocrine tumor type II	RET
von Hippel-Landau disease	VHL
Retinoblastoma	rb
Li-Fraumeni syndrome	p53
Melanoma	P16, CDK4

Hereditary nonpolyposis colon cancer syndrome

Hereditary nonpolyposis colon cancer (HNPCC) syndrome is caused by a mutation in the MMR genes responsible for repair of DNA replication errors, termed DNA mismatch repair genes. During synthesis of new DNA strands, the DNA polymerase enzyme may create mismatches or loop-outs, which deform the DNA double helix. This is most likely to occur in segments of the DNA where there are simple tandem repeats or microsatellites. Repair of the DNA nucleotide mismatch involves at least six proteins, all of which are necessary to ensure that DNA mismatches are excised and repaired. The MMR enzymes recognize the abnormality and repair it by nucleotide excision, re-synthesis and ligation. If any of the six MMR genes is mutated, DNA repair is hampered and abnormal copies of genes are transmitted to the next generation of daughter cells. These mutations contribute to genomic instability and increase the likelihood of critical genes acquiring mutations. MMR gene mutations are associated with early onset of cancer development and multiple cancers, as in the HNPCC syndrome. About 2-4% of colorectal cancers are due to inheritance of a mutated MMR repair gene.

MULTI-STEP PROCESS OF CARCINOGENESIS

Several gene mutations are necessary for the full development of a cancer. Genomic instability, oncogene activation and loss of tumor suppressor genes cooperate in creating the full blown cancer. The multi-step process has been well worked out in colon cancer development. The Vogelstein's model of adenoma-carcinoma sequence is depicted in Figure 2.7.

Figure 2.7 Multi-step process of development of colon cancer

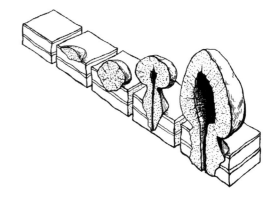

Colon cancer starts with a mutation in the APC (adenomatous polyposis coli) gene, followed by alterations in several other genes. Initially, the neoplastic cells are indistinguishable morphologically from their normal counterparts, but over time abnormal features, such as differences in shape and size, and nuclear changes become obvious. These abnormal cells proliferate and form outgrowths in the colon, called polyps. The polyps gradually enlarge and as further mutations accumulate, the cells begin to display traits of frank malignancy with invasion and destruction of the adjacent normal tissues, formation of new blood vessels (angiogenesis), and eventually the breaking away of cells, which travel through the blood vessels to other parts of the body (metastasis).

Chapter 3

HALLMARKS OF CANCER

KEY POINTS

- The fundamental property of cancer is an abnormal increase in cell number due to increased cell proliferation and/or decreased cell death
- All cell types can undergo malignant transformation, but epithelial cells are most susceptible
- Cancers arise from single cells – clonal origin
- Several cellular genes (tumor suppressor genes and oncogenes) must be mutated to lead to a full-blown malignant state
- Progressive accumulation of mutations leads to sub-clones with different phenotypic characteristics
- Cancer formation occurs in a stepwise fashion with invasion and metastasis being key features of malignancy
- Cancers that are clinically detectable are at a biologically advanced stage of their natural history

BIOLOGY OF CANCER

There are four cardinal features of malignancy.

Inappropriate cell proliferation

In a healthy adult, organs like liver, lung or skin are in a steady state, i.e. rates of cell birth and cell death are equal so that there is no increase in cell number over time. In a cancer, however, the homeostatic mechanisms that maintain the appropriate number of cells in normal tissues are defective. As a consequence, new cell production or cell birth exceeds cell death, resulting in a net increase in cell number. The increase in cell population is the result of an imbalance between cell proliferation, due to successive mitoses of the neoplastic cells, and

cell attrition, due primarily to programmed cell death or apoptosis.

The uncontrolled accumulation of abnormal cells in an organ results in the disruption its function. Organs, such as the liver, may be infiltrated and replaced by malignant cells, or hollow structures, such as the bronchus, may be blocked. Compromise of the function of vital organs is the primary cause of death from cancer. It is important to note that there are over 200 discrete cell types in the human body, but not all are equally susceptible to cancer development. Cells in some tissues, like heart myocytes or nerve cells, may persist throughout life without dividing, and cancers in such tissues are uncommon. Cancers are most common in tissues with rapid cell turnover, especially those exposed to environmental carcinogens (e.g. skin, gut or lung), or whose proliferation is regulated by hormones (e.g. breast or prostate).

Angiogenesis

All cells require oxygen and nutrients for survival and these are supplied by the vasculature. During organogenesis, there is a coordinated growth of vessels to ensure that all cells in a tissue are within 100-200 microns of a capillary blood vessel, since the diffusion of oxygen and solutes through the intercellular spaces is limited. Once a tissue is formed, the vasculature is generally quiescent, and the growth of new blood vessels or angiogenesis is transitory and controlled. Physiological conditions during which angiogenesis occurs in the adult are restricted to the uterine changes during the menstrual cycle and wound healing.

A critical property for an incipient neoplasm is the recruitment of new blood vessels from pre-existing ones. Neoplasms larger than 2 mm in diameter stimulate the in-growth of blood vessels (angiogenesis) from the surrounding normal tissues into the expanding mass. Angiogenesis is controlled by both positive and negative regulators, secreted by the tumors and their associated stroma. The angiogenic peptides secreted by tumors are similar to those released during normal physiological functions, such as wound healing. Two of the most potent angiogenic inducers are vascular endothelial growth factor (VEGF) and basic fibroblast growth factor (bFGF). Inhibitors of angiogenesis include thrombospondin-1, angiostatin and endostatin. There are more than 20 angiogenic inducer factors and a similar number of inhibitor proteins. The ability to promote angiogenesis occurs via an "angiogenic switch" during neoplastic development. This causes an imbalance between the angiogenesis inducers and inhibitors. A common strategy for this shift is the increased expression of VEGF and bFGF through altered gene transcription by the neoplastic cells. Alternatively, expression of the inhibitors is down-regulated. The mechanisms responsible for the shifts in the balance between the angiogenic regulators are not fully understood, but there is some evidence that they are linked to oncogenes and tumor suppressor genes. For example, the ras protein regulates VEGF expression, while p53 protein activates thrombospondin-1.

The formation of new tumor vasculature occurs through endothelial cell proliferation, migration and tubule formation. The tumor blood vessels are distinct from those in normal tissues. They are tortuous, dilated, leaky, and may end in blind loops. Also, the walls of normal vessels are formed by endothelial cells, but tumor vasculature can contain tumor cells as part of the vessel. Unlike normal vessels, tumor vessels require the continued presence of angiogenic factors to maintain their stability.

Invasion and metastasis

Many cells are in contact with an extracellular matrix (ECM) whose proteins form a highly organized 3-dimensional matrix. The basement membrane, which underlies epithelial tissues, is a specialized form of ECM. Cell interaction with the ECM is important for growth and differentiation of cells. This is mediated through interactions with cell adhesion molecules (CAMs), which are trans-membrane proteins with extracellular and intracellular domains. There are two classes of cell adhesion molecules: integrins and cadherins.

Integrins are a family of membrane proteins expressed by all cells. They bind to a number of molecules in the ECM, allowing them to sense their extracellular environment. They regulate a variety of cell functions, including cell proliferation and apoptosis during embryonic development as well as postnatally. They are also part of the signal transduction complexes.

Cadherins are a family of over 20 membrane proteins that mediate cell-cell adhesion. A major epithelial cadherin is E-cadherin. In some poorly differentiated cancers, the expression of E-cadherin is reduced, and this facilitates the detachment of cells from the main cancer.

Normally, the ECM stabilizes the cellular microenvironment through interactions with CAMs. Alterations in CAMs allow the dissociation of cells in a cancer and facilitate their mobility. In addition, within the matrix are proteinases and proteinase inhibitors. A balance exists between these, but in malignant states, aberrant proteolysis upsets the balance, leading to degradation of the basement membrane and ECM to remove the physical barrier to cell migration. As a result, the cancer invades adjacent tissues (Figure 3.1). The malignant cells then spread along tissue planes, across body cavities, and through the lymphatic and blood systems.

Figure 3.1 Schematic representation of progression of cancer from early stage (in situ) to invasive stage with disruption of the basement membrane

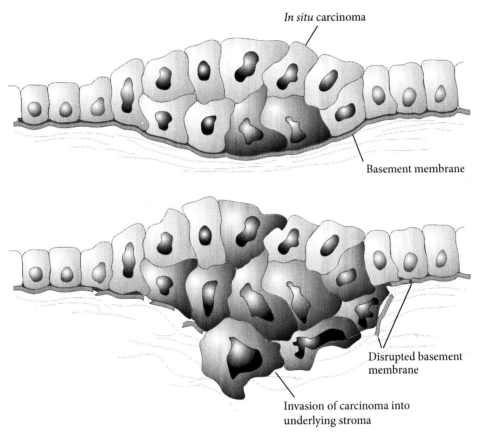

In situ carcinoma

Basement membrane

Disrupted basement membrane

Invasion of carcinoma into underlying stroma

The penetration of a cancer cell through the wall of a lymphatic or blood vessel permits its dissemination through the body. These are major routes of spread of cancer. Individual cancer cells, or a small clump of cells, may detach from the primary cancer and circulate in the lymph or blood system as an embolus. As the cancer cells circulate through the vasculature, they become arrested in the capillaries of the liver or lungs. Following their arrest in the microcirculation, the cancer cells exit the vasculature and establish new sites of growth, called metastases, in distant organs. Different cancers preferentially metastasize to specific organs. This may, in part, be due to CAMs, which are responsible for the anchoring of cells in tissues. As cancer cells travel through the blood stream, they encounter changing microenvironments with novel matrix components. By adapting to these new matrix substrates through shifts in the spectrum of integrins, the cells are able to colonize distant organs.

Genomic instability

A number of genes responsible for cancer development have been identified, and in many cases they are mutated versions of genes that are involved in normal physiological processes, such as control of the cell cycle, transmission of growth signals, and regulation of cell differentiation and cell death. Spontaneous mutations usually occur at a low frequency: 1 in 10^5-10^6 cell divisions. As the cell moves through the cell cycle, checkpoints operate at critical junctions to ensure that any DNA damage is repaired. In cancer, malfunction of specific components of the genomic caretaker system results in the accumulation of mutations. A good example is the mismatch repair (MMR) gene system, which is associated with a hereditable form of colon cancer (hereditary non-polyposis colon cancer syndrome). MMR is responsible for repairing nucleotide mismatch during DNA replication, and in the presence of a mutated MMR gene, the cell has a high nucleotide mutation rate. This leads to an increased rate of mutation at oncogene and tumor suppressor gene loci throughout the tumor cell genome. Another example is the p53 tumor suppressor gene. If there is DNA damage, the normal p53 protein stops the cell cycle at the G1-S checkpoint, allowing DNA repair to take place; alternatively, if the DNA damage is excessive, it triggers apoptosis. In the presence of a mutated p53 gene, a cell with DNA damage can traverse the G1-S checkpoint.

A mutation in a single gene is incapable of inducing transformation to a fully malignant cell, and several mutations in different classes of genes are required. As a neoplasm grows, more and more mutations accumulate and the cells become genetically unstable, giving rise to several phenotypic traits that allow the emergence of other virulent properties, such as invasion of adjacent tissues and metastasis to distant sites. Increasing genomic instability as a cancer develops is a hallmark of oncogenesis.

CLONAL EVOLUTION OF CANCER

Cells have one of three options: divide, differentiate or die. Cells capable of perpetually dividing are undifferentiated, and are referred to as "stock cells" or "stem cells." On the other hand, cells that are differentiated are "end cells" and are capable of only a limited number of cell divisions. When a stem cell divides, the daughter cells have two choices: they can either become new stem cells or differentiated cells (Figure 3.2). To maintain homeostasis, a stem cell gives rise to a new stem cell and a differentiated cell; in this way, the stem cell pool is replenished, while the differentiated cell undergoes a few more cell divisions and eventually dies. The pattern of gene expression distinguishes a stem cell from a differentiated cell, and which path the individual cell takes depends on the interaction of signals, including contact with other cells, interactions with extracellular matrices, endocrine hormones, and paracrine growth and differentiation factors.

Figure 3.2 Options for stem cell division. A – cell division leads to one stem cell and one differentiated cell; B – both daughter cells become differentiated with consequent "loss" of a stem cell from the pool; C – two new stem cells are produced with "gain" of a stem cell

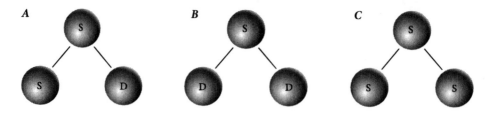

Neoplastic conversion begins with a gene mutation caused by errors in DNA replication or induced by carcinogenic exposure. The mutation provides the cell with a selective growth advantage over its neighbours. This cell becomes the "parental" cell, or tumor stem cell, from which a clone develops. As cell proliferation continues, further genetic events occur with the emergence of new sub-lines with additional growth advantage. An important consequence of this is that a cancer is composed of cells that are heterogenous for a wide variety of phenotypic characteristics (Figure 3.3). These include differences in cell size and shape (morphology and histology), karyotype, cell surface antigens, intracellular concentrations of enzymes and tumor cell markers, such as estrogen receptor.

Figure 3.3 Clonal development of a cancer

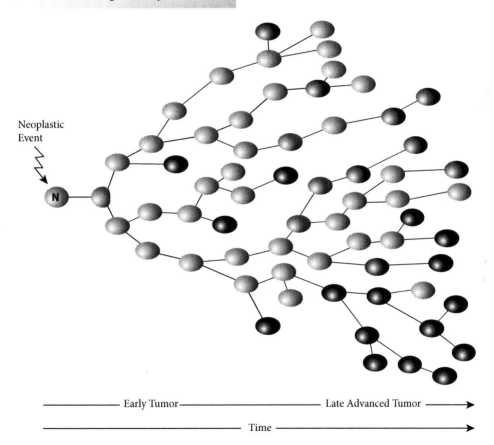

Neoplastic Event

N

——— Early Tumor ——————————— Late Advanced Tumor ———→

——————————————— Time ———————————————→

GROWTH PATTERNS OF CANCER

As in normal cells, the cell cycle of a cancer cell is divided into four phases. G1 is the phase during which RNA and proteins are synthesized for a variety of different cell functions. During S phase, DNA is replicated. G2 is the phase between the completion of DNA synthesis and the beginning of the nuclear changes that occur in preparation for chromosomal condensation. During M phase or mitosis, the mitotic spindle forms, and cell cleavage occurs with the formation of two daughter cells, each with a full complement of chromosomes. A cell may leave the cycle of proliferation and enter a quiescent state, called G0. Cells in G0 can be recruited to re-enter the cell cycle when the conditions are right.

The cell cycle time, also called generation time, is the time required for a cell to complete one cell cycle. Contrary to what was generally believed, cancer cells do not have a short cell cycle time. The average cell cycle time of most normal human cells is about 12-24 hours, whereas that of cancer cells can be as long as 48-72 hours. In addition to individual cell proliferation, tissue growth is an important consideration. Doubling time refers to the time required for a tissue to double in size or cell number. Although the cell cycle and tissue doubling times might be expected to be equal, the doubling time of a clinical cancer depends on two measures of tissue growth: growth fraction and cell loss fraction.

Growth fraction refers to the percentage of the total cell population that is cycling. This is the best measure of tissue growth. The tumor growth fraction is generally small, and the proportion of cells in S phase is 3-15% for many cancers; most cells are in G0 phase. Even though higher rates of cell proliferation may be present in fast-growing cancers, the rate of cell proliferation in cancers is usually less than that of some normal renewing tissues, such as the bone marrow. Thus, the accumulation of cells in cancers is not due to a more rapid rate of cell proliferation, but other factors are at play. There is a defective maturation process of the cancer cells, and an imbalance between new cell production and cell loss.

Cell loss fraction represents the percentage of newly produced daughter cells that die. This number is high in cancer, and 75-90% of new cells die.

A conceptual model of tumor growth can be developed (Figure 3.4). Not all cells in a cancer are proliferating at the same time. A cycling cell is a member of the proliferative compartment or growth compartment. In a typical breast cancer, for example, the proliferative compartment is <20%, although it can range from 4% to 80%. A cell in prolonged G0 or arrested G2 is in the non-proliferative compartment or quiescent compartment. Finally, cells are constantly dying by apoptosis or necrosis. This cell loss fraction is an important determinant of cancer growth. The degree of imbalance between production of new tumor cells and cell death determines the rate at which a cancer grows. When cell birth exceeds cell death, growth occurs. Growth also reflects average cell size, vasculature, content of extracellular matrix, edema, hemorrhage, etc., but these are of secondary importance.

Figure 3.4 Schematic representation of different cell compartments in a cancer

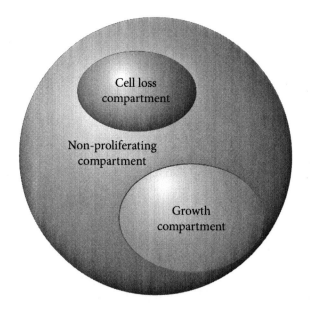

Cancer growth follows a general pattern. Growth is initially rapid, proceeding in an exponential manner, and then progressively decreases. This pattern of growth best fits a Gompertzian curve (Figure 3.5). Two major mechanisms account for the retardation in growth rate over time. First, there is a progressive decrease in the growth fraction. This is not caused by a stable change in individual cells, but is due to decreased cell responsiveness to growth stimuli, such as hormones or growth factors. Second, there is an increase in programmed cell death, or apoptosis, as well as necrosis. In most clinical cancers, areas of necrosis are evident. This may be due to major chromosomal defects or abnormal segregation of chromosomes during mitosis, which are incompatible with cell survival. Also, cancers have abnormal blood vessels and rupture of these with hemorrhage

and thrombosis is common. In addition, poor oxygenation and lack of nutrients are other factors responsible for cell death.

An important feature of Gompertzian growth is that to attain a mass with a diameter of one centimeter (10^9 cells), which is the usual threshold of clinical detection, the original cancer cell has undergone 30 doublings. By then, growth is no longer exponential. A further 10 doublings produce a mass of 10^{12} cells, weighing 1 kg, which is the limit of tolerance for the host. Estimates using the Gompertzian model suggest that, for most human cancers, growth occurs over a few years. It is noteworthy that by the time a cancer becomes large enough to be clinically detectable or cause symptoms, most of its growth has already occurred, and the exponential phase is over.

Figure 3.5 Gompertzian growth pattern of cancer

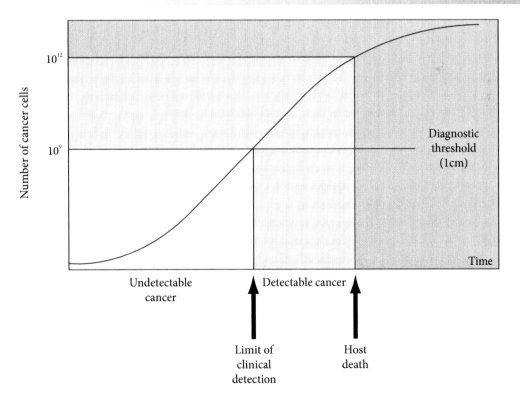

CLINICAL PROGRESSION OF CANCER

Epithelial cancers develop in a stepwise manner from a pre-malignant state to a frankly malignant tumor. A clear histological and genetic evolution has been defined for some cancers. For example, colorectal cancer progresses from mucosal dysplasia, through enlarging polyps to invasive cancer. This progression can take a few years. Similarly, breast cancer commonly arises in the mammary ductal epithelium, and progresses from dysplasia to carcinoma *in situ* to invasive cancer. An obvious implication of this pattern of growth is the opportunity to intervene early through screening. In the case of colon cancer, for example, this permits the removal of pre-malignant colonic polyps or allows the diagnosis of cancer at an early stage when treatment is more effective.

Once a cancer has become invasive, it has the potential to metastasize to regional lymph nodes and to distant organs. There are four major patterns of spread of cancer: by direct local invasion, through the lymphatics, through the blood stream, and across the celomic cavities, such as the pleural, pericardial or peritoneal space.

Chapter 4

CANCER PATHOLOGY

KEY POINTS

- Cancer is a family of diseases classified according to the tissue and cell of origin: carcinoma, sarcoma, lymphoma/leukemia, germ cell tumors and glial tumors
- Benign and malignant tumors display different traits
- *In situ* cancer is distinct from invasive cancer
- Cancers are graded by their degree of differentiation
- An accurate pathological diagnosis is essential for all cancers

INTRODUCTION

Cancer is not a single disease, but a family of diseases. The first step in the pathological assessment of a cancer is to determine the organ or tissue from which it arises. For example, cancer of the stomach is different from cancer of the colon. Further, cancers arising within a single organ can be of different histological types. For example, cancers of pancreas may arise from the cells lining the pancreatic ducts (adenocarcinomas) or from the islet cells (neuroendocrine tumors). These have different causes, different modes of spread and different clinical courses. Therefore, a precise pathological diagnosis is essential in the assessment of a patient in order to assign the correct prognosis and guide appropriate therapy.

DEFINITION OF COMMON TERMS

Hyperplasia: An increase in the number of cells in an organ or tissue in response to a stimulus. When the stimulus is removed, the hyperplasia regresses.

Hypertrophy: An increase in the size of cells within an organ. This process occurs in response to a stimulus. When the stimulus is removed, the cells return to normal size.

Atrophy: A reduction in either the size of cells or the number of cells within an organ. This process is reversible when it represents part of a response to an external stimulus or it can be part of the normal aging process.

Dysplasia: A pre-malignant change in cells (usually in the epithelium) characterized by disorderly growth and morphologic changes in the cell nuclei. Dysplasia may be graded as low, medium or high grade depending on the severity of the abnormality.

Metaplasia: A reversible change in which one cell type is replaced by another cell type. The most common epithelial metaplasia is the transformation from columnar to squamous epithelium in the respiratory tract due to chronic irritation.

Tumor: Literally, a swelling of any sort. However, the term is often used to describe a neoplastic mass.

Hamartoma: A tumor-like mass consisting of excessive but focal growth of tissues that are native to the organ in which it occurs. It is generally considered to be developmental in origin.

Neoplasm: An abnormal mass of tissue, the growth of which exceeds and is uncoordinated with that of normal tissues. The neoplasm persists after removal of the stimuli which evoke the change. Neoplasms may be benign or malignant.

Cancer: A generic term for all malignant neoplasms.

CLASSIFICATION OF NEOPLASIA

Neoplasia is subdivided into benign and malignant tumors. All neoplasms, whether benign or malignant, are made up of two basic compartments: proliferating neoplastic cells, which form the parenchyma, and supporting stromal cells. The stromal cells comprise connective tissue and blood and lymphatic vessels; they are not neoplastic and are derived from normal host tissues that the tumor recruits for its own use. When large quantities of fibrous tissue are present, the tumor is said to be scirrhous or desmoplastic.

A malignant tumor present within an organ may arise from that organ (a primary tumor) or it may represent a metastatic deposit (a secondary tumor) from a cancer of another organ. Certain organs, especially the lungs, liver, bone and brain, are common sites of metastases, and this possibility should always be considered, particularly if multiple lesions are present.

The distinction between primary and secondary cancers is important, since secondary cancers display similar biological characteristics and response to treatment as the primary tumor from which they arise.

FEATURES OF NEOPLASIA

Benign tumors grow slowly and push against adjacent tissues, but they do not invade or destroy them. As a result, their growth remains localized and circumscribed, and they do not metastasize. This behavior makes them rarely fatal, and they can be cured by surgical removal. Histologically, the cells of benign tumors closely resemble those of its tissue of origin. Some benign tumors can be precursors of malignant neoplasms. For example, colonic adenoma can give rise to carcinoma. Other benign types of tumor, such as lipoma, do not undergo malignant transformation.

In contrast to benign tumors, malignant tumors grow rapidly. They directly invade and destroy adjacent organs, and they have the ability to metastasize, i.e. spread to other parts of the body. This latter behavior is the most characteristic feature of a malignant tumor. Metastases occur via the lymphatic channels to regional lymph nodes, the blood stream to distant organs, or across serous membranes (peritoneum, pleura or pericardium) forming tumor implants.

SPREAD OF CANCER

Lymphatic spread

The lymphatic system is part of the circulatory system and it is made up of a vast network of lymphatic channels. The chief function of the lymphatics is to collect excess tissue fluid, or lymph, which eventually drains into the blood system. The superficial lymphatic channels are in the skin and subcutaneous tissues. These drain into deeper lymphatic channels in the deep fascia between the muscles and subcutaneous tissues. The lymphatic channels eventually collect into larger lymphatic vessels that come together to form either the right lymphatic duct or the thoracic duct. The right lymphatic duct drains lymph from the right side of the head and neck, the right upper limb and the right chest region, and the right half of the thoracic cavity. The thoracic duct drains the rest of the body. The lymphatic system is connected with lymph nodes that are scattered throughout the body.

Passage through the lymphatic channels is the most common mode of spread for most cancers, especially those that arise in epithelial tissues. The pattern of lymph node involvement is dictated by the natural lymphatic drainage. For example, cancers arising in the outer half of the breast usually spread to the ipsilateral axillary lymph nodes, while those in the inner half spread to the internal mammary chain of lymph nodes.

Blood-borne spread

Venous spread is another common mode of dissemination of cancers arising from epithelial tissues and connective tissues. Similar to lymphatic spread, it follows the natural routes of drainage. For example, cancers of the gastrointestinal tract spread via the portal vein to the liver. Direct invasion of the veins may occur in some cancers, such as renal cell cancer, which may invade the renal veins. Arterial invasion is uncommon.

Transcelomic spread

Transcelomic spread across the body cavities and surfaces occurs when the neoplastic cells gain access to these sites. The peritoneal and pleural cavities are common sites of this pattern of cancer dissemination. For example, ovarian cancer typically spreads across the peritoneal cavity, with seeding of the cancer throughout the peritoneal surface. Similarly, lung cancer can spread across the pleural cavity.

NOMENCLATURE OF NEOPLASMS

The nomenclature of neoplasms is determined by the organ (or tissue) from which they arise and their cell of origin. Within the body, the major tissues are as follows:

- Epithelium: skin, the lining of the gut, urinary tract and lung, and solid organs, e.g. liver, kidney and pancreas
- Lymphoid and blood-forming tissues: lymph nodes, spleen, bone marrow and thymus
- Central nervous system (glial cells)
- Germ cells: testis and ovary
- Connective tissue: muscle, fat, bone, cartilage and blood vessels

Benign tumors of the epithelium or connective tissues are generally designated by attaching the suffix –oma to the cell of origin. For example, a benign tumor of fat cells is lipoma. Malignant tumors of the epithelium are called carcinomas, and those of connective tissues are called sarcomas. Malignant tumors of the lymphoid tissues and blood cells have various names, and they are collectively referred to as malignant lymphomas and leukemias, respectively. There are several categories of malignant tumors of the central nervous system and germ cells. Table 4.1 lists some of the common neoplasms arising in the different tissues.

IN SITU AND INVASIVE CANCER

An important distinction needs to be made between carcinoma *in situ* and invasive epithelial carcinoma. Epithelial neoplastic growth starts as dysplasia. Dysplasia does not inexorably progress to cancer, and mild to moderate changes that do not involve the full thickness of the epithelium may revert to normal if the inciting stimulus is removed. Over time, the dysplastic cells may become more abnormal, and as they accumulate, they involve the entire thickness of the epithelium, pushing against the underlying basement membrane. Such a lesion is considered to be a pre-invasive neoplasm and is referred to as carcinoma *in situ*. The term carcinoma *in situ* is synonymous with high grade dysplasia. Carcinoma *in situ* displays most of the cellular morphological changes of cancer cells, but it is not invasive and, therefore, cannot metastasize. By molecular analysis, car-

Table 4.1 Common neoplasms by tissue of origin

Tissue of origin	Benign tumors	Malignant tumors
Epithelial tumors		
Squamous	Squamous cell papilloma	Squamous cell carcinoma
Glands or ducts	Adenoma	Adenocarcinoma
Transitional	Transitional cell papilloma	Transitional cell carcinoma
Liver	Adenoma	Hepatocellular carcinoma
Skin	Papilloma	Squamous cell carcinoma
		Basal cell carcinoma
		Malignant melanoma
Connective tissue tumors		
Bone	Osteoma	Osteosarcoma
Cartilage	Chondroma	Chondrosarcoma
Fat	Lipoma	Liposarcoma
Smooth muscle	Leiomyoma	Leiomyosarcoma
Skeletal muscle	Rhabdomyoma	Rhabdomyosarcoma
Blood vessel	Angioma	Angiosarcoma
Fibrous tissue	Fibroma	Fibrosarcoma
Blood cells and lymphoid tumors		
Lymphoid tissues	–	Lymphoma
Marrow granulocytes	–	Myeloid leukemia
Marrow lymphocytes	–	Lymphocytic leukemia
Plasma cells	–	Myeloma/plasmacytoma
Germ cell tumors		
Testis	–	Seminoma
		Embryonal carcinoma
Central nervous system tumors		
Glial cells		Gliomas

cinoma *in situ* has fewer mutations than invasive cancer. Most, but not all, carcinomas *in situ* will eventually progress to invasive carcinoma.

TUMOR GRADE

In general, neoplasms, both benign and malignant, resemble the tissues from which they arise. The differentiation of a tumor is the extent to which the neoplastic cells resemble their normal counterparts, both morphologically and functionally. Tumor grade refers to the degree of differentiation of the neoplasm.

• Grade 1 (well differentiated) neoplasms closely resemble the normal tissues from which they are derived

• Grade 2 (moderately differentiated) denotes that the neoplasms are similar to the normal tissues, but they do not resemble them as closely as Grade 1 neoplasms

• Grade 3 (poorly differentiated) only slightly resemble the tissues from which they are derived, and these neoplasms may have unspecialized cells

Sometimes, Grades 1 and 2 are combined into a low grade category, and Grade 3 designated as high grade. Patients with Grade 3 cancers generally have a poorer prognosis than those with Grade 1 or Grade 2 cancers. Malignant neoplasms that are composed of primitive-appearing, undifferentiated cells are said to be anaplastic; these tend to be aggressive cancers.

The assessment of tumor differentiation takes into account the following features:
- Variation in cell shape and size (pleomorphism)
- Increased nuclear DNA content (hyperchromatism)
- Increased nuclear size and irregular contour
- Increase in the number of mitoses
- Loss of orientation of the cells in relation to the basement membrane (loss of polarity)

PATHOLOGICAL ASSESSMENT

An accurate pathological assessment is essential for good treatment. This requires an adequate sample of tissue, or biopsy, from the cancer, complemented by a complete clinical profile. Obtaining a tissue diagnosis can be achieved by several means:
- Cytology of body fluids, such as sputum, urine, pleural fluid, ascitic fluid or cerebrospinal fluid
- Cytology of tissue scrapings which are superficial cells removed from a body surface, such as cervix, vagina or bronchus, by scraping or brushings
- Fine needle aspirate (FNA) is the insertion of a fine needle into a cancer with aspiration of cells for microscopic examination. This may be done by direct palpation of superficial cancers, such as peripheral lymph nodes, or under ultrasound or CT scan guidance for deeper cancers, such as a liver mass
- Core needle biopsy removes a core of tissue by a biopsy needle, usually under local anesthesia. More tissue is obtained than with an FNA, permitting more accurate diagnosis

- Incision biopsy is the removal of a small piece of the cancer, usually from its edge, by a scalpel or by a punch biopsy
- Excision biopsy is the removal of the entire cancer with a narrow margin of normal surrounding tissue. While it allows for a more accurate diagnosis, the size of the cancer may limit the ability to repair the surgical defect. For large cancer an incision biopsy is carried out, and once the diagnosis is established, a formal surgical procedure is planned to remove the cancer *in toto*

The pathologist can provide useful information about the neoplasm that is critical to decisions about treatment. These include:
- Benign versus malignant neoplasm
- Tissue of origin
- Primary versus secondary cancer
- Tumor differentiation or grade
- Extent of disease or stage
  - tumor size and macroscopic appearance
  - extent of local invasion: organ capsule, blood and lymphatic vessels, perineural spaces
  - number of lymph nodes removed and number involved
  - excision margins of the tumor (complete [R0 resection], or incomplete with microscopic involvement [R1 resection]) (Note: incomplete excision with macroscopic residual disease [R2 resection] is documented during surgery)
- Immunochemical markers (e.g. estrogen receptor status)

BREAST NEOPLASIA AS AN EXAMPLE OF TUMOR NOMENCLATURE

The breast is made up of epithelial tissues (ducts and lobules) and connective tissues (fat, fibrous tissue and vessels). During pregnancy and lactation, the lobules expand and secrete milk, which is carried by the ducts to the nipple. Near the lobules, the ducts are small in caliber, but as they approach the nipple, they are fewer, but larger. Within the lobules is loose fibrous connective tissue, which accommodates physiological expansion during pregnancy and lactation; in the extra-lobular sites is denser fibrous connective tissue, which provides structural support.

Benign mixed tumors, arising from the stromal and epithelial tissues, are common; they are termed fibroadenomas. Malignant variants of mixed tumors, called malignant cystosarcoma phyllodes, may also occur, but are rare. The majority of malignant breast cancers are epithelial in origin, arising either in the ducts or lobules. Breast cancer starts in the duct or lobule and, initially, it is confined within the basement membrane. During this phase of growth, the neoplasm is referred to as carcinoma *in situ* or, more specifically, intraductal or intralobular carcinoma. In the later stages, the neoplastic cells break through the basement membrane and invade the surrounding connective tissues. At this stage, it becomes infiltrating ductal or infiltrating lobular carcinoma. Infiltrating cancer has the potential to spread through the lymphatics to axillary lymph nodes or through the blood stream to distant organs (bone, lungs, liver and brain).

In addition to the basic histology, information about stage of the cancer can be ascertained, including the tumor and nodal status. Also, certain prognostic markers are routinely tested for in the more common breast carcinomas; they include the tumor grade and special markers (estrogen and progesterone receptors, and HER-2 gene amplification).

Table 4.2 *Classification of breast neoplasms*

	Benign tumors	In situ *tumors*	*Malignant tumors*
Ductal carcinoma	Papillary adenoma	Intraductal carcinoma	Infiltrating ductal
Lobular carcinoma	–	Intralobular carcinoma	Infiltrating lobular
Stromal tumors	Angioma	–	Angiosarcoma
Mixed tumors	Fibroadenoma	–	Cystosarcoma phyllodes

Chapter 5

CANCER STAGING

KEY POINTS

- Cancers are staged by a universal staging system (TNM system) based on the primary tumor (T), nodal status (N), and metastasis (M)
- Staging provides important information for therapeutic decisions and allows assignment of prognosis

ELEMENTS OF THE TNM STAGING SYSTEM

The stage of a cancer refers to the extent of the cancer in the body and where it is located. The commonly used system is the TNM (**T**umor, **N**ode, **M**etastasis) system developed by the International Union Against Cancer (UICC). The elements of the TNM system are based on a set of rules that are adapted for specific primary sites. The three components of the system are as follows:

- T – extent of the primary or original tumor
  Increasing size and local extent of the primary tumor are designated as Tis (*in situ*), T1, T2, T3 and T4. If the primary cannot be assessed the designation Tx is used. If there is no evidence of the primary, it is noted as T0
- N – absence or presence of regional nodal metastasis
  If the nodes are negative, they are designated N0. Increasing involvement of the regional nodes is referred to as N1, N2 or N3. If the regional nodes cannot be assessed, the designation is Nx
- M – absence or presence of distant metastasis
  If no distant metastasis is present, the designation M0 is used. M1 refers to the presence of distant metastasis. If distant metastasis cannot be assessed, the designation is Mx

TNM CLASSIFICATION

There are two major categories of TNM classification: clinical and pathological.

Clinical classification is based on information obtained by clinical examination, laboratory tests, imaging studies, endoscopy, biopsy or surgical exploration. The information gleaned from these sources provides a useful guide to treatment, and also allows the prognosis to be determined.

Pathological classification is based on the clinical data, supplemented by additional information obtained from surgery and pathological examination of the cancer. The pathological classification is designated by the prefix "*p.*"

After assignment of the T, N and M status, cancers are usually grouped into different stages from I to IV. The details of this vary from one tumor site to another and can be ascertained by reference to standard charts or from the TNM Staging Manual.

Staging is done at the time of initial diagnosis of cancer. This assigned stage of the cancer does not change over time even if the cancer progresses. If the cancer recurs at a later date and more treatment is planned, restaging of the cancer may be done, using the same system. However, this must be identified by the prefix "*r*" and it is recorded separately from that done at diagnosis.

The information of the TNM Stage of cancer at diagnosis forms the basis of clinical decision making and data analysis. Staging provides vital data to:

- Determine treatment
- Allow prediction of prognosis
- Evaluate the efficacy of treatment for individual stages of the cancer

- Allow comparison of treatment results from one cancer centre to another
- Contribute to continuing investigation of cancer

As an example, the detailed TNM Staging system for breast cancer is as follows:

TNM categories

Primary tumor (T)

TX — Primary tumor cannot be assessed

T0 — No evidence of primary tumor

Tis — Carcinoma *in situ*

- Tis (DCIS) — Intraductal carcinoma *in situ*
- Tis (LCIS) — Lobular carcinoma *in situ*
- Tis (Paget's) — Paget's disease of the nipple with no tumor; tumor-associated Paget's disease is classified according to the size of the primary tumor

T1 — Tumor 2 cm or less in greatest dimension

- T1mic — Microinvasion 0.1 cm or less in greatest dimension
- T1a — Tumor more than 0.1 but not more than 0.5 cm in greatest dimension
- T1b — Tumor more than 0.5 cm but not more than 1 cm in greatest dimension
- T1c — Tumor more than 1 cm but not more than 2 cm in greatest dimension

T2 — Tumor more than 2 cm but not more than 5 cm in greatest dimension

T3 — Tumor more than 5 cm in greatest dimension

T4 — Tumor of any size with direct extension to (a) chest wall or (b) skin

- T4a — Extension to chest wall
- T4b — Edema (including *peau d'orange*) or ulceration of the breast skin, or satellite skin nodules confined to the same breast
- T4c — Both (T4a and T4b)
- T4d — Inflammatory carcinoma

Note: Dimpling of the skin, nipple retraction, or any other skin change except those described for T4b and T4d may occur in T1-3 tumors without changing the classification.

Regional lymph nodes (N): Clinical classification

NX — Regional lymph nodes cannot be assessed (e.g. previously removed)

N0 — No regional lymph node metastases

N1 — Metastasis to movable ipsilateral axillary lymph nodes(s)

N2 — Metastasis to ipsilateral axillary lymph node(s) fixed or matted, or in clinically apparent ipsilateral internal mammary nodes in the absence of evident axillary node metastases

- N2a — Metastasis to ipsilateral axillary lymph node(s) fixed to one another (matted) or to other structures
- N2b — Metastasis only in clinically apparent (as detected by imaging studies [excluding lymphoscintigraphy] or by clinical examination or grossly visible pathologically) ipsilateral internal mammary nodes in the absence of evident axillary node metastases

N3 — Metastasis to ipsilateral infraclavicular lymph node(s) with or without clinically evident axillary lymph nodes, or in clinically apparent ipsilateral internal mammary lymph node(s) and in the presence of clinically evident axillary lymph node metastases, or metastasis in ipsilateral supraclavicular lymph nodes with or without axillary or internal mammary nodal involvement

- N3a — Metastasis to ipsilateral infraclavicular lymph node(s)
- N3b — Metastasis to ipsilateral internal mammary lymph node(s) and clinically apparent axillary lymph nodes

- N3c — Metastasis in ipsilateral supraclavicular lymph nodes with or without axillary or internal mammary nodal involvement

Distant metastasis (M)
MX — Distant metastasis cannot be assessed
M0 — No distant metastasis
M1 — Distant metastasis

Stage groupings

Stage	0	— Tis N0 M0
Stage	I	— T1 N0 M0 (including T1mic)
Stage	IIA	— T0 N1 M0; T1 N1 M0 (including T1mic); T2 N0 M0
Stage	IIB	— T2 N1 M0; T3 N0 M0
Stage	IIIA	— T0 N2 M0; T1 N2 M0 (including T1mic); T2 N2 M0; T3 N1 M0; T3 N2 M0
Stage	IIIB	— T4 N0 M0; T4 N1 M0; T4 N2 M0
Stage	IIIC	— Any T N3 M0
Stage	IV	— Any T Any N M1

Chapter 6

GENERAL APPROACH TO THE CANCER PATIENT

It is helpful to approach the diagnosis of cancer in a systematic manner. In general, for a particular cancer, the following information is useful in the overall assessment:

- Incidence: does the cancer occur commonly or uncommonly?
- Age: is there an age of peak incidence (e.g. young vs. older persons)?
- Gender: is it more common in men or in women?
- Predisposing or risk factors: are there known risk factors?
- Pathology: what is the common histological type?
- Pathways of spread: what is the characteristic pattern of spread?

SYMPTOMS AND SIGNS

The symptoms and signs caused by a cancer are nonspecific and may be caused by conditions other than a malignancy. Nonetheless, these do depend on the site of origin of the cancer and its possible spread to other organs. Approaching the problem in this manner can help make the diagnosis.

Effects of the primary tumor

As the primary cancer enlarges, it disrupts the function of the organ from which it originates. For example, hollow structures, such as the colon or bronchus, may be blocked, leading to colicky pain or dyspnea, respectively; visceral organs, such as the liver, can be destroyed, leading to hepatic insufficiency. Extension of the cancer into the surrounding tissues can cause further symptoms. The invasion of the pelvic sidewalls by a rectal cancer, for example, causes pelvic pain.

Effects of secondaries or metastases

Involvement of the regional nodes by a cancer results in their enlargement. If this occurs rapidly, discomfort or pain is common. Massive nodal enlargement may also lead to compression or displacement of underlying structures. Metastases to visceral organs are responsible for their progressive dysfunction and eventual failure.

The common sites of metastases for cancer include the lungs (dyspnea, cough), liver (abdominal discomfort, anorexia, weight loss, jaundice, ascites), bone (pain, fracture), and brain (headaches, seizures, muscle weakness, visual disturbances).

Systemic effects of malignancy

These are caused by production of biologically active substances, such as hormones or cytokines (e.g. anorexia-cachexia syndrome).

APPROACH TO THE CANCER PATIENT

Each cancer has its own natural history, depending on its anatomic site of origin, patterns of spread and the speed with which it spreads. As an example, these guidelines can be applied to rectal cancer.

History

The primary cancer causes pain or discomfort on defecation, tenesmus, mucus discharge and bleeding per rectum. As the cancer enlarges, there is obstruction of the rectum, and the patient can experience lower abdominal crampy pain. Pelvic discomfort may occur due to extension of the cancer into the pararectal tissues and pelvic sidewalls. Metastasis to liver causes upper abdominal discomfort, anorexia, jaundice and ascites. General effects are due to anemia (fatigue, malaise), and weight loss may occur.

Examination

The primary is palpable as a rectal mass. Metastases in the liver lead to hepatomegaly and ascites, and there may be a palpable left supraclavicular node. The general effects of the cancer may manifest as pallor, icterus or weight loss.

Assessment of Performance Status

A reliable measure of the systemic effects of a malignancy on patients can be determined through a rating of their performance status. This is simple to assess clinically through the effects of the illness on the functioning of the individual, and there is a generally good correlation between the performance score and patient survival. Two scales are commonly used.

Eastern Cooperative Oncology Group (ECOG) Performance Status Score

0 - Asymptomatic; able to carry out all normal activities without restriction
1 - Minimal symptoms present; able to carry out work of a light or sedentary nature
2 - Ambulatory and capable of all self-care; confined to chair or bed <50% of waking hours
3 - Capable of limited self-care; confined to chair or bed >50% of waking hours
4 - Completely disabled; unable to carry out any self-care; totally confined to chair or bed
5 - Dead

Karnofsky Performance Status (KPS) Score

100 - Normal; no complaints
90 - Able to carry on normal activities; minor symptoms
80 - Normal activities with effort; some symptoms of disease
70 - Cares for self; unable to carry out normal activity or do active work
60 - Requires occasional assistance, but able to care for most needs
50 - Requires considerable assistance and frequent medical care
40 - Disabled; requires special care and assistance
30 - Severely disabled; hospitalization indicated although death not imminent
20 - Very sick; hospitalization necessary; active supportive treatment necessary
10 - Moribund; fatal process progressing
0 - Dead

In general, patients with ECOG performance status >2 or Karnofsky score <70 do not tolerate intensive cancer treatments.

TUMOR MARKERS

Tumor markers are molecules which indicate the presence of a cancer. They are generally not sensitive or specific enough to be useful as a screen for early disease, but they are good in other respects.

• Aid diagnosis
In the appropriate clinical setting, the measurement of serum tumor markers can support the diagnosis. For example, elevation of alpha-fetoprotein in a patient with known cirrhosis and a liver lesion on imaging study indicates a hepatocellular carcinoma.

• Assess prognosis
High levels of tumor markers can be predictive of an adverse outcome. High levels of human

chorionic gonadotrophin (hCG) in testicular cancer patients indicate a poor prognosis.
• Predict response to treatment
A decrease in tumor marker levels is an indication of a favorable response to treatment. A decrease of serum levels of carcinoembryonic antigen (CEA) in patients receiving chemotherapy for metastatic colorectal cancer predicts for a good tumor response.
• Detect early relapse of cancer
A major role of tumor markers is the monitoring of patients who have undergone potentially curative resection of their cancer. For example, a rise in serum CEA level after a complete surgical resection of a colorectal cancer is a reliable indicator of disease recurrence.
• Distinguish cancer types
Tumor markers can distinguish between the different types of cancer. For example, epithelial membrane antigens and common leucocyte antigen are useful in differentiating epithelial cancers from lymphoid malignancies.

A number of tumor markers are in common clinical use (Table 6.1).

PATHOLOGY

The following simple classification is always worthwhile in the assessment of cancers affecting any organ, since it minimizes the likelihood of missing the diagnosis:
• Benign
• Malignant
  ◆ primary
  ◆ secondary
It is mandatory to confirm the malignant nature of the lesion. This always requires a tissue diagnosis, since radiological or clinical features are not always sufficient by themselves.

STAGING

Once the diagnosis of a cancer is confirmed, it is necessary to establish the extent of the disease. The specific tests required to determine the extent of the cancer are guided by knowledge of the pattern of spread for the particular cancer. The information gathered by clinical, imaging and pathological assessment is used to assign the TNM stage of the cancer.

Table 6.1 Tumor markers in common clinical use

Tumor marker	Main tumor types	Other tumor types
Alpha-fetoprotein	testis, liver	
CA15-3	breast	
CA19-9	stomach, pancreas	colorectum, lung
CA125	ovary	
CEA	colorectum	other GI cancers, breast, lung
Chromogranin A	carcinoid tumor neuroendocrine tumor	
HCG	germ cell tumors (testis and ovary) malignant gestational tumor	
PSA	prostate	
Urinary Bence-Jones protein	myeloma	
Urinary 5HIAA	carcinoid tumor	
VMA	pheochromocytoma neuroblastoma	

Implications of lymph node metastasis

For many epithelial cancers, involvement of the regional lymph nodes can be detected by clinical examination, imaging studies or on surgical removal. Metastases to the lymph node are rarely life threatening in their own right, and frequently the involved nodes are removed as part of the surgical procedure. However, the presence of lymph node metastases is a sign that the cancer may already be disseminated, and the patient has a higher than usual risk of harbouring microscopic metastases elsewhere. Because of this, the presence of lymph node metastases is often used as an indication for additional postoperative treatment to deal with the disseminated microscopic metastases.

TREATMENT

In general, the treatment of cancer can be curative, adjuvant, maintenance or palliative.

Curative treatment

Curative treatment is the complete ablation of the cancer.

- Surgery is the main treatment modality for the majority of cancers
- Radiation can be curative in some cancers like laryngeal cancer
- Chemotherapy can produce cures in a few chemo-sensitive cancers like testicular cancer

Adjuvant treatment

A major problem in cancer is the presence of undetected metastatic disease at the time of initial diagnosis. The continued growth of these "micro-metastases" later becomes manifest as cancer recurrences. The observation of the natural history of different cancers after primary treatment has provided a good indication of the probability of recurrent disease over time in relation to the stage at initial diagnosis. To deal with the micro-metastases that may be present at diagnosis, additional therapy, called adjuvant therapy, can be given in conjunction with the primary treatment to improve cure rates. For example, adjuvant chemotherapy or hormone therapy is given after surgery for high-risk breast cancer patients, such as those with axillary lymph node metastasis. The treatment given in the adjuvant setting may not be curative when there are obvious metastases, and the efficacy of adjuvant therapy is likely due to the increased sensitivity of microscopic amounts of disease to radiation, chemotherapy or hormone therapy. Adjuvant therapy is given soon after the main treatment for a limited period, e.g. 4-6 months.

Maintenance therapy

In some patients whose cancer shrink or disappear completely after the main treatment, maintenance drug therapy is given to delay relapse of the cancer and improve overall patient survival. Maintenance therapy is generally given for protracted periods, e.g. 12 months or longer. There are some uncertainties about the duration and even the need for maintenance therapy in solid tumors. This arises in part from a lack of a clear understanding of its mechanism of action. Several hypotheses have been proposed, one or more of which may be active in any individual patient:

- The continuous presence of low doses of the anticancer drug kills slowly dividing tumor cells as they re-enter the cell cycle
- Maintenance therapy suppresses the proliferation of residual tumor cells until senescence or apoptosis occurs
- Maintenance therapy modifies the host

immune response, enabling it to destroy residual tumor cells

Palliative treatment

Palliative treatment may be appropriate when the cancer is incurable. The primary goal is to relieve symptoms and, thus, improve the quality of the patient's life; prolongation of life is secondary. Several treatment modalities may be used depending on the specific situation.

- Surgical resection of a cancer may be advised even in the presence of metastatic disease. For example, resection of a colon cancer can relieve the symptoms of bowel obstruction due to the primary cancer, and is, therefore, worthwhile even in the presence of liver metastases
- Radiation therapy can be given to an advanced primary cancer or metastatic deposits that are painful or bleeding
- Hormonal therapy can cause regression of advanced breast or prostate cancer and, thus, relieve symptoms
- Chemotherapy may be used to palliate the symptoms caused by some advanced cancers by reducing their volume
- Analgesics or nerve blocks are useful for pain control in patients with advanced cancer

CANCER IN THE ELDERLY

The greatest risk factor for the development of cancer is increasing age, and this is especially true for the common malignancies, such as breast, prostate, colorectal and lung cancers. More than one-half of all cancers are diagnosed in people over the age of 67 years. There is no evidence that cancer arises by a different mechanism in the elderly compared with younger individuals, and the increasing incidence of cancer with advancing age may reflect the

longer cumulative exposure to cancer-causing agents coupled with the longer period of continuous cell turnover.

The management of cancer in elderly persons is often complicated by co-morbid illnesses. Nonetheless, elderly patients can have a good life expectancy, and it is important to assess how their co-morbidity influences tolerance to cancer treatment and how they are likely to fare afterwards. A few areas where attention is required include:

- Delay in diagnosis

Symptoms of cancer are often nonspecific and their occurrence in the elderly can be attributed to other causes. For example, rectal bleeding may be due to hemorrhoids or diverticular disease, both of which are more common older individuals, and this may lead to a delay in diagnosis of a colorectal cancer, which may also present with rectal bleeding. The similarity between the symptoms of benign conditions and cancers can cause uncertainty in the correct diagnosis. A high index of suspicion for cancer is, therefore, required for persistent, symptoms to allow early diagnosis.

- Incomplete investigation and staging

There is a tendency to incompletely investigate and stage elderly patients on the presumption that these procedures are not likely to influence treatment. Most early cancers are curable by surgery, and prompt attention to early symptoms and appropriate work-up can identify patients who will benefit from surgical or other therapeutic interventions.

- Inadequate treatment

The decision to treat elderly patients by radical surgery or with intensive chemotherapy regimens is not always easy. At the core of the issue is the patient's life expectancy and how this is affected by co-morbid illnesses, such as heart disease or chronic lung disease. It is more important to consider the patient's "biological" age rather than the "chronological" age. An assessment of the functional status of the patient can provide useful information to guide decisions about treatment. This assessment should take into account the patient's performance status, co-morbid conditions, physical mobility, mental status and social situation.

In general, radiation therapy has a good therapeutic/toxicity ratio, and age by itself is not a contraindication to treatment. Operating on the elderly, however, requires meticulous preoperative evaluation, careful intra-operative monitoring and specialized postoperative care. Considerable progress has been made in the surgical care of older patients undergoing cardiac or orthopedic surgery, and similar anesthetic guidelines can benefit cancer patients.

The use of chemotherapy for the elderly is a more difficult decision. There is a tendency to withhold more aggressive chemotherapy regimens and use a "gentler" approach for older patients. This may be appropriate in some situations. For example, the use of oral chemotherapy (etoposide) in older patients with small cell lung cancer produces results that compare satisfactorily with the more aggressive combination chemotherapy protocols. On the other hand, combination chemotherapy regimens designed for younger patients can also improve the outcome in elderly patients with certain lymphomas. In general, however, there are limited data on the outcome (e.g. survival or quality of life) of intensive chemotherapy protocols in this population, although this is now being addressed in clinical studies.

There are some important considerations when giving chemotherapy to patients, which are especially relevant in the elderly. These include interactions with other drugs the patient may be taking, and possible reduced metabolism and differences in pharmacological disposition of cancer drugs. Nonetheless, those who have cancer for which effective treatment is available should undergo a full assessment to determine their suitability for treatment. The final decision about treatment must take in account the wishes of the patient.

ASSESSMENT OF RESPONSE TO TREATMENT

Monitoring the response of a cancer to treatment is an important part of the clinical assessment of patients. This allows the identification and selection of new treatments for further evaluation in clinical trials, and also guides everyday clinical decisions about treatment of individual patients. Tumor responses can be assessed by several means, including clinical examination, for example documenting changes in the size of palpable disease like peripheral lymph nodes, tumor marker measurements, and imaging studies. Imaging studies provide a reliable, objective measure of tumor dimensions, and they are the preferred method of assessment.

In assessing the response to treatment, the percentage change in tumor size before and after treatment is measured. A common method to measure tumor response is the RECIST (Response Evaluation Criteria in Solid Tumors) system. In essence, this measures the change in the sums of the longest diameters of the lesions. Table 6.2 shows the definitions of RECIST criteria.

Table 6.2 RECIST criteria of tumor response

Response criteria	Change in the sum of longest diameters
Complete response (CR)	Disappearance of all lesions for least 4 weeks
Partial response (PR)	>30% reduction in sum of longest diameters of lesions
Stable disease (SD)	Neither PR or PD criteria met
Progressive disease (PD)	>20% increase in the sum of longest diameters of lesions or appearance of a new lesion

While disappearance of all cancer is the ultimate goal of cancer treatment, this may not be attained in many cases. Nonetheless, improvement of symptoms and prolongation of life can be achieved when there is shrinkage of the cancer. Increasingly, it is being recognized that a clinical benefit can still be obtained when treatment brings about stabilization of the size of the cancer.

QUALITY-OF-LIFE ASSESSMENT

In addition to tumor response, the assessment of quality of life (QOL) of patients is helpful. This is a multidimensional evaluation that takes into account the patient's perception of their well-being. QOL is subjective and its evaluation is done through a self-administered questionnaire. Four domains are usually measured:
- Physical health, namely bodily status and function
- Psychological health
- Occupational status
- Social relationships

PROGNOSIS

Prognosis generally depends on four main factors.
- Site of the cancer

Different cancers have different natural histories, from slow growing (e.g. carcinoid tumor of the small bowel) to rapidly growing (e.g. small cell lung cancer).
- Pathologic factors

The pathological determinants of prognosis are the histological type and the degree of differentiation of the cells. As the molecular basis of malignancy becomes more clearly understood, other parameters are increasingly being used. For example, breast cancers in which the HER-2 oncogene is amplified have a worse prognosis.

- Stage of disease

Early stage or localized disease, in general, has a more favorable prognosis than late stage disease with metastasis.
- General condition of the patient

A significant proportion of the common cancers occur in elderly persons, who may have concomitant medical illnesses, such as chronic lung disease or congestive heart failure. These co-morbid medical conditions can, by themselves, affect the life expectancy of a patient as well as influence the delivery of treatment, such as chemotherapy. A patient's performance status score at diagnosis is a useful prognostic indicator.

FOLLOW-UP ASSESSMENT

The follow-up assessment of the cancer patient fulfills several objectives.

Detection of a curable cancer recurrence

Some cancers are potentially curable when they recur after initial diagnosis and treatment. Hence, careful follow-up evaluation to find these recurrences at an early stage is important. This applies to the following malignancies:
- Hodgkin's lymphoma
- Testicular cancer
- Local recurrence of breast cancer treated by lumpectomy
- Nodal recurrence of head/neck squamous cell cancer
- Local or nodal recurrence of anal squamous cell cancer after radiation
- Nodal recurrence of malignant melanoma
- Local recurrence of prostate cancer after primary radiation therapy

Occurrence of a second primary cancer

Patients with certain types of cancer are at a high risk for a second primary cancer. This may be attributable to a "field" effect on the whole organ by the carcinogenic process, such as exposure to a toxin. An increased risk for a second primary cancer is present in patients with cancers of the skin, head/neck, colorectum, breast and lung.

Familial cancer clustering

In some families, there is clustering of certain cancer types. Follow-up assessment of these patients through appropriate surveillance methods will allow the detection of cancer at an early stage. Cancers of the breast, ovary, uterus and colorectum are well recognized to occur in some families.

Assessment of late effects of treatment

Cancer treatments are associated with several acute and late side effects and the follow-up of patients permits the recognition and management of these. This is particularly important in children, in whom late treatment effects include growth retardation, impairment of cognitive function, infertility, hypothyroidism and hypopituitarism. Some chemotherapy drugs and radiation therapy can also induce cancers at a later date.

The specific tests and frequency with which they are done depend on the cancer type. In general, if the detection of a recurrence or the finding of a new primary can be managed effectively by further surgery, radiation or chemotherapy, intensive follow-up is useful. On the other hand, if no effective treatment is available in the event of a recurrence, follow-up testing can be less rigorous.

Chapter 7

PRINCIPLES OF CANCER TREATMENT

GENERAL PRINCIPLES OF CANCER THERAPY

Three major treatment modalities are available for cancer: surgery, radiation therapy and systemic therapy (chemotherapy, hormone therapy and targeted therapy). When given for potential cure, surgery and radiation therapy are used for relatively localized cancers. Except in very rare cases, neither can be expected to cure disseminated disease, although either may be used to relieve symptoms in that situation. Systemic therapy has the potential to cure disseminated disease as well as provide symptomatic relief.

The choice of treatment requires a consideration of several factors.

- Site of the cancer
- Histological type of the cancer
- Size and extent of the cancer and its potential for spread
- Short- and long-term complications of treatment
- Patient's age and physical and psychological state
- Patient's wish

SURGERY

For most cancers, surgery is the mainstay of curative therapy. The aims of curative surgery are to remove the cancer in its entirety and to repair the defect. Surgical resection of cancer is usually done with concomitant removal of adjacent tissue that may contain metastases. Even if a curative resection cannot be achieved, surgery plays an important role in palliation of cancer-related symptoms, such as abdominal cramps due to bowel obstruction from a cancer. It is also beneficial in the local control of the disease to avoid subsequent complications. For example, a breast cancer eroding into the skin can cause a painful, bleeding ulcer with cellulitis. A simple mastectomy may be an effective way to deal with this problem. The decision for surgery depends on a number of factors:

- Type of cancer

Certain cancers, such as small cell lung cancer, are usually metastatic at presentation even though there may be no overt signs of metastasis on clinical examination or imaging studies. Removal of an apparently localized small cell lung cancer is frequently followed by the rapid emergence of metastasis in regional lymph nodes and extra-thoracic sites, such as the liver, bone and brain. Hence, radical surgery has no role in the management of this cancer.

- Chances of a complete resection

Although a cancer may be localized, its local extent into adjacent tissues can preclude its complete removal. Rectal cancer can occasionally infiltrate into the pelvic sidewalls. Attempts to resect such a cancer are likely to be unsuccessful, since malignant disease will be left in the pelvis, and this will eventually regrow and lead to further complications.

- Available alternative treatment

In some cancers, equally effective alternative treatments may be available. If these produce less morbidity, they are preferred. For example, squamous cell cancer of the anus often presents as a localized cancer that can be completely resected, but this requires a permanent colostomy. Radiation can produce results comparable with surgery without the need for a colostomy, and it is, therefore, the preferred treatment.

- Treatment-related morbidity

When effective alternative treatment, such as radiation therapy, is available, the morbidity of surgery must be considered. Basal cell cancer of the skin is a highly curable type of cancer by either surgery or radiation therapy. Radiation therapy is the preferred treatment if the cancer occurs on the nose or lip because of the better cosmetic result.

• Effect of the cancer on the patient's life expectancy

Certain cancers run an indolent course and in elderly patients they may be unlikely to produce any significant symptom or be the cause of death. Extensive surgery to remove the primary cancer in these instances would not lead to improved quality or length of life.

• Patient's physical and psychological state

Patients, especially the elderly, may not be fit for radical surgery because of co-morbid medical conditions. For example, prostate cancer occurs commonly in older men, who may have other significant medical illnesses, such as cardiac or lung diseases, which put them at increased risk for surgical complications. Radiation therapy may be advised for localized prostate cancer in these situations.

• Incomplete surgical resection combined with other treatment modalities

In some cancers, the complete removal of all gross disease is not possible, but a "de-bulking" operation with resection of as much as possible disease may be part of a planned multimodality approach to treatment. For example, ovarian cancer usually spreads through the peritoneal cavity, often precluding complete surgical resection. In selected cases of ovarian cancer, de-bulking the cancer surgically followed by chemotherapy improves patient survival.

RADIATION THERAPY

Radiation is energy and comes in two forms: photons and particles. Photons are "energy packages" that do not have mass or charge, but behave like particles or waves when they interact with each other or with matter. X-rays and γ-rays are examples of photon radiation. Particle radiation comprises electrons, protons and neutrons. When radiation is absorbed by matter, energy is transferred. If this transfer of energy is high, it causes the ejection of orbital electrons from atoms in the matter. The consequence is a loss of electrons by the atom which, therefore, becomes charged or ionized. Hence, this type of radiation is called ionizing radiation. The ionization of atoms and the further effects of the ejected electrons cause molecular damage to tissues and are responsible for the biological effects of radiation. Radiation therapy is the application of ionizing radiation to treat cancer. For clinical use, the energy of radiation in the range of 50kV to 25MV is employed.

The amount of energy transfer is used as a measure of the radiation dose. Originally, the unit of measure was the roentgen, but this was replaced by the rad, which is defined as the dose of radiation resulting in an energy deposition of 100 ergs per gram of matter. The rad was subsequently replaced by the SI unit, called the Gray. One Gray is equivalent to 100 rads. In common practice, the unit used is the centiGray, or cGy, which equals one rad.

When cancer cells are irradiated, their DNA is damaged. Cells with double-strand breaks in the DNA molecule die when they undergo mitosis unless they are successful in repairing the damage; this is referred to as mitotic cell death. Some cell types, such as lymphocytes, can die after radiation without undergoing mitosis, a process termed interphase cell death.

In order to maximize the therapeutic ratio (chance of cure/risk of damage) radiation is usually given in a series of small daily treatments, called fractions. Fractionation enhances the biological effects of radiation through a few mechanisms, commonly referred to as the "4 Rs" of radiation.

• Repair

After delivery of a dose of radiation, the molecular and cellular damage incurred is repaired. Normal cells have a greater capacity for repair; thus, by giving multiple small fractions with sufficient time (6-24 hours) in between for normal cells to repair the damage, the therapeutic ratio is enhanced.

• Repopulation

In both cancer and normal tissues, surviving cells proliferate during the course of radiation. This is known as repopulation, and it is an important factor influencing both cancer control and normal tissue recovery. The overall duration of fractionated radiation is planned to ensure that repopulation of the normal tissue is complete. Conventional radiation is given on a daily basis over 3-5 weeks for most cancers.

• Redistribution

Cycling cells are more sensitive to radiation than those that are in the resting phase (G0), possibly because G0 cells are more capable of repairing potential lethal damage. As cells are killed during the course of radiation, some of the surviving cells will be recruited into the cell cycle to repopulate the tissue or cancer. This redistribution of cells makes the cancer more sensitive to fractionated treatment compared with a large, single dose.

• Re-oxygenation

Hypoxic cells in large cancers are more resistant to radiation. Some of the surviving cells may gain access to oxygen as the cancer shrinks. This re-oxygenation can result in the cells becoming more sensitive to subsequent radiation treatment.

Radiation therapy is a major form of cancer treatment, and about 50% of cancer patients receive it at some time in the course of their disease. There are three methods by which radiation therapy is delivered:

• Teletherapy

This is commonly referred to as external beam radiation, and it is the usual method of radiation therapy. A source, such as an X-ray generator, cobalt-60 unit or linear accelerator, outside the body is used to generate the energy, which is delivered to a prescribed anatomic site.

• Brachytherapy

Brachytherapy is the placement of a radiation source in contact with the body. For example, radioactive gold seeds can be inserted into a malignant prostate gland to deliver radiation.

• Isotope therapy

This refers to the administration of radioactive isotopes either orally or by intravenous injection. The isotope is selectively taken up by a specific cancer where its subsequent decay releases radiation. For example, oral radioiodine (Iodine-131) is a common method of treatment for certain thyroid cancers.

Clinical uses of radiation therapy

Radiation therapy has wide clinical application and it is prescribed either alone or in combination with surgery or chemotherapy.

• Curative treatment

Radiation can cure certain cancers, such as laryngeal cancers.

• Alternative to surgery

Radiation is not limited by the same anatomical constraints as surgery, and it may be advised in certain situations where it allows preservation of organ function. For example, the treatment of anal cancer by radiation therapy is more likely to preserve anal sphincter function than surgery. In addition, radiation therapy can produce a better cosmetic outcome than surgery, and it is favored in those situations, such as skin cancers, when it provides comparable results in terms of long-term patient survival.

• Preoperative down-staging of cancer

Radiation therapy may be used in conjunction with surgery to maximize the chance of cure. For cancers that invade adjacent structures, radiation therapy can be given to "down-stage" the cancer to permit complete surgical resection. When used for this purpose, radiation is sometimes combined with chemotherapy as a radiosensitizer; for example, radiation is combined with chemotherapy in the preoperative treatment of locally advanced rectal cancer.

• Postoperative adjuvant therapy

When there is a high risk of local relapse after potentially curative surgery, radiation is offered to prevent recurrence. For example, breast cancer patients who undergo a lumpectomy are treated with radiation to the breast.

• Palliative radiation

Radiation therapy is an effective measure for control of symptoms caused by unresectable or metastatic cancer. For example, it can control bleeding from ulcerating cancers or pain due to bone metastasis.

• Urgent/emergency situations

There are a number of situations where radiation is urgently indicated: spinal cord compression, brain metastases with increased intracranial pressure, bronchial obstruction, superior vena cava syndrome or impending bone fractures.

Side effects of radiation therapy

Radiation therapy produces potentially harmful changes in the radiated normal tissues surrounding the cancer, but these can be limited by careful attention to technique and the prescribed dose.

• Acute radiation damage

An acute inflammatory reaction in the tissues being radiated develops within two weeks of the start of treatment, and usually begins to subside 2-3 weeks after the end of treatment.

This reaction is relatively nonspecific and the symptoms are predictable, depending on the tissues receiving radiation. Tissues containing large populations of proliferating cells are more susceptible to acute radiation damage. These include the gastrointestinal mucosa, skin and bone marrow. The radiation effects manifest clinically as nausea/vomiting, cramps and diarrhea (GI); warmth, redness or pruritis (skin); and fatigue, bleeding or infections (bone marrow). While the acute side effects are usually self-limiting, they can occasionally be severe, and the patient may need supportive care until they heal.

• Late radiation damage

Late radiation damage predominantly involves stromal tissues, such as connective tissue and small blood vessels. The effect is usually not clinically apparent for several months after completing treatment, and it may not appear for years. The primary cause of late radiation damage is the gradual loss of small blood vessels, parenchymal cell dysfunction and fibrosis. These late complications can be serious and they are the major dose-limiting factor in radiation therapy. The damage may be aggravated by concurrent diseases that affect small blood vessels, such as autoimmune diseases like rheumatoid arthritis.

SYSTEMIC TREATMENTS

Traditional systemic therapy comprises cytotoxic chemotherapy and hormone treatment. More recently, there is a growing list of new agents, referred to as targeted therapy, consisting of molecules that modulate cell signal transduction. Systemic therapy has the potential to cure some disseminated cancers, but it is used chiefly for the palliation of advanced cancer and as adjuvant therapy.

CHEMOTHERAPY

Tumor cell heterogeneity and cancer chemotherapy

Chemotherapeutic drugs kill cells according to first-order kinetics; this means that a given dose kills a constant fraction of cells in a cancer, not a constant number of cells. This implies that curability depends on the size of the cancer (cell population), the drug concentration, and number of cycles of treatment delivered. This concept has been the basis for giving adjuvant chemotherapy after surgery or radiation to deal with the microscopic burden of cancer.

A major obstacle to the cure of cancers by chemotherapy resides in their biochemical heterogeneity. Although cancers develop from single neoplastic cells, they are genetically unstable, and clinical cancers display a remarkable degree of biochemical diversity that encompasses resistance to the commonly used cancer drugs. This drug resistance is mediated by a wide range of cellular proteins. It is not un-

common for chemotherapy to bring about an initial marked regression of a clinical cancer, only for it to re-grow despite continuing treatment. This results from the initial killing of drug-sensitive sub-clones of cancer cells, followed by growth of the surviving drug-resistant sub-clones (Figure 7.1). In order to minimize the emergence of drug-resistant sub-clones, different classes of drugs with different modes of action are usually combined to treat cancers.

Another important consideration in the use of chemotherapy to cure cancer is the cancer stem cell. Most of the cells in cancer are committed to differentiation pathways and have a limited life span whereas the cancer stem cells form only a small sub-population of the cancer. Nevertheless, the stem cells have the potential to regenerate the cancer cell population. A cure can only be achieved if the cancer stem cell population is eradicated.

Table 7.1 shows the chemo-sensitivity of various types of cancer to the currently available drugs.

Table 7.1 Chemo-sensitivity of different cancers

High sensitivity	Moderate sensitivity	Low sensitivity
Germ cell tumor (testis)	Breast	Melanoma
Hodgkin's lymphoma	Ovary	Liver
Acute leukemias	Colorectum	Prostate
Lymphomas	Chronic leukemia	Soft tissue sarcoma
Ewing's sarcoma	Stomach	Pancreas/biliary system
Lung cancer (small cell)	Esophagus	Kidney
	Head/neck	
	Multiple myeloma	
	Lung cancer (non-small cell)	
	Bladder	

Chemotherapeutic drugs

Many chemotherapeutic drugs are now in common use and they are grouped by their mechanisms of action. The choice of drugs for a

particular cancer type depends on the demonstration of their efficacy in clinical trials.

• Alkylating agents
Alkylating drugs contain an alkyl group that

Figure 7.1 Emergence of drug-resistant sub-clone following chemotherapy

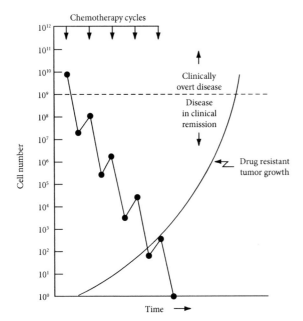

binds to electrophilic sites of DNA, causing cross-links between the strands of DNA, which impede its replication. They are among the most commonly used cancer drugs and include several families:

- Cyclophosphamide and chlorambucil for lymphomas, chronic lymphocytic leukemia and breast cancer
- Nitrosoureas (e.g. BCNU and CCNU), lipid soluble drugs which attain high CNS concentrations, for brain tumors
- Busulphan for chronic myelogenous leukemia
- DTIC (dimethyl triazeno imidazole carb-oxamide) for melanoma and soft tissue sarcomas

- Platinum compounds

Platinum compounds are an important group of cancer drugs. They produce intra-strand and inter-strand cross-links in DNA, which disrupt its function and replication. Two commonly used analogues are cisplatin and carboplatin, which are used for treatment of a number of cancer types – germ cell tumors, lung, upper GI tract, ovary, bladder, head/neck cancers, and sarcomas. A third analogue is oxaliplatin, which is active in colorectal cancer and gastro-eso-phageal cancers.

- Anti-metabolites

The anti-metabolites disrupt critical inter-mediary metabolism of tumor cells by blocking enzymes or serving as pseudo-substrates for important cellular macromolecules, especially DNA. They are widely used in the treatment of childhood malignancies, acute leukemias and lymphomas, and for palliation of several common cancers. Figure 7.2 shows the mode of action of some anti-metabolites.

- Fluoropyrimidines, e.g. 5-fluorouracil (5FU), bind to thymidylate synthase in the presence of reduced folates to inhibit the synthesis of thymidine. 5FU is the most commonly used anti-metabolite, and it is an important drug for the treatment of GI tract, breast and head/neck cancers
- Methotrexate is a commonly used anti-metabolite that blocks the enzyme dihydro-folate reductase (DHFR). DHFR is required for the metabolism of reduced folates, which serve as sources of methyl groups for the synthesis of thymidine and other molecules necessary for DNA synthesis. Methotrexate is used for treatment of acute leukemia, breast cancer and head/ neck cancers
- Cytosine arabinoside or Ara-C is a fraud-ulent nucleoside made up of the purine cytosine linked to a sugar molecule, arabinose. It is incorporated into DNA as Ara-CTP and inhibits DNA replication and repair. Its primary use is for acute myelogenous leukemia

• Gemcitabine is a cytidine analogue which, like Ara-C, becomes incorporated into DNA and interferes with its replication. It has a broad spectrum of activity, including cancers of the pancreas, breast, lung, bladder and ovary

• Fludarabine is an adenosine analogue which has several modes of action. It becomes incorporated into DNA, inhibits DNA polymerases involved in DNA synthesis and repair, and also interferes with RNA function. It is an important drug for the treatment of chronic lymphocytic leukemia

Figure 7.2 Diagram of the sites of action of some anti-metabolites

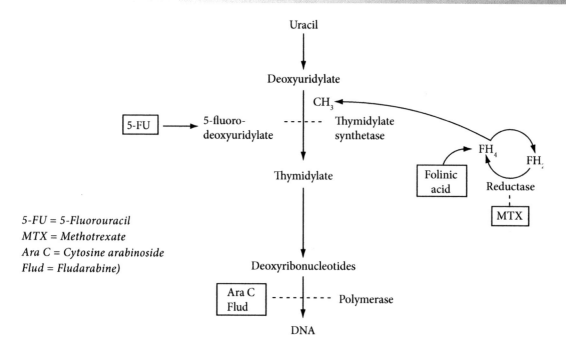

5-FU = 5-Fluorouracil
MTX = Methotrexate
Ara C = Cytosine arabinoside
Flud = Fludarabine)

• Antitumor antibiotics
Antitumor antibiotics are derived from *Streptomyces* species. Their clinical use is limited to a few specific cancers.

  • Actinomycin D inhibits RNA and protein synthesis. It is used mainly for the treatment of childhood cancers, particularly soft tissue sarcomas and neuroblastoma
  • Mitomycin C is a unique molecule that functions as an alkylating agent, but it also generates reactive oxygen molecules. It is mainly used to treat superficial bladder cancer where it is instilled directly into the

bladder. It is also useful in some other cancers, such as anal cancer
• Bleomycin has a unique mechanism of action with formation of ferrous iron-oxygen-bleomycin complex that cleaves DNA, producing single- and double-strand breaks. Bleomycin is an important drug in the curative treatment of testicular cancer and lymphoma
• L-asparaginase is an enzyme that converts L-asparagine, a nonessential amino acid, to L-aspartic acid. Most normal cells can synthesize L-asparagine, but lymphoid

malignancies lack this ability, and are, therefore, susceptible to treatment with this drug.

• Topoisomerase inhibitors

Topoisomerases are nuclear enzymes that make nicks in the strands of the DNA molecule during replication. This is essential because as the DNA double helical molecule uncoils, torsion builds up. By making nicks in the strands, the topoisomerases reduce the tensional strain in the DNA molecule. They are also responsible for repairing the nicks. Two classes of these enzymes exist: topoisomerase I makes single-strand nicks, and topoisomerase II makes two-strand nicks. The topoisomerase inhibitors interact with these enzymes and block their action.

  ◆ Anthracyclines are a class of topoisomerase II inhibitors, which form a complex with topoisomerase II. Additional antineoplastic effects of anthracyclines are the generation of reactive oxygen, which interferes with mitochondrial function, and the induction of apoptosis. Three anthracyclines in routine use are doxorubicin, epirubicin and daunorubicin, which are among the most active drugs for the treatment of lymphomas and myeloid leukemia. They are also used to treat a wide variety of cancers, including breast, gastric and hepatocellular cancers, some childhood cancers, and osteogenic sarcoma

  ◆ Podophyllotoxins are a second class of topoisomerase II inhibitors. Etoposide is used in the treatment of testicular cancer, small cell lung cancer, lymphoma and lymphoid leukemia

  ◆ Camptotecins are topoisomerase I inhibitors. Two agents of this class in clinical use are irinotecan and topotecan for colorectal and ovarian cancers, respectively

• Anti-microtubule agents
  ◆ Vinca alkaloids disrupt the formation of the mitotic spindle and prevent the cell from completing mitosis. Three drugs of this class are vincristine, vinblastine and vinorelbine, which form part of the drug combinations used for treatment of several cancers, including testicular cancer, lung cancer, lymphoma and leukemia

  ◆ Taxanes are another class of anti-microtubule agents. Paclitaxel is the main drug of this class. It interacts with the microtubules and stabilizes them, unlike the vinca alkaloids which prevent their assembly into the spindle. The result is that the microtubules do not dissolve, and the dynamic balance between their formation and dissolution is upset. As a consequence, mitosis is disrupted. Paclitaxel is used for the treatment of ovarian, lung, breast and prostate cancers. A second agent of this class is docetaxel, a semi-synthetic taxane, which is also active in these cancers

Blood-brain barrier

A clinically relevant issue in cancer chemotherapy is the presence of a blood-brain barrier. Cerebral capillary endothelial cells differ from endothelium at other sites because of tight intercellular junctions which limit the passage of molecules. Hence, the passage of drugs across the capillary walls is restricted. This is particularly true for molecules >200 kDa, and those that are not lipid soluble. The clinical consequence for chemo-responsive cancers is that a complete remission can be attained for systemic disease, but brain metastases are less likely to be eradicated. As an example, the successful treatment of childhood leukemia with chemotherapy is often followed by the emergence of overt brain metastasis at a later date.

Recognition of this has led to the practice of giving prophylactic cranial radiation and intrathecal chemotherapy to those who have a complete systemic remission of their disease. A similar barrier exists between the blood and testis, referred to as the blood-testis barrier. The testes are "sanctuary" sites, where chemotherapy drugs do not reach high concentration levels. Complete eradication or cure of a primary testicular cancer by chemotherapy is, therefore, not as reliably achieved as for metastatic deposits in the abdomen or lungs.

Common side effects of chemotherapy

Many chemotherapeutic drugs are given at 3-week intervals to allow recovery of the susceptible tissues, especially the bone marrow. They have several side effects and recognition of these is important to reduce the morbidity they produce.

• Fatigue

Fatigue is the most common side effect of chemotherapy and its severity can vary from mild lack of energy to intense tiredness that may interfere with the patient's routine daily activities. There is no specific treatment, but patients should be encouraged to remain active. Contributing factors, such as anemia, need to be corrected, and metabolic causes, such as diabetes, treated. Cancer patients may also suffer from depression and this requires appropriate treatment.

• Nausea and vomiting

These are common symptoms which usually occur within hours of chemotherapy. For highly emetogenic drugs, like cisplatin or irinotecan, pre-treatment with dexamethasone and a serotonin receptor antagonist, such as ondansetron, can be effective in reducing the acute onset of nausea and vomiting. Nausea and vomiting may also be delayed, occurring 24 hours after chemotherapy. Aprepitant is a new anti-emetic that blocks the neurokinin-1 receptor in the brain and reduces acute and delayed nausea and vomiting.

• Myelosuppression

Myelosuppression is a serious side effect, and most chemotherapeutic drugs cause a transient decrease in the blood cell counts, particularly the neutrophil counts. This occurs about 7-14 days after chemotherapy, and hematologic recovery is usual by 21 days. Patients who experience a fever (>38.5°C) should be carefully evaluated to rule out an infection, since this requires prompt treatment with antibiotics in the face of neutropenia. Severe neutropenia ($<1.0 \times 10^9$/L) carries a significant risk of infection and septic complications. Granulocyte colony-stimulating factor (G-CSF) can shorten the duration of neutropenia. Less common is thrombocytopenia, and the risk of bleeding is significant when the platelet counts fall below 20×10^9/L. Anemia is not uncommon with most chemotherapy regimens, and the hemoglobin should be maintained at a reasonable level (>100 g/L) by red blood cell transfusion.

• Stomatitis

Stomatitis is common particularly with the anti-metabolites, such as 5FU or methotrexate. It comes on a few days after chemotherapy and usually resolves within a week. Severe stomatitis is treated with local anesthetic agents.

• Diarrhea

Diarrhea is especially common with irinotecan and 5FU chemotherapy. The diarrhea usually occurs within a few days to a week after chemotherapy. Severe diarrhea can lead to hypovolemia, and when it is associated with neutropenia, life-threatening complications can occur. Mild to moderate diarrhea is treated with opioid anti-diarrheal agents, such as loperamide. More severe diarrhea requires prompt intravenous fluid replacement. Octreotide is effective in reducing the severity and duration of chemotherapy-induced diarrhea.

Irinotecan also causes a unique type of diarrhea that is mediated through a cholinergic mechanism. The diarrhea occurs during the administration of the drug or within 24 hours, and it is often associated with lacrimation, sweating, abdominal cramps and, occasionally, hypotension. Atropine is an effective treatment for this.

• Peripheral neuropathy
Peripheral neuropathy is common with the vinca alkaloids and platinum compounds. It is dose-related and slow recovery occurs on discontinuation of the drug. Paresthesia or a "pins-and-needles" sensation in the toes and fingers is the first sign. If the drug is continued, progressive motor impairment, usually heralded by loss of the ankle reflexes, can result. The neuropathy associated with oxaliplatin is aggravated by cold exposure.

• Nephropathy
Nephropathy is a potential complication with cisplatin chemotherapy. High doses of cisplatin (>40 mg/m²) are given with intravenous fluids and furosemide to induce a diuresis.

• Cardiomyopathy
Cardiomyopathy may occur with the anthracyclines. This is dose-related and it is more common when the cumulative dose of doxorubicin is >400 mg/m2. Congestive heart failure is the consequence of anthracycline-induced cardiomyopathy.

• Pulmonary fibrosis
Pulmonary fibrosis may occur with several chemotherapeutic agents, but it is particularly common with bleomycin. Administration of oxygen, such as may be given during surgery, can aggravate the condition, and it is contraindicated in cases of bleomycin-induced pulmonary fibrosis.

• Hair loss
Hair loss is a common side effect of many chemotherapeutic agents. The anthracyclines and irinotecan cause alopecia, whereas the taxanes produce loss of all body hair. Most other agents can lead to varying degrees of hair loss. It is usually reversible.

• Gonadal damage and sterility
Several chemotherapy drugs, especially the alkylating agents, procarbazine, vinblastine and cytosine analogues, can cause sterility. Young men may consider sperm banking before the start of treatment. It is also possible to store eggs and this is an option for young women; another possibility is *in vitro* fertilization and storage of the embryo.

HORMONE THERAPY

Hormones produced by the ovaries, testes and adrenal glands can regulate the growth of breast, uterine and prostate cancers. The manipulation of hormone secretion by medical or surgical means plays an important part in the management of patients with these cancers.

Suppression of estrogens

• Suppression of ovarian function
Estrogen produced by the ovaries influences the growth of breast and uterine cancers. Removal of the ovaries or suppression of estrogen synthesis by gonadotrophin releasing hormone (GnRH) agonists (e.g. goserelin) decreases the levels of estrogen, and this can retard the growth of these cancers.

• Selective estrogen receptor modulators (SERMs)
SERMs competitively inhibit the binding of estrogen to estrogen receptors. A major drug of this class is tamoxifen, whose actions are complex, and it also has partial estrogen agonist activity. In the uterus, tamoxifen displays es-

trogenic properties, and this effect is important, since prolonged treatment can lead to uterine hyperplasia and an increased risk of uterine cancer. Raloxifene, which has less pro-estrogenic action on uterine tissue, is an alternative drug.

• Aromatase inhibitors

After menopause, as ovarian function declines, the relative proportion of estrogens synthesized in extra-gonadal sites increases. Estrogen suppression in postmenopausal women is best achieved by inhibition of the enzyme aromatase, which converts androgenic precursors of adrenal origin (testosterone and androstenedione) to estradiol and estrone in adipose tissue, liver, muscle and brain. Aminoglutethimide is an older aromatase inhibitor, which has been supplanted by agents, such as anastrozole, letrozole and exemestane, which have less side effects. These are now an important class of drugs used in the hormone management of breast cancer.

Progestational agents

Progestational agents are effective in suppressing tumor growth in uterine and breast cancers. The mechanism of action of progestational agents is unclear.

Suppression of androgens

Like estrogen in breast cancer, production of androgen by the testes promotes the growth of prostate cancer. Suppression of androgen levels can control prostate cancer and this is achieved in a few ways.

• Suppression of testicular function

Androgen levels can be reduced by the surgical removal of the testes. Inhibition of testicular production of testosterone by luteinizing hormone releasing hormone (LHRH) agonists, like leuprolide, can also suppress androgen levels.

• Anti-androgen agents

Non-steroidal anti-androgens compete with natural androgens for binding to the androgen receptor. The anti-androgens now in use in Canada and the United States include flutamide, bicalutamide and nilutamide. Cyproterone acetate, a steroidal anti-androgen, is used in Europe.

IMMUNOTHERAPY

The immune system was seen as a surveillance mechanism to detect and kill cancer cells. In some cancers, such as melanoma or renal cell cancer, spontaneous regression of the disease may infrequently occur, and this was attributed to the immune system. However, in situations where the immune system is suppressed for prolonged periods, the development of the common cancers is unusual; more frequent is the occurrence of malignancies, like Kaposi's sarcoma, for which a viral etiology is suspected. This has led to the idea that the immune system may play more of a role in increasing the host response to cancers.

Immunotherapy is presently limited in clinical practice. Two general methods of modulating the immune system to heighten the host response are available: nonspecific modulation and specific modulation.

• Nonspecific biological response modifiers

Two classes of compounds are used to induce or augment the immune response to cancer: interferons and interleukins.

Interferons are normally produced by the body, especially in response to viral infections. Three distinct types of interferons are known: IFN-α, IFN-β and IFN-γ. Their mechanisms of action against cancer are wide, including immunological effects, anti-angiogenesis and cell cycle regulation. They are modestly effective against some cancer types, such as chronic myelogenous leukemia, hairy cell leukemia, melanoma, Kaposi's sarcoma, renal cell cancer and carcinoid tumor.

Interleukin-2 (IL-2) is the major member of this class. It is a glycoprotein secreted by lymphocytes with direct effects on T-lymphocytes, B-lymphocytes, monocytes/macrophages and natural killer (NK) cells. In a few cancers, particularly renal cell carcinoma and melanoma, IL-2 by itself or in combination with other cytokines produces tumor responses in about 20% of patients with a small survival advantage in patients with good performance status. However, the toxicity of IL-2 limits its clinical use.

• Specific biological response modifiers

Specific biological response modifiers include a variety of molecules directed against tumor-associated antigens or tumor cells modified to increase their immunogenicity. An important agent of this class is the anti-CD20 antibody. B-lymphocytes undergo an orderly developmental process that includes the expression of CD20, a specific cell surface receptor. Rituximab is an anti-CD20 antibody that binds to CD20, causing B-cell depletion through one or more antibody-dependent mechanisms:

- Fc receptor gamma-mediated antibody-dependent cytotoxicity
- Complement-mediated cell lysis
- Growth arrest
- B-cell apoptosis

Although CD20 is present on normal lymphocytes and B-cell lymphomas, the body quickly replenishes the normal lymphocytes. Rituximab is used to treat non-Hodgkin's lymphomas.

TARGETED THERAPY

Targeted cancer therapy is an emerging field and the list of targeted agents is growing rapidly. A targeted agent is defined as a medication that blocks the growth of cancer cells by interfering with specific signal pathways that are uniquely disrupted in cancer cells. The classification of the targeted drugs is not well-established and

subgroups have overlapping modes of action. A pragmatic classification is into three groups: angiogenesis inhibitors, cell signal transduction modulators and pro-apoptotic agents.

Angiogenesis inhibitors

Angiogenesis is necessary for cancer growth, and cancers as small as 2 mm induce angiogenesis through the angiogenic switch (see Chapter 3). There are three generations of angiogenesis inhibitors.

• First generation angiogenesis inhibitors

These include drugs like interferon and thalidomide. Their toxicity and modest efficacy limit their clinical use.

• Second generation angiogenesis inhibitors

The prototype of this class is bevacizumab, a monoclonal antibody directed to vascular endothelial growth factor (VEGF). Bevacizumab binds to circulating VEGF, and in combination with chemotherapy it improves response rates and prolongs patient survival in patients with advanced cancers, such as colorectal, breast and lung cancers.

• Third generation angiogenesis inhibitors

These are tyrosine kinase inhibitors that act at the intracellular sites of VEGF receptor and other angiogenesis receptors. Sunitinib and sorafenib are small molecule tyrosine kinase inhibitors that target the VEGF receptors, among others.

Signal transduction modulators

Molecules that modulate cell signal transduction are increasingly being tested as cancer treatment. They can be subdivided into two groups: those that act at the level of the surface receptors or those that act along the intracellular signal pathways. Figure 7.3 shows a portion of the cell signal pathways that can be targeted.

Figure 7.3 Schematic diagram of a small section of the cell signal network

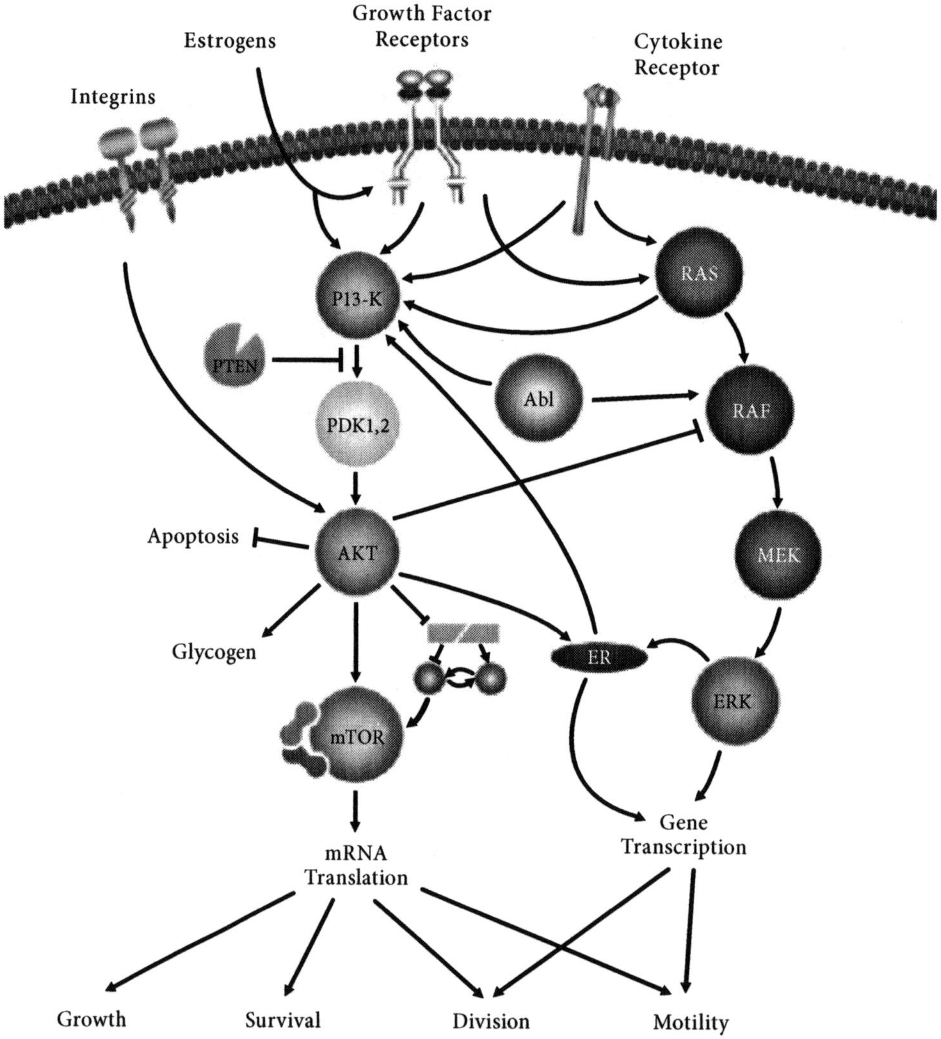

• Molecules targeting growth factor receptors

Epidermal Growth Factor Receptor or EGFR
The EGFR family is the most studied target for drug therapy. It comprises four members: HER-1 (also known as EGFR), HER-2, HER-3 and HER-4. EGFR is a trans-membrane molecule with an extracellular portion and an intracellular portion. Activation of EGFR causes activation of the ras signal cascade. Downstream of this are several intracellular kinases, including MAPK, Akt and JNK pathways, that promote cell proliferation.

Over-expression of EGFR occurs in a broad range of epithelial cancers, including those of the head/neck, breast, colorectum, kidney and bladder. Cetuximab is a monoclonal antibody which binds to the extracellular portion of EGFR, preventing the receptor from being activated. It is an effective second-line treatment for colorectal cancer and non-small cell lung cancer. It is also used alone or with radiation for head/neck cancers. Panitumumab is another monoclonal antibody directed towards EFGR, which is active in advanced colorectal cancer. A third generation EGFR antibody, nimotuzumab, is under investigation for colorectal cancer, and is widely used in Asia for head/neck cancers.

HER-2 receptor is a trans-membrane tyrosine kinase receptor that is over-expressed in 20% of breast cancers as well as other cancers. Trastuzumab is a monoclonal antibody which binds to the extracellular segment of the HER-2 receptor and inhibits its downstream phosphorylation cascade. It may also inhibit angiogenesis. It is used for HER-2-positive breast cancer in both the adjuvant and metastatic settings.

• Molecules targeting intracellular signal pathways

Small molecule tyrosine kinase inhibitors
In addition to drugs that target the extracellular domain of cell surface receptors, several small molecules, called tyrosine kinase inhibitors, have been designed to bind the intracellular phosphorylation sites of the receptor to prevent phosphorylation when the receptor is activated by its ligand.

Imatinib is a tyrosine kinase inhibitor that selectively inhibits the c-kit receptor. Deregulation of c-kit is implicated in some cancers, such as gastrointestinal stromal tumors (GISTs). GISTs frequently have mutations in c-kit tyrosine kinases, which result in downstream signalling that leads to rapid cell proliferation. Imatinib brings about complete and partial remissions in up to two-thirds of patients with GISTs. It is also an effective treatment for chronic myeloid leukemia, in which there is a bcr-abl translocation with the resulting fusion protein (bcr-abl) having tyrosine kinase activity.

Gefitinib and erlotinib are small molecule inhibitors of EGFR. They are active in adeno-carcinoma/bronchiolo-alveolar lung cancers, especially in women, who are non-smokers and are of Asian origin; this may be related to specific mutations in the tyrosine kinase domain of the receptor. Erlotinib is also an active agent in combination with gemcitabine for pancreatic cancer.

Lapatinib is a dual receptor tyrosine kinase inhibitor against EGFR and HER-2. It binds to the intracellular phosphorylation sites of the receptors. It is an active drug in breast cancer.

Other small molecule tyrosine kinase inhibitors that have shown useful clinical activity include sorefinib for hepatocellular cancer and renal cancer, and sunitinib for renal cancer.

mTOR inhibitors
mTOR (mammalian target of rapamycin) is a downstream serine/threonine kinase that regulates cell proliferation, motility and survival, especially when the tumor suppressor gene PTEN is mutated. Temsirolimus and everolimus are active drugs for renal cell cancer. Everolimus also shows activity in pancreatic neuroendocrine tumors.

Pro-apoptosis agents

The ability to avoid apoptosis is one of the hallmark features of cancer cells, and drugs that promote apoptosis are in development as cancer therapy. Proteasome inhibitors are an example of this class of drugs. In normal cells, proteasomes regulate protein expression by degradation of ubiquitinylated proteins. They also clean the cell of abnormal or misfolded proteins. The main function of the proteasome is to degrade unneeded or damaged proteins by proteolysis. The 26S proteasome plays a central role in the regulation of proteins involved in cell regulation and apoptosis, such as cyclins, cyclin-dependent kinases and inhibitors, c-myc and nuclear factor kappa B. Bortezomib is the first therapeutic proteasome inhibitor, which causes cancer cells to undergo apoptosis by interfering with proteins. It is used as second-line treatment for multiple myeloma.

GENE THERAPY

The identification of specific genes associated with cancer provides the opportunity to develop new treatment strategies. The goal of gene therapy is the introduction of genetic information into the cell to correct or reverse the defects which contribute to the development of cancer. This new field of cancer treatment remains experimental.

• Inhibition of oncogene transcription

Inhibition of oncogene transcription may be achieved by nucleotide sequences, which bind to promoters of known oncogenes. For example, the adenoviral gene E1A inhibits transcription of HER-2 promoter.

• Inhibition of oncogene translation

Oncogene translation may be inhibited by nucleotide sequences complementary to the relevant mRNA. These sequences are called anti-sense oligonucleotides. An example is the use of an oligonucleotide sequence to the bcl-2 oncogene, which is mutated and over-expressed in some lymphomas.

• Restoration of tumor suppressor gene function

Tumor suppressor gene function is lost in cancers with the result that cell cycle checkpoints are abolished, apoptotic pathways are interrupted, and DNA repair mechanisms disrupted. Tumor suppressor gene function may be restored by transduction with wild type gene. The p53 gene is mutated in many cancers, and its function can be restored by using a vector, such as liposomes or an attenuated virus with an intact p53 gene, to infect p53-deficient cancer cells. This strategy is being explored in some cancers.

CLINICAL TRIALS IN NEW DRUG DEVELOPMENT

New cancer drugs are evaluated through clinical trials, which are designed to answer a defined set of questions. Clinical trials are carried out in three sequential phases, and the results, although based on a small sample of the population, are then used in drawing up guidelines for treatment of the larger population.

Phase I trials

Once a new molecule is identified in preclinical studies to have potential anticancer activity, it is tested in a Phase I trial. In this, there is no comparative treatment, and it is not a randomized trial. A Phase I trial is conducted in a small number of patients, usually for whom there is no available efficacious treatment. The aims are to determine toxicity, investigate pharmacokinetic and pharmacodynamic profiles, and identify the maximal tolerated dose (MTD) of the drug. Possible antitumor activity may also be documented although this is not the principal objective. If the safety of the drug is confirmed, a Phase II trial is set up, using the dose schedule established in the phase I studies.

Phase II trials

Phase II studies determine whether the new drug has sufficient anticancer activity to be worthy of large scale studies. Phase II studies are usually two-staged trials. In the first stage, a cohort of patients are treated and if no tumor response is seen, the study is discontinued; if, however, there is a tumor response, the study is continued. The first step in the design of a Phase II trial is to set the minimum acceptable level of tumor response, for example a 20% response rate may be chosen as the threshold. If no response is observed in 14 patients, then the probability of getting a 20% response is low. If at least one response is seen, then the probability of getting a >20% response is 5% or more, and a second cohort is enrolled to determine the true response rate. About 40-60 patients may be required to establish the response rates achieved by a new drug. The two primary endpoints of Phase II trials are documentation of antitumor activity, expressed in term of response rates, and further confirmation of the toxicity profile of the drug.

Phase III trials

After a drug has been found to have a predefined level of activity in Phase II trials, its relative efficacy is determined in Phase III clinical trials. In these, the new treatment is compared with the standard therapies, and patients are randomly assigned to the different treatment arms. This potentially applies to every stage of a cancer. For example, a new drug may be tested against one in regular use for advanced stages of a cancer or a new adjuvant treatment may be compared with that in standard clinical practice. If the new drug proves to be better than the standard treatment, it is incorporated in treatment guidelines. Phase III trials are, therefore, the most important for assessing the efficacy of a new treatment. In the design of these trials, the outcome measure is defined at the outset. This may be overall patient survival, disease-free survival, time to tumor progression or other measures of efficacy.

Overall survival
This is the ultimate indicator of treatment success or failure. Some studies use cancer-specific survival analysis by censoring deaths from other causes.

Disease-free survival (DFS)
The effect of treatment may be defined by other events. One such measure is the period during which a patient has no manifestation of cancer.

Time to tumor progression (TTP)
The period during which the cancer is controlled by treatment may be assessed. In palliative treatment, this may be an appropriate measure of the effect of treatment.

Chapter 8

BREAST ONCOLOGY

CLASSIFICATION OF BREAST MASS

Benign

- Cyst
  smooth, discrete mass that is slightly mobile; cysts are present in women of childbearing age, with increasing frequency as menopause approaches
- Fibroadenoma
  rubbery, mobile mass, occasionally multiple, in young women
- Fibrocystic mass
  thickened prominent area of breast tissue that fluctuates in size in relation to menstrual cycles, reducing in size or completely disappearing after each menstrual cycle
- Galactocele
  may be indistinguishable from a cyst; aspiration of typical milky fluid confirms the diagnosis

Malignant

Primary
- Carcinoma
  firm, irregular mass that may be immobile; skin or muscle involvement produces a dimpling or puckering overlying the mass
- Sarcoma
  uncommon; presents as a large, fast-growing, painless mass
- Lymphoma-rare

Secondary – uncommon
- Direct invasion from chest wall cancers (history of thoracic cancer may be present)
- Metastatic deposit from other cancer (prior history of cancer, especially melanoma)

BREAST CARCINOMA

INCIDENCE

Breast cancer is the most common cancer in women in most of the developed countries, and it accounts for about 15% of all cancers in Canada and the US. It is second to lung cancer as the leading cause of cancer-related deaths among women. There are large regional differences in the incidence of breast cancer; e.g. Japan is a low incidence region, whereas Canada and the US are high incidence regions. Japanese women who migrate to Hawaii or USA have an increasing risk of breast cancer with each subsequent generation, raising the possibility of an environmental factor, such as diet.

Breast cancer is uncommon before the age of 30, and it shows a sharp increase in incidence between the ages of 30 to 50. After age 50, the incidence continues to increase, but at a slower rate. This may reflect the effects of ovarian hormones which cease at the menopause.

RISK FACTORS

- Age
The incidence of breast cancer increases with age. For example, the risk by age 40 is 1/200, by age 60 it is 1/25, and by age 85 it is 1/9.
- Hereditary factors
  - Positive family history of breast cancer
  - Inherited mutations (See section on Hereditary Breast Cancer)
- Prior history of breast cancer
A history of *in situ* or invasive breast cancer increases the risk of breast cancer in the contralateral breast.
- Endogenous endocrine factors
  - Early age of menarche (below 12 years) and late age of menopause

- Late age of first birth (>32 years of age)
- Nulliparity: an increased number of ovulatory cycles are suggested to be responsible for the increased risk
- Exogenous endocrine factors

Hormone replacement therapy (HRT) in postmenopausal women or oral contraceptive use in premenopausal women is associated with a small increase in the risk of breast cancer. In the case of HRT, there may be some interaction with family history. Although oral contraceptives do not substantially increase the risk of breast cancer, prolonged use, especially prior to the first-term pregnancy, may be associated with an increased risk of developing breast cancer before the age of 45.

- Environmental factors
  - Region of birth
  - Diet: increased caloric intake, fat, meat and alcohol are associated with a slightly increased risk for breast cancer. On the other hand, high intake of fibre, fruits and vegetables, antioxidant vitamins (A, C and E), and phyto-estrogens may reduce the risk
  - Exposure to radiation: an increased incidence of breast cancer is noted among atomic bomb survivors as well as in women who received radiation therapy to the thorax, such as for Hodgkin's lymphoma
- Obesity and increased body mass index in postmenopausal women

Table 8.1 summarizes the relative risk for breast cancer.

PATHOLOGY

Macroscopic

The most common location is the upper outer quadrant of the breast, but cancers can occur at any location where there is breast tissue, from the axillary tail to infraclavicular area to the midline. The cancer is frequently hard or firm, usually painless, and may be gritty.

Table 8.1 Estimated relative risk (RR) for breast cancer

Risk Factor	RR
Increased age	15
Family history in first degree relatives	2-4
Endogenous endocrine factors	
Late age at first birth	4
Nulliparity	4
Late menopause	3
Early menarche	2
Exogenous endocrine factors	
Oral contraceptive	1.8
Hormone replacement therapy	1.4
Irradiation to chest	5
Obesity	3

Microscopic

Breast cancer begins as an abnormal proliferation of cells in the epithelial lining of the ducts. Initially, this is confined to the superficial areas above the basement membrane (*in situ* disease). At this stage, the cancer cannot spread. Breaching of the basement membrane with invasion of the deeper layers occurs later. Almost all breast cancers are adenocarcinomas. About 80% are of ductal origin while the remainder are lobular (10%), medullary (5%) or tubular (5%) carcinomas.

Tumor Grade

Grade 1
- Good tubular formatiom
- Little nuclear pleomorphism
- Few mitotic figures

Grade 2
- A little tubular formation
- Moderate nuclear pleomorphism
- Some mitotic figures

Grade 3
- Little or no tubular formation
- Marked nuclear pleomorphism
- Many mitotic figures

Special tests

• Estrogen/progesterone receptor

Tumors that express estrogen (ER) or progesterone (PgR) receptor have a more indolent course than those that are receptor-negative. Determining the receptor status of a breast cancer is, therefore, an important part of the initial evaluation.

• HER-2 protein over-expression

HER-2 gene amplification occurs in about 20% of invasive breast cancer. Amplification generates additional gene copies, which become transcribed to mRNA and translated to the surface receptor protein. HER-2 receptor is an important growth factor receptor, and its over-expression is associated with a poor prognosis. Testing for HER-2 gene amplification or the receptor protein over-expression is now done routinely.

Spread

Direct extension to the skin and subcutaneous tissues produces dimpling, ulceration and, occasionally, retraction of the nipple. Deeper extension may involve the pectoral muscles, serratus anterior muscle and eventually the chest wall.

Lymphatic drainage of the breast follows the blood vessels:

(a) Along the tributaries of the axillary veins to the axillary lymph nodes.

(b) Along the perforating branches of the internal mammary vessels, which pierce each intercostal space, to the lymph nodes along the internal mammary chain. Although the lymph vessels lying between the lobules of the breast communicate freely, there is a tendency for the lateral half of the breast to drain to the axilla, and the medial half to drain to the internal mammary chain. In late stages of the disease, other nodes may be involved, such as the infraclavicular or supraclavicular nodes, mediastinal nodes, cervical nodes and the contralateral axillary nodes.

Blood-borne spread to distant organs. Although breast cancer can metastasize to almost any organ in the body, the common sites are lungs, liver, bone and brain.

Transcelomic spread to the pleura (pleural effusion), peritoneum (ascites) or pericardium (pericardial effusion) can occur in advanced stages of the disease.

Prognostic factors

The following factors have an adverse effect on prognosis:

• Lymph node metastasis
• Large size of the tumor (>2 cm)
• Lymphatic or vascular invasion
• Absent estrogen and progesterone receptors
• Poor tumor differentiation (high grade tumor)
• HER-2 over-expression

Lymph node involvement is a major prognostic factor, but categories of women with node-negative cancers are also at high risk. Discrimination of risk within node-negative disease remains challenging. Tumor size, hormone receptor status, histological grade and lymphovascular invasion (LVI) are the most important prognostic factors. Over-expression of HER-2 is another important prognostic and it is associated with an increase in relative risk of mortality of approximately 2. Young age (<35 years) appears to be an independent prognostic factor for both early node-negative and node-positive disease.

HEREDITARY BREAST CANCER

Most women with breast cancer do not have a positive family history for the disease. However, the occurrence of several cases of breast and ovarian cancers in a family, or bilateral breast cancers, especially at a relatively young age, increases the chances that an inherited gene mutation, such as a BRCA gene, is involved. About 5-7% of patients with breast cancer have a known germ-line mutation.

BRCA genes

Mutations of the tumor suppressor genes, BRCA-1 on chromosome 17 and BRCA-2 on chromosome 13, are associated with hereditary breast cancer. In cancers from women with one altered germ-line BRCA-1 or BRCA-2 gene, the normal copy is lost in the cancer cells. Sporadic breast or ovarian cancers have mutated BRCA-1 or BRCA-2 genes less than 10% of the time. Approximately 1 in 800 individuals carries a BRCA mutation. In individuals of Ashkenazi Jewish decent, the rate is more than 1 in 100. Other populations, e.g. French Canadian, Dutch and Scandinavian, have specific mutations that are passed down through the generations. Over 100 mutations have been identified in the BRCA-1 gene, although some are more commonly found in affected families. The large majority of mutations are frame-shift or nonsense sequence changes that lead to premature truncation of the peptide. A minority, about 5%, are missense mutations. There are also polymorphisms of unknown significance. Likewise, multiple mutations have been detected in BRCA-2, and about half of these are unique for specific families. There is some question as to whether specific breast cancer risk is different depending on where in the gene the mutation occurs.

The relative risk for breast or ovarian cancer in BRCA-1-linked families is high compared with the general population. The cumulative incidence of breast cancer by age 50 is 2% for the general population, compared with over 50% in the BRCA-1-linked kindred. By age 70,

this risk increases to 85%. Similarly, the lifetime cumulative risk for ovarian cancer is about 1.5% for the general population, whereas for BRCA-1-linked families it is over 60%.

In addition to breast and ovarian cancer risks, some families have an increased relative risk for other cancers: colon (4-fold increase), prostate (3-fold increase), and pancreas (8-fold increase). Also, inheritance of a mutated BRCA-2 gene is associated with male breast cancer. The breast cancer risk for a male carrier of a BRCA-2 mutation is about 6% by age 70.

Individuals with a strong family history of breast/ovarian cancers are candidates for genetic screening for mutated BRCA-1 and BRCA-2 genes. Before any genetic screening of the individual or family members is undertaken, genetic counselling is important so that they are cognizant of the implications of identification of a specific genetic mutation.

Loss of p53 suppressor gene

Loss of the p53 tumor suppressor gene (chromosome 17), known as Li-Fraumeni syndrome, is also associated with a high risk of breast cancer. This is rare.

SCREENING

Mammography

Mammograms can detect cancers as small as 0.5 cm, and can identify *in situ* as well as invasive cancers. Mammography screening enables earlier detection of breast cancer when treatment is more effective. Annual screening by mammography can reduce mortality by 25-40% in women between 40 and 79 years of age. This translates into a reduction in all-cause mortality of 2% for women older than 50 years. (See also Chapter 1.)

• Mammographic features of cancer

For screening, two views of each breast are taken to include as much of the breast tissue as possible: craniocaudal and mediolateral oblique. There are two main findings: mass lesion and abnormal calcifications.

A mass lesion

A mass may be benign (a cyst or a fibroadenoma) or a cancer. Benign lesions are usually smooth in outline, whereas cancer has indistinct borders or is spiculated, indicative of invasion of the adjacent normal breast tissues by malignant cells. An ultrasound can help distinguish a cyst from a solid mass.

Abnormal breast micro-calcifications

Fine calcifications may be indicative of an underlying malignancy. Calcium deposits are dystrophic calcification secondary to necrotic tumor cells. Micro-calcifications associated with breast cancer occur as fine, irregular particles in a ductal pattern with linear forms or small foci of clustered pleomorphic calcifications. Widespread calcifications within the breast are more difficult to evaluate. These may be due to benign conditions, such as sclerosing adenosis, or widespread *in situ* carcinoma. Figure 8.1 shows a mammogram with pleomorphic micro-calcifications; this is due to an intraductal carcinoma.

• Limitations of mammography

A mammogram can miss a cancer in certain situations:

- ◆ In premenopausal women with radiologically dense breast tissue
- ◆ A lesion located in the extreme periphery of the breast
- ◆ A huge lesion that is interpreted radiologically as an overall increase in breast density
- ◆ Cases of lobular breast carcinoma

Ultrasonography

Approximately 90% of cancers are detected as masses or pleomorphic micro-calcifications on mammograms. Ultrasonography can further characterize the abnormality and it is useful to distinguish a fluid-filled cyst from a solid mass. Solid masses require tissue biopsy, since ultrasonography cannot conclusively distinguish a benign from a malignant mass. Ultrasonography is also useful in women with a palpable breast mass but normal mammogram. This is especially helpful in women with dense breasts. A palpable mass should always be fully evaluated by a fine needle aspirate even if the ultrasound is normal.

Figure 8.1 Mammogram showing pleomorphic micro-calcifications (in the circled area) in the breast

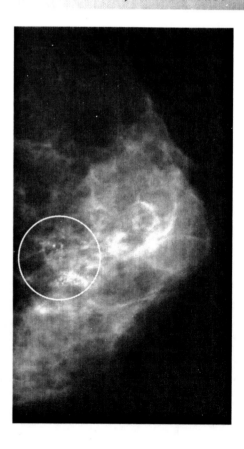

SURVEILLANCE OF WOMEN WITH BRCA MUTATIONS

Because of the high risk for developing breast or ovarian cancer, women with BRCA mutations should undergo cancer surveillance. The three elements of surveillance for breast cancer are breast self-examination, clinical examination and radiological imaging.

- Breast self-examination monthly from age 18
- Starting at age 25, clinical examination of the breast and regional nodes by a trained practitioner every 6 months
- Annual mammograms, starting 5-10 years before the earliest breast cancer diagnosed in the family, but not younger than age 30
- Annual MRI of the breasts
- Annual breast ultrasound in specific cases

Another option that may be considered in a high-risk individual is removal of the breasts as a preventive measure (bilateral prophylactic mastectomies). Prophylactic mastectomies will decrease the risk of developing cancer by 99%. The disturbance in body image, impact on sexuality, and risks and morbidity of surgery need to be considered in the decision-making process. At present, there are no specific recommendations for or against prophylactic mastectomy, and this is usually a personal decision.

Patients with BRCA mutations are also at risk for ovarian cancer. There is no proven screening test for ovarian cancer. Fewer than 50% of early stage ovarian cancers produce elevated CA125 titre (a serum tumor marker elevated in ovarian cancer). The positive predictive value of transvaginal pelvic ultrasound is low. Surgical removal of the ovaries (bilateral salpingo-oophorectomy) is recommended for women when their childbearing is complete, usually by their late thirties or early forties.

CLINICAL FEATURES

Local features: Many breast cancers are now detected by screening mammography in areas where this is widely practised. Otherwise, the most common presentation for a woman with breast cancer is a self-detected, asymptomatic breast lump. Breast lumps are a common clinical finding, and about 80% are benign. In premenopausal women, a period of observation for four weeks may be appropriate in some circumstances to determine whether there is a cyclic involution during the menses. All suspicious breast lumps must, however, be carefully evaluated to rule out a breast cancer and this requires histological confirmation. Less common presentations include breast pain, indrawing of the nipple, a blood-stained discharge or an axillary mass. Uncommonly, a rash is present at the nipple (Paget's disease).

Lymphatic spread occurs primarily to the ipsilateral axillary lymph nodes. There can also be spread to the internal mammary nodes, especially for cancers in the inner half of the breast. In more advanced cases, the supraclavicular and infraclavicular nodes may be involved.

Blood-borne metastatic disease is uncommon at initial diagnosis. It is more likely a manifestation of later progression of the cancer. Symptoms include:

- bone pain or pathological fracture without obvious trauma
- cough or shortness of breath due to lung metastases or pleural effusion
- abdominal pain or discomfort due to liver metastases
- back pain with leg numbness or weakness from spinal cord compression
- neuropathic pain resulting from spread into the brachial plexus
- symptomatic hypercalcemia

Physical examination may reveal a thickening or nodularity or a dominant mass. An uncommon presentation is inflammatory cancer (2%), which is associated with redness, heat and swelling of the breast with or without an underlying mass. Examination of the patient with a breast mass should be done in an orderly manner:

- Inspection for evidence of nipple retraction or elevation, puckering, *peau d'orange* or redness and thickening of the skin
- Palpation begins with the normal breast, followed by the affected breast for evidence of any abnormality. In the case of a vague thickening of the breast, it is helpful to compare the affected breast with the mirror image area of the opposite breast. A symmetrical thickening is more likely benign. The axillary nodes are then examined, followed by other nodal areas: infraclavicular, supraclavicular, cervical and contralateral axillary nodes. The description of a breast mass should include its location (left or right; detailed location using quadrant, clock face or distance from the nipple); size and depth; tenderness, mobility or fixation to either deep structures or skin and subcutaneous tissues; contours (smooth or irregular); texture (soft, hard or rubbery); any overlying skin changes (redness, ulceration, *peau d'orange*)
- The presence of metastatic disease is assessed by a general examination with particular attention to the skeleton, chest, liver and pelvis

Approach to the patient with a palpable breast abnormality

Breast lumps are common, and almost 1 in 2 women will consult their doctor during their lifetime about a breast problem. The clinical assessment and work-up of breast lumps can be challenging. In the vast majority of cases, these are due to benign conditions. Nonetheless, a systematic approach is necessary to ensure that a small breast cancer is not overlooked. There are two presenting clinical features: a vague area of thickening/nodularity or a dominant mass.

- Thickening or nodularity of the breast

In premenopausal women, the hormonally responsive breast tissues respond to the cyclic changes in hormone levels with cycles of proliferation and involution. An important initial step in a woman who finds a thickening or nodularity in her breast is to determine the timing of the abnormality in relation to the menstrual cycle. If there is a low index of suspicion of a cancer based on the physical findings, the rate of change of the abnormality, recent history of trauma, hormone use, her age, family history or prior personal history of cancer, close follow-up clinical evaluation may be appropriate. A reassessment should be done on days 5, 6 or 7 (follicular phase) of the next menstrual cycle. An abnormality that persists through the cycle requires further evaluation.

In a postmenopausal woman with a thickening in her breast, it is usually appropriate to undergo follow-up evaluation in 4-6 weeks when there is a low index of suspicion for breast cancer. However, if the thickening is new or if there is progression of the abnormality, further evaluation by mammography, ultrasonography, or both, is required. If these are normal, regular follow-up examination is indicated. If, however, the abnormality progresses, a biopsy is required despite the mammogram being normal.

The most common cause of nodularity is fibrocystic change, especially if it is tender. In young women, the upper outer quadrants and axillary tails are most frequently involved. It is worth noting that older women have a bilateral firm ridge of tissue (infra-mammary ridge) as a normal variant.

• Dominant palpable breast mass

Breast cancer generally presents as a firm or hard, irregular, non-tender mass, but it is sometimes impossible to rule out a malignant tumor on clinical grounds alone. Evaluation of a breast mass in a woman begins with an assessment of her cancer risk. If the risk is low, premenopausal women should be re-examined on days 5, 6 or 7 of the next menstrual cycle. If the mass persists or if it has any feature of a malignancy, further evaluation is essential. Any suspicious breast mass in a woman of any age should be evaluated by mammography and ultrasonogaphy, followed by a fine needle aspirate (FNA) or core needle biopsy. A negative mammogram should not lead to a delay in biopsy when there is a high suspicion of a cancer, since 10% of breast cancers are not detected by mammograms. The diagnostic accuracy of clinical examination, mammography and FNA, referred to as the triple test, of a dominant breast mass is 99%. Nonetheless, if there is any concern of the nature of the mass despite the triple test, an open biopsy should be done.

Approach to the patient with an abnormal mammogram

The increasing use of screening mammography has resulted in the detection of suspicious breast lesions, which are not clinically palpable. These can present a dilemma, and the desirability to diagnose a small cancer needs to be balanced with the avoidance of unnecessary biopsies and procedures, which can cause patient anxiety and be costly. When the index of suspicion of a cancer is high, further evaluation is advised. More refined mammography projections, FNA cytology and core biopsy of the lesion are acceptable procedures to confirm the diagnosis. Core needle biopsy is the best option to distinguish between a benign and a malignant lesion.

INVESTIGATIONS

• Complete blood count
• Serum biochemistry: liver enzymes, alkaline phosphatase, creatinine, calcium
• Tumor markers: CA15-3, CEA
• Bilateral mammograms are required to exclude a synchronous primary in the involved breast or the contralateral breast
• Chest x-ray
• Bone scan if the alkaline phosphatase is elevated or there is bone pain or the primary tumor is large (>5 cm)
• Imaging study of the liver if there is hepatomegaly or the liver enzymes are elevated
• CT scan of the brain if there are neurological symptoms

STAGING

The TMN staging is described in Chapter 5.

TREATMENT

Surgery

Partial or total mastectomy with axillary node dissection is the standard treatment for breast cancer. For unifocal cancers <5 cm, a breast-conserving partial mastectomy or lumpectomy with ipsilateral axillary node dissection is appropriate treatment, and this gives a better cosmetic result, provided it is combined with postoperative radiation to the breast. Lumpectomy refers to any breast-conserving operation; the aim is to remove the cancer with a wide margin of surrounding normal tissue. An axillary nodal dissection is carried out as part of the overall treatment, but the nodes also provide important prognostic information. In addition to the presence of lymph node metastasis, the number of involved nodes (1-3, 4-9, >10) is important in determining prognosis.

Sentinel lymph node biopsy
The sentinel node is the first node that receives lymph from the cancer, and the histological status of this node, namely, whether or not it contains malignant cells, may be predictive of axillary nodal involvement. The sentinel node is identified by injecting a dye or radio-labelled technetium in the tumor area and tracking its flow to the first node. If this node is removed and found to contain no cancer, there is a high probability (>90%) that no other regional lymph nodes are involved, and, therefore, no further surgery is necessary. On the other hand, if the node is positive, full axillary dissection is required.

Postoperative adjuvant therapy

After surgery, other therapeutic modalities, such as radiation, hormones or chemotherapy, are given as adjuvant therapy to women at high risk for recurrent breast cancer. The aim of adjuvant therapy is the eradication of any remaining cancer cells at the primary site as well as any systemic micro-metastases. The success of postoperative adjuvant therapy is measured by its ability to prolong the disease-free interval and, ultimately, overall patient survival.

• Adjuvant endocrine therapy
The basis of adjuvant endocrine therapy is to prevent endogenous estrogen from stimulating the growth of remaining cancer cells, specifically those that have hormone receptors. Cancers that do not make hormone receptors are not dependent on estrogen for growth, and hormone therapy is, therefore, ineffective in such patients.

Tamoxifen is a standard option for adjuvant therapy for both premenopausal and postmenopausal women with ER-positive breast cancer. Five years of adjuvant tamoxifen pro-duce a 9% reduction in mortality (26% vs. 35%). (In addition, adjuvant tamoxifen results in a 39% reduction in the risk of contralateral breast cancer in women with ER-positive or ER-unknown disease.)

Aromatase inhibitors (anastrazole or letrozole) are as effective as tamoxifen for adjuvant hormone therapy for postmenopausal women, and are increasingly preferred to tamoxifen. The sequential use of tamoxifen and aromatase inhibitors improves disease-free survival compared with tamoxifen alone, and an aromatase inhibitor should be considered as a component of adjuvant hormone therapy in postmenopausal women with hormone receptor-positive breast cancer.

The optimal adjuvant hormone therapy for menstruating women is uncertain and trials of various adjuvant therapy strategies in young women are in progress. The available hormone therapies for premenopausal women include tamoxifen and ovarian function suppression either by permanent ovarian ablation or temporarily by use of a GnRH agonist, such as goserelin or triptorelin.

• Adjuvant chemotherapy
Adjuvant chemotherapy benefits both premenopausal and postmenopausal women although the absolute magnitude of benefit is greater in younger women compared with older women. For women under 50 years, chemotherapy reduces the risk of disease relapse and death by 37% and 30%, respectively. For women aged 50-69, the risk of relapse or death is decreased by 19% and 12%, respectively. For women aged 70 years and older, the benefits of chemotherapy are less certain because few studies included women in this age group.

The need for postoperative adjuvant chemotherapy is determined by certain risk factors: tumor size, nodal status, hormone receptor status and HER-2 status of the tumor. In general, adjuvant chemotherapy is the standard of care for women with high-risk hormone receptor-negative tumors. For women with hormone receptor-positive cancer, the addition of chemotherapy to hormone therapy is recommended for those with positive lymph nodes as well as for those with high risk features even though the nodes are not involved. In addition, HER-2-positive tumors respond to targeted therapies, such as trastuzumab, and this is now combined with chemotherapy (see below). Tumors that lack estrogen receptors, progesterone receptors and are HER-2 negative comprise about 10-15% of breast cancers. These "triple negative" cancers are resistant to endocrine therapy and existing targeted therapies, and seem to have a worse outcome than other subtypes of breast cancers. Chemotherapy is the treatment of choice.

Several adjuvant chemotherapy choices are available, usually based on an anthracycline or a taxane, and are given for 4-6 months.

• Targeted therapy
The monoclonal antibody, trastuzumab, directed against HER-2 cell surface receptor can shrink tumors when used alone or combined with chemotherapy in patients with cancers that over-express the HER-2 receptor. In the adjuvant setting, trastuzumab with chemotherapy results in a 50% reduction in the odds of recurrence and a 30% reduction in the odds of death. Trastuzumab is now given concurrently with chemotherapy and is continued for up to 12 months.

Selection of adjuvant systemic therapy
Increasingly, the selection of treatment is being determined by the status of the tumor (Table 8.2). The benefits of adjuvant therapy for individual patients can be predicted by an on-line program "Adjuvant!Online" which takes into consideration several clinical and pathological factors.

Table 8.2 Summary of guidelines for adjuvant systemic therapy

◆ ER/PR positive, HER-2 negative tumors	
Premenopausal:	Chemotherapy Tamoxifen or ovarian ablation/suppression
Postmenopausal:	Chemotherapy Aromatase inhibitor (alone or after initial treatment with tamoxifen)
◆ HER-2 positive, any ER/PR or menopausal status	
Trastuzumab in combination with chemotherapy	
◆ ER negative, PR negative, HER-2 negative (triple negative) Chemotherapy (anthracycline, cyclophosphamide and a taxane)	

• Adjuvant radiation
Postoperative adjuvant radiation to the breast is now standard for women who have undergone a lumpectomy or partial mastectomy. If four or more axillary lymph nodes are positive, the lymph node bearing areas are treated as well. Following mastectomy, radiation is given to the chest wall and lymph nodes for cases with positive nodes.

Treatment of metastatic disease

Women with metastatic breast cancer are candidates for systemic therapy with hormones, chemotherapy and/or targeted therapies to relieve symptoms and prolong life. In deciding on the appropriate treatment, a number of factors are taken into account. A long interval between the initial diagnosis of the breast cancer and the appearance of overt metastasis (disease-free interval), hormone receptor-positive tumors, and soft tissue or bone metastasis predict a more indolent course with a relatively long survival time. In these circumstances, endocrine therapy is suitable. On the other hand, patients with a short disease-free interval, hormone receptor-negative tumors or involvement of vital organs, such as liver or lung, have a shorter survival time, and they require treatment with a more rapid onset of action. Chemotherapy is the choice in such patients.

• Endocrine therapy

The time to response to hormones is about 4-12 weeks. ER-positive tumors show a 60-70% response with a median duration of response of 12-15 months. For premenopausal women, initial options include tamoxifen or ovarian function suppression (oophorectomy or a GnRH agonist), or a combination of ovarian suppression plus tamoxifen. Combined endocrine therapy results in higher response rates and a longer time to progression, and it possibly has a small beneficial impact on overall survival. Premenopausal women, who progress after initial tamoxifen therapy, can be considered for ovarian function suppression as an alternative to chemotherapy. An aromatase inhibitor, such as anastrazole or letrozole, is often introduced immediately following oophorectomy.

For postmenopausal women, an aromatase inhibitor is now favored over tamoxifen as the first choice for advanced disease. On progression of disease, another hormonal agent, such as megestrol or fulvestrant, can be offered. Oophorectomy and GnRH agonists are ineffective treatments for postmenopausal women.

• Chemotherapy

Because hormone therapy has a more favorable side effect profile, it should be considered as initial therapy for metastatic breast cancer. However, chemotherapy and targeted therapies are appropriate once a hormone-responsive tumor becomes hormone-refractory, and for women who have rapidly progressive, symptomatic visceral metastases.

The overall response rate to chemotherapy is 40-70% with complete remission in 5-10% of cases. The median time to response is two weeks, and the median duration of response is 6-12 months. Active drugs include the taxanes, doxorubicin, epirubicin, fluorouracil (or capecitabine), methotrexate, cyclophosphamide, gemcitabine and vinorelbine. Combination chemotherapy may be an appropriate first-line choice for symptomatic patients or those with rapidly progressive visceral metastases because of the greater likelihood of an objective response. Because of the lack of an appreciable survival difference and quality-of-life benefit, therapy with serial single agents is a reasonable alternative to combination chemotherapy regimens, especially in the second-, third- or fourth-line treatment setting.

• Targeted therapy

Trastuzumab alone or in combination with chemotherapy is effective in HER-2-positive metastatic breast cancer. In combination with chemotherapy, it improves survival of patients. A trastuzumab-containing regimen is therefore recommended as first-line therapy to women with HER-2-positive metastatic breast cancer. The usual regimens include trastuzumab plus a taxane with or without carboplatin. If a taxane agent is contraindicated, trastuzumab plus vinorelbine could also be considered. The use of trastuzumab is associated with a small risk (1-4%) of cardiotoxicity; hence, it is not combined with an anthracycline. Lapatinib is a dual erbB-1/2 tyrosine kinase inhibitor that affects both the epidermal growth factor receptor (EGFR, also called erbB-1) and HER-2 (also called erbB-2). It is usually given in combination with capecitabine for patients with HER-2-positive breast cancer who had received prior therapy with an anthracycline, a taxane and trastuzumab.

Choice of chemotherapy and targeted therapy for metastatic breast cancer

The choice of drugs depends on whether the patient received previous adjuvant chemotherapy and the HER-2 status of the tumor (Table 8.3). There is no standard regimen and the goal is to design a treatment plan for the individual patient that systematically applies different treatment options to achieve the best outcome. After first-line treatment, other chemotherapy regimens are usually given as second- or third-line treatment options.

Table 8.3 Choice of drugs for advanced breast cancer based on prior adjuvant chemotherapy and HER-2 status

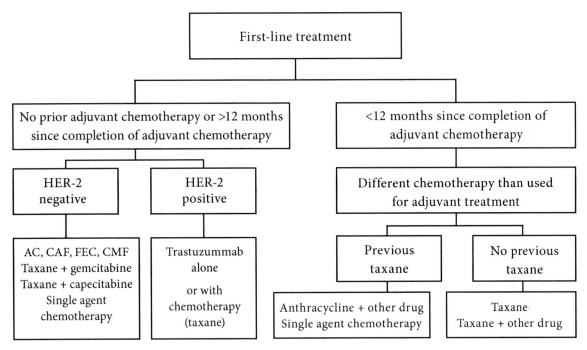

AC = cyclophosphamide-doxorubicin
FEC = cyclophosphamide-epirubicin-FU
CAF = cyclophosphamide-doxorubicin-FU
CMF = cyclophosphamide-methotrexate-FU

• Radiation therapy
Radiation therapy is useful for palliation of patients with metastatic disease, especially those with painful bone metastasis, soft tissue metastases, spinal cord compression or brain metastasis.

• Bisphosphonates
Bisphosphonates, such as pamidronate, clodronate or zoledronate, are useful in the treatment of hypercalcemia and bone pain even when bone metastases are not detected. In patients with bone metastases, they reduce bone pain and the risk of pathological fractures.

SPECIAL SITUATIONS

Carcinoma *in situ*

• Lobular carcinoma *in situ (LCIS)*
LCIS is usually diagnosed incidentally when a breast biopsy is done for benign disease. It is more common in premenopausal women and is

often bilateral. LCIS is usually undetectable clinically and does not show up on a mammogram. Its presence indicates a high risk for the later development of an infiltrating carcinoma in either or both breasts. The risk to each breast is approximately equal and approaches 15% within 10-15 years. Patients can be given the option of either careful follow-up or bilateral mastectomy. Tamoxifen or raloxifene reduces the risk of developing invasive ER-positive cancer by one-half, and is, therefore, another option.

• Ductal carcinoma *in situ* or DCIS
DCIS is being diagnosed with increasing frequency as a result of mammography screening. About 12% of all newly diagnosed breast cancers and at least 20% of those detected by mammography are DCIS. The typical mammographic finding is multiple abnormal clusters of calcification. Invasive and DCIS share the same risk factors. DCIS is also a component of the inherited breast-ovarian cancer syndrome due to mutations in the BRCA genes, and it tends to occur at a younger age in women with inherited BRCA mutations. DCIS originates in the epithelial cells lining the lactiferous ducts, and can spread through a large area of segmental ducts with multiple tumor foci within the connected ducts. There is no invasion of the ductal basement membrane, and the disease, therefore, does not metastasize. However, if left untreated, DCIS develops into invasive carcinoma in the ipsilateral breast in 25-35% of women over 10 years. Clinically, a breast lump may be palpable in about 60% of patients with DCIS.

Treatment is designed to maximize control of the local disease while minimizing treatment morbidity. Total mastectomy provides a cure rate of 98-99%. Patients with localized disease are candidates for breast conserving therapy, provided a 10-mm margin of clearance can be achieved. Although the rate of local recurrence is higher with breast conserving surgery, survival after local recurrence is excellent. If adequate margins of clearance cannot be obtained, radiation may be considered. The use of tamoxifen to reduce the risk of breast cancer recurrence after breast conserving surgery is not conclusively proven in this setting.

Inflammatory breast cancer

This is uncommon and comprises 2% of all breast cancers. Clinically, there is ill-defined erythemia, tenderness, induration and edema of the skin of the breast. The clinical features mimic a breast abscess. Histologically, there is invasion of the lymphatics in the skin by cancer cells. Inflammatory breast cancers are aggressive with a high risk of local recurrence and distant metastases.

Paget's disease of the breast

Paget's disease represents invasion of the epidermis of the nipple and areola by large, pale cancer cells (Paget's cells). It is associated with 1-2% of breast cancers, especially in older women. It often presents as a rash, resembling eczema. Paget's disease occurs on the nipple and areola whereas eczema is confined to the areola and may be bilateral. There is an underlying ductal carcinoma (invasive or DCIS), and a breast lump may be palpable in half the patients. A full thickness skin biopsy confirms the diagnosis. Treatment is a total mastectomy followed by adjuvant therapy, depending on the ER status of the tumor and menopausal status of the woman.

Breast cancer during pregnancy

Breast cancer rarely develops in pregnant or lactating women: two breast cancers occur in every 10,000 pregnant women. Nonetheless, any enlarging breast mass should be assessed to rule out a cancer even if there are no identifiable risk factors. Breast cancers that arise in this setting tend to be more aggressive with a poor prognosis. Mammograms can be done safely, and FNA of a palpable abnormality confirms the nature of the mass. Treatment of breast cancer during pregnancy is problematic. Options include a therapeutic abortion if the pregnancy is in the first trimester, followed by standard breast cancer management. Surgery should be done as soon as possible, preferably after the first trimester. Diagnosis during the second or third trimester must take into consideration the viability of the fetus and the need to start anticancer therapy.

Male breast cancer

Cancer of the male breast is rare and accounts for <1% of all breast cancers. Inheritance of a mutated BRCA-2 gene predisposes to the development of breast cancer in men. Most are infiltrating ductal adenocarcinomas and the treatment is similar to female breast cancer. Mastectomy and axillary node dissection is standard with postoperative radiation therapy given because of the closeness to the underlying pectoralis muscle. Most are ER-positive tumors and, thus, patients benefit from hormone therapy. Chemotherapy is required for high-risk cancers or ER-negative cancers.

FOLLOW-UP EVALUATION

The primary goal of follow-up of breast cancer patients is to detect a new breast cancer or curable recurrent disease. Potentially curable conditions include:

- New breast cancer in the contralateral breast. This occurs with a frequency of 0.5-1% per year

- Local recurrence in a breast previously treated by partial mastectomy. The frequency of this is 1% or less per year
- Local recurrence on the chest wall or, occasionally, in the regional nodes
- Second cancers, primarily those of the colon, ovary or uterus

The follow-up evaluations include:
- Clinical examination every 6 months for 5 years, then yearly. Particular attention is paid to the affected breast or mastectomy site, regional nodal area, liver, lungs and spine for signs of recurrent disease
- Breast self-examination
- Annual mammograms are recommended, bilateral for women with breast-conserving surgery, and unilateral for women with mastectomy
- Routine screening for metastatic disease is not generally recommended in the absence of signs or symptoms

OUTCOME

Five-year breast cancer-specific survival in a cohort of 12,988 women in British Columbia is shown in the Table 8.4.

Table 8.4 Five-year survival by age groups

Age group (years)	50-64	65-74	75-84	>85
Stage I	95%	95%	93%	82%
Stage II	83%	81%	79%	68%
Stage III	58%	55%	53%	34%
Stage IV	21%	15%	21%	25%

Chapter 9

THORACIC ONCOLOGY

CLASSIFICATION

Benign
- Adenoma
- Carcinoid
- Hamartoma
- Leiomyoma
- Hemangioma

Malignant

Primary
- Bronchogenic carcinoma
- Mesothelioma

Secondary
- Carcinoma: breast, esophagus, kidney and rectum
- Melanoma
- Sarcoma

CARCINOMA OF THE LUNG

INCIDENCE

Lung cancer is the most common malignancy worldwide. In Canada and the US, it is by far the leading cause of cancer-related deaths in both men and women. There has been a decline in the incidence in men since the mid-1980s, and in the past decade it has begun to level off in women. Lung cancer rates parallel cigarette smoking prevalence rates, and about 85% of lung cancers are attributed to active cigarette smoking or exposure to second-hand smoke. Recently, the incidence of adenocarcinoma has been increasing relative to the other subtypes. This is thought to be related to the use of filters with less tar, but the nitrosoamine content remains high.

RISK FACTORS

- Tobacco smoking

More than 3,000 chemicals have been identified in tobacco smoke. The major carcinogens are the polycyclic aromatic hydrocarbons and nitrosoamines. They are activated by Phase I enzymes in the lungs, and they bind to DNA, causing gene mutations. Non-smokers who are exposed to cigarette smoke also inhale numerous carcinogens. The passive inhalation of cigarette smoke leads to an increase in the incidence of lung cancer; this is especially true for non-smokers who live with smokers. The cancer risk declines after smoking cessation. However, the risk remains substantial for long-term heavy smokers, who give up smoking after the age of 50 years.

- Occupational exposure

A number of environmental toxins have been identified: asbestos, radon gas (underground mining and indoor exposure), bis(chloromethyl) ether, polycyclic aromatic hydrocarbons, chromium, nickel, silica and arsenic.

- Infection

Among non-smokers, infections with papillomavirus and other viruses may play a role.

- Genetic factors

The lifetime risk of lung cancer for a one pack-a-day smoker is approximately 16% in men and 10% in women. Genetic polymorphisms of enzymes, particularly those of the cytochrome P450 family (Phase I enzymes) that convert pro-carcinogens to active carcinogens, glutathione-s-transferases (Phase II enzymes) that detoxify carcinogens, as well as DNA repair capacity, may determine an individual's susceptibility to lung cancer.

PREVENTION AND SCREENING

Because the overwhelming cause of lung cancer is inhalation of cigarette smoke, reduction in smoking would result in a decrease in the number of lung cancer cases. A number of compounds, such as COX-2 inhibitors, LOX inhibitors, and botanical food supplements like green tea, are being investigated as possible chemopreventive agents.

No proven screening technique is presently available. Newer detection techniques, such as improved sputum cytology examination methods, plasma proteomic markers, fluorescence bronchoscopy for localization of small preinvasive cancer, and spiral chest CT scan are promising, but their role in population screening has not yet been established.

PATHOLOGY

Macroscopic

Most lung cancers arise in the bronchial epithelium and grow circumferentially and longitudinally along the bronchus. They present as submucosal infiltrates or endobronchial lesions, which cause narrowing of the bronchus. About 50% of lung cancers are visible at bronchoscopy. Local hemorrhage and necrosis may be evident. The lung segments distal to the obstruction may be collapsed, and secondary infection is common.

Microscopic

Four main histological types of lung cancers are identified:
- Small cell lung carcinoma (20%)
- Adenocarcinoma (40%)
- Squamous cell carcinoma (30%)
- Large cell carcinoma (10%)

From a therapeutic standpoint, it is convenient to divide lung cancers into two subgroups: small cell lung cancer and non-small cell lung cancer, which comprises the three other histological types.

Spread

Locally along the bronchus, often causing bronchial occlusion and lobar collapse. The cancer can also extend to the pleura, pericardium, recurrent laryngeal nerve, esophagus, brachial plexus, cervical sympathetic nerves and diaphragm.

Lymphatic to intralobar, hilar and mediastinal (subcarinal, paratracheal and subaortic) nodes. More distal nodes (supraclavicular or cervical) can be involved and this is almost always an indication of distant spread.

Blood-borne to bone, liver, skin and brain. Metastasis to the adrenal glands occurs in a high proportion of cases. Metastases within the lungs can occur from a variety of mechanisms: airborne spread, retrograde lymphatic spread and blood-borne spread.

Transcelomic across pleural and, less commonly, pericardial spaces.

CLINICAL FEATURES

Local growth of the cancer in the large airways causes cough, breathlessness, wheeze or stridor. Hemoptysis occurs frequently; this is usually blood-streaked sputum and massive hemoptysis is uncommon. Local invasion of adjacent structures produces chest pain or hoarseness (recurrent laryngeal nerve involvement). A malignant pleural effusion may also be responsible for dyspnea. Post-obstructive pneumonia may occasionally be the presenting complaint. Cancers arising in the lung apex can invade the brachial plexus, leading to pain which radiates down the arm to the medial aspect of the forearm (Pancoast syndrome).

Lymphatic involvement of the mediastinal nodes can occasionally lead to dysphagia or superior vena cava (SVC) syndrome.

Secondary deposits can occur in the skeleton (bone pain or fracture), liver (jaundice or upper abdominal discomfort), brain (neurological symptoms), and adrenal glands (uncommonly, adrenocortical failure may result).

The general effects include the anorexia-cachexia syndrome, fatigue, weakness, and paraneoplastic syndromes. Paraneoplastic syndromes occur in 10% of small cell lung cancer, and less frequently in non-small cell lung cancer. The most common syndrome is inappropriate ADH syndrome, leading to low serum sodium levels. Other paraneoplastic syndromes are ectopic ACTH production and Eaton-Lambert myasthenic syndrome. Hypercalcemia due to ectopic parathyroid hormone production is sometimes associated with squamous cell carcinoma, but not with small cell lung cancer.

Examination may be unremarkable in the minority of patients whose lung cancer is detected incidentally by a chest x-ray. Usually, patients have evidence of pneumonic consolidation; clubbing of the fingers may be present and the fingers are nicotine-stained. The supraclavicular nodes, which are in continuity with the regional nodes, can be enlarged. Involvement of the cervical sympathetic nerves at T1 leads to Horner's syndrome (ptosis, miosis, enophthalmos and loss of hemi-facial sweating). There may be evidence of distant metastatic disease to liver (hepatomegaly), bone (tenderness or pathological fractures), or brain (neurological signs).

DIAGNOSIS

A chest x-ray is a quick, non-invasive method for the initial assessment of a lung neoplasm. The characteristic features include a discrete mass, sometimes with cavitation, associated with hilar adenopathy, consolidation or

collapse of the lung, and a pleural effusion. Erosion of the ribs may be evident and the hemi-diaphragm can be elevated due to involvement of the phrenic nerve by mediastinal infiltration. Figure 9.1 depicts the chest x-ray findings of a non-small cell lung carcinoma of the left lung.

Figure 9.1 Chest x-ray showing a mass in the left upper lobe with associated left tracheobronchial and hilar lymphadenopathy and a small left pleural effusion

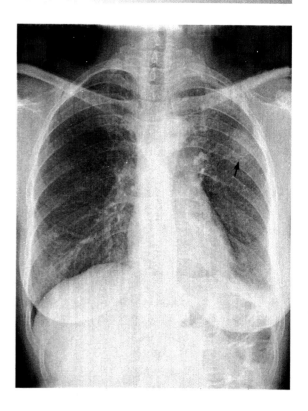

The diagnosis of lung cancer requires cytological or histological confirmation. Several procedures are available to establish this and one or more of these may be necessary.

• Sputum cytology

Three daily pooled sputum samples taken in the early morning or induced sputum by inhalation of hypertonic saline are recommended. A post-bronchoscopy sample when the patient is coughing vigorously can also be useful. The yield for central cancers is about 80%, but much less for peripheral ones.

• Fine needle aspirate or biopsy

If there is a pleural effusion, a palpable supra-clavicular node or liver lesions, the diagnosis can be confirmed by cytology or histology of material obtained from these sites.

• Bronchoscopy

Most lung cancers are diagnosed by trans-bronchial biopsy or cytology. Centrally located cancers, such as squamous cell carcinoma, often present as endobronchial masses. Small cell lung cancer infiltrates submucosally and may be visible at bronchoscopy. More peripheral tumors may not be evident at bronchoscopy, but they can be diagnosed by fluoroscopy-guided trans-bronchial biopsy or cytology.

• Mediastinoscopy/mediastinotomy

Mediastinoscopy and mediastinotomy (for assessment of the anterior mediastinal nodes in cases of left upper lobe cancers) are important for staging of the mediastinal nodes, which are often involved with metastasis. An endoscopic ultrasound-guided needle biopsy can also be performed.

• Trans-thoracic needle biopsy

This is useful for peripherally located cancers. It is usually done with x-ray fluoroscopy or CT guidance.

• Thoracoscopy

Thoracoscopy can be helpful for diagnosis of difficult cases. It is also a staging procedure for the diagnosis of pleural disease or malignant effusion in a patient who is otherwise a candidate for radical surgery.

• Open lung biopsy

This is the most invasive diagnostic procedure, which is used when other measures have failed to establish the diagnosis.

SMALL CELL LUNG CANCER

STAGING

The staging system for small cell lung cancer recognizes two stages:

• Limited stage (35%), defined as disease confined to one hemi-thorax and the ipsilateral supraclavicular lymph nodes

• Extensive stage (65%), which includes disease at all other sites. The presence of a pleural effusion, whether cytologically positive or negative, puts the cancer in this stage

This is a practical staging system. Limited stage small cell lung cancer can be encompassed in a reasonable field of radiation therapy. The separation between these two stages has considerable prognostic significance.

INVESTIGATIONS

• Complete blood count
• Serum biochemistry: liver enzymes, LDH, electrolytes, creatinine
• Chest x-ray
• CT scan of the chest for limited stage disease to facilitate radiation planning
• CT of abdomen
• CT scan of the head
• Bone scan
• Bone marrow aspirate and biopsy if the blood counts are abnormal
• Pulmonary function tests if there is concern about the toxicity of thoracic radiation due to

poor pulmonary reserve

If a patient has extensive stage disease apparent at presentation or on initial work-up, all of these tests or procedures are not necessary.

TREATMENT

Small cell lung cancer has a marked tendency to metastasize early, and it is regarded as a systemic disease at the outset even if overt metastases are not evident. It is sensitive to chemotherapy and combination chemotherapy is the mainstay of treatment. Several drugs are active in the treatment of small cell lung cancer. The most commonly used regimen is the combination of cisplatin and etoposide. Elderly patients may be treated with oral etoposide with satisfactory results.

In limited stage disease, combination chemotherapy produces tumor response rates of 80-90%, and about half of these are complete responses. Four to six cycles of treatment are usually given. Radiation therapy is given to the primary cancer and the mediastinal nodes to reduce local or nodal recurrent disease. In addition, there is a high rate of relapse of disease in the brain, a chemotherapy sanctuary site, and prophylactic cranial radiation is recommended for patients who achieve a systemic remission. The median survival time for limited stage patients is 18 months, with about 20% patients being long-term survivors.

Patients with extensive stage disease are treated with combination chemotherapy, such as cisplatin-etoposide, or single agent chemotherapy, such as oral etoposide, if they are elderly or infirm. Patients who respond to chemotherapy are also treated with prophylactic cranial radiation and often a consolidative course of radiation to the primary site of disease in the lung. The median survival time for extensive stage patients is 9 months with few long-term survivors.

Patients who relapse after chemotherapy and who are fit with a good performance status (ECOG<2) may be treated with second-line chemotherapy, such as topotecan.

Because of the systemic nature of the disease at presentation, surgery is not considered the standard of care in the management of small cell lung cancer. When surgery is done, it should be followed by chemotherapy and radiation to address micro-metastases.

NON-SMALL CELL LUNG CANCER

STAGING

The TNM staging system is used. This is based on the anatomic routes of spread of the cancer.

T1 - Tumor <3 cm diameter, surrounded by lung or visceral pleura, without invasion more proximal than lobar bronchus

    T1a - Tumor <2 cm in diameter

    T1b - Tumor >2 cm in diameter

T2 - Tumor >3 cm but <7 cm, with any of the following features:
- involves main bronchus >2 cm distal to carina
- invades visceral pleura
- associated with atelectasis or obstructive pneumonitis that extends to the hilar region but does not involve the entire lung

    T2a - Tumor <5 cm

    T2b - Tumor >5 cm

T3 - Tumor >7 cm or any of the following:
- directly invades any of the following: chest wall, diaphragm, phrenic nerve, mediastinal pleura, parietal pericardium, main bronchus <2 cm from carina (without involvement of carina)
- atelectasis or obstructive pneumonitis of the entire lung
- separate tumor nodules in the same lobe

T4 - Tumor of any size that invades the mediastinum, heart, great vessels, trachea, recurrent laryngeal nerve, esophagus, vertebral body, carina, or with separate tumor nodules in a different ipsilateral lobe

N0 - No regional lymph node metastases

N1 - Metastasis in ipsilateral peribronchial and/or ipsilateral hilar lymph nodes and intrapulmonary nodes, including involvement by direct extension

N2 - Metastasis in ipsilateral mediastinal and/ or subcarinal lymph node(s)

N3 - Metastasis in contralateral mediastinal, contralateral hilar, ipsilateral or contralateral scalene, or supraclavicular lymph node(s)

M0 - No distant metastasis

M1 - Distant metastasis

   M1a - Separate tumor nodule(s) in a contralateral lobe; tumor with pleural nodules or malignant pleural or pericardial effusion

   M1b - Distant metastasis

Stage Groupings

Stage IA	T1a-T1b N0 M0
Stage 1B	T2a N0 M0
Stage IIA	T1a-T2a N1 M0
	T2b N0 M0
Stage IIB	T2b N1 M0
	T3 N0 M0
Stage IIIA	T1a-T3 N1 M0
	T4 N0-N1 M0
Stage IIIB	T4 N2 M0
	T1a-T4 N3 M0
Stage IV	any T any N M1a-1b

Goldstraw, P, Crowley, J, Chansky, K, et al. The IASLC Lung Cancer Staging Project: Proposals for the revision of the TNM stage groups in the forthcoming (seventh) edition of the TNM classification of malignant tumours. J Thorac Oncol 2007; 2:706.

INVESTIGATIONS

- Complete blood count
- Biochemistry: electrolytes, calcium, creatinine, liver enzymes
- Chest x-ray
- CT scan of the chest and abdomen
- Bone scan if bone symptoms are present
- CT scan of the head if neurological symptoms are present or if the disease is Stage II or worse
- PET scan to detect extra-thoracic spread
- Pulmonary function tests in patients for radiation or surgery

If the patient has metastatic disease apparent at presentation, all of these staging tests are not necessary.

TREATMENT

Surgery

The cornerstone of treatment for non-small cell lung cancer is surgery although only about 30% of patients are suitable candidates. Early stage disease that is potentially resectable includes Stage I and Stage II cancers. Some patients with Stage III disease with involvement of ipsilateral or subcarinal mediastinal nodes (Stage IIIA) may be candidates for resection, usually as part of a combined modality approach with chemotherapy and radiation. Involvement of contralateral mediastinal, hilar or supraclavicular nodes (Stage IIIB), or the presence of metastatic disease (Stage IV) rules out surgical resection. Patients with malignant pleural effusion are unresectable and are not appropriate candidates for radical surgery.

The aim of surgery resection is removal of the primary cancer with clear margins along with the draining peribronchial and hilar nodes. Mediastinal nodes are also removed or sampled. A lobectomy is the most commonly performed surgery, but more radical resection (bilobectomy or pneumonectomy) may be required for more extensive cancers. In selected patients, a partial lobectomy (wedge resection) may be performed.

Radiation therapy

Radiation therapy may be advised for patients with early stage lung cancer that is technically resectable if there are medical contraindications for surgery, such as coexisting heart or pulmonary disease. For Stage III disease, radiation is used in conjunction with surgery and chemotherapy as part of a multimodality treatment. Although this approach has more systemic toxicity and esophagitis, the 5-year survival rate is 30% in patients with good performance status (ECOG 0 or 1) and minimal weight loss (<5% in the preceding 3 months).

Postoperative adjuvant radiation for completely resected non-small cell lung cancer decreases local recurrences, but this is not standard practice.

Radiation is also useful for palliation of painful bone metastasis, symptoms from brain metastases, superior vena cava obstruction, hemoptysis, and dyspnea due to bronchial obstruction.

Chemotherapy

Postoperative adjuvant chemotherapy
Postoperative adjuvant chemotherapy improves survival in early stage and is standard care for Stages II and IIIA non-small cell lung cancer with a 10-15% survival benefit at 5 years. The chemotherapy regimens include cisplatin with vinorelbine, gemcitabine or docetaxel. Among these, cisplatin-vinorelbine has the most supporting evidence.

Chemotherapy for advanced disease
Non-small cell lung cancer is less responsive to chemotherapy than small cell lung cancer. In locally advanced Stage IIIB or unresectable Stage IIIA lung cancer, concurrent chemotherapy and radiation is the standard treatment.

In Stage IV or recurrent non-small cell lung cancer, which represents the largest population of patients, palliative chemotherapy can modestly improve median survival time and quality of life compared with best supportive care in patients with good performance status (ECOG 0 or 1). Chemotherapy usually consists of cisplatin or carboplatin in combination with docetaxel, paclitaxel, gemcitabine or vinorelbine. Patients with ECOG performance status 2 or elderly patients over age 70 years may benefit from single-agent chemotherapy, such as gemcitabine or vinorelbine, or combination chemotherapy, but the benefit is small, and the decision to treat must be considered on an individual basis. Patients who are sicker (ECOG 3 or 4) do not benefit from chemotherapy.

Second-line chemotherapy for fit patients, who have recurrent or progressive disease after treatment with a platinum-based regimen, also improves quality of life and survival. Docetaxel or pemetrexed is the usual choice of drugs in this setting, although targeted agents are treatment options (see below).

Targeted therapy

Targeted therapy is emerging as a new treatment option for lung cancer patients. The epidermal growth factor receptor (EGFR) is known to play a key role in cellular growth and differentiation of lung cancer cells. Erlotinib, which inhibits tyrosine kinase activity of EGFR, is a useful second- or third-line drug in non-small cell lung cancer. Predictors of response to an EGFR inhibitor have been difficult to define. Some patients have mutations or over-express EGFR and may be more sensitive to these agents. In addition, there is a suggestion that women, non-smokers, those of Asian origin, and adenocarcinoma or bronchioalveolar type of lung cancer may be more likely to respond to EGFR inhibitors. Similarly, gefitinib is an active drug in the second-line setting. In Stage IV disease, the addition of bevacizumab, an inhibitor of angiogenesis, to conventional chemotherapy has shown efficacy in selected patients.

Endobronchial therapy

Several local modalities are available for palliation of central bronchial tumors.
• Brachytherapy
Brachytherapy or endobronchial radiation may be useful in the palliation of symptoms, mainly hemoptysis, cough or dyspnea.
• Electrocautery or Argon Plasma Coagulation
Electrocautery or argon plasma coagulation is used for coagulation and de-bulking endobronchial tumors. In patients with superficial squamous cell carcinoma, these modalities may also be potentially curative.
• Photodynamic therapy
Photodynamic therapy involves the administration of a photosensitizing agent, e.g. Photofrin, which selectively accumulates in the cancer. A red laser light activates the Photofrin to produce a photochemical reaction that destroys the cancer. It may be potentially curative for small, early bronchial cancers confined to the bronchial wall, but its main value is the treatment of inoperable patients with early cancer or those with multiple bronchial cancers.
• Stents
Stents are silicone or metallic tubes which may be used to maintain a patent airway in patients who have extrinsic compression of the airway by tumor or lymph nodes.

Table 9.1 summarizes the general approach to management and outcome for non-small cell lung cancer. The overall prognosis is poor even for completely resected Stage I or Stage II

Table 9.1 Summary of management and outcome for non-small cell lung cancer

Stage	Principal treatment modalities	5-year survival
I	surgery	65%
II	surgery + chemotherapy	40%
IIIA	surgery + chemotherapy or radiation + chemotherapy	30%
IIIB	radiation + chemotherapy	15%
IV	chemotherapy	<5%
Overall	–	14%

SECONDARY TUMORS

The lung is second to the liver as a site for metastasis from other cancers. Spread may be either the result of blood-borne metastases or retrograde lymphatic permeation from involved mediastinal nodes, causing lymphangitic carcinomatosis. A chest x-ray should be done in all cases of cancer to rule out lung metastasis.

APPROACH TO MANAGEMENT OF SOLITARY LUNG LESIONS

Routine chest x-rays for other reasons may bring to attention a solitary lung nodule. The investigation of this should begin with a comparison with any previous chest x-rays, if available. A lesion that is old, especially if it has been present for two or more years, with no change in size is likely not malignant. Central calcification is typical of benign lesions. A new lung lesion or one that is increasing in size should be considered malignant. PET imaging can be helpful to differentiate between a malignant and benign nodule. However, false negative scans can occur with small lesions or in bronchioalveolar carcinoma. False positive scans can occur with inflammatory or infectious nodules. The diagnosis should be confirmed cytologically or histologically prior to treatment.

MESOTHELIOMA

INCIDENCE

Mesothelioma is an uncommon cancer of the pleura and peritoneum. It is predominantly a disease of men in the age group 50-70 years. The incidence appears to be increasing, by as much as 50% in the past decade.

RISK FACTORS

• Exposure to asbestos

The chief risk factor for mesothioloma is asbestos exposure. The average lag time from first asbestos exposure to diagnosis is 40 years. Occupational exposure accounts for 80% of all cases. Individuals at risk include miners, builders, tile workers, insulation workers and naval dockworkers. Spouses of asbestos workers are also at increased risk due to fibres carried on clothing. There are two types of asbestos, based on their shape and size: chrysotile (curly fibres) and amphibole (rod-like fibres). Of these, amphibole fibres are responsible for mesothelioma.

• Infective process

A possible association with Simian virus 40 has been suggested.

SCREENING AND PREVENTION

The risk for mesothelioma is high in those exposed to asbestos. The role of regular chest x-ray as a screening test for these individuals is unclear. Smoking increases the risk for lung cancer, but not mesothelioma, in patients exposed to asbestos. They should, therefore, be advised to stop smoking.

Because of the recognized association of mesothelioma with asbestos exposure, its use is now limited in industry. Care must be taken in renovation of older buildings in which asbestos is present; this includes isolation of the working area and use of respirators.

Patients with mesothelioma who were exposed to asbestos at work may be entitled to compensation.

PATHOLOGY

Macroscopic

Mesothelioma arises from the mesothelial cells of the pleura and, less commonly, peritoneum. In rare cases, it can originate in the pericardium or tunica vaginalis of the testis.

Multiple small tumor nodules are present on the visceral and parietal surfaces of the pleura. They coalesce to form plaques that spread into the fissures and intralobular septa. The lungs eventually become encased and a bloody pleural effusion collects.

Microscopic

There are two predominant cell types: epithelial (glandular) and spindle (sarcomatous). The epithelial cell type is more common, making up about two-thirds of cases. The sarcomatous variety is more aggressive. Asbestos fibres can be found in the underlying lung tissues.

Spread

Local growth is the primary mode of spread. The pleural space is obliterated and the tumor invades the adjacent structures: chest wall, pericardium and contralateral hemi-thorax. Invasion through the diaphragm leads to involvement of the peritoneal space and abdominal organs. *Lymphatic spread and blood-borne spread* are uncommon.

CLINICAL FEATURES

Local growth is responsible for the common symptoms. Most patients experience increasing dyspnea and chest discomfort, usually for a few months. A dry cough may be present, but there is no hemoptysis, unlike lung cancer.

Generalized symptoms include anorexia, weight loss and fever.

Examination reveals reduced expansion of the chest associated with percussion dullness and reduced breath sounds. Finger clubbing may be present.

Adverse prognostic factors

- Poor performance status
- Advanced stage
- Leucocytosis
- Male gender
- Sarcomatous histology
- Presence of chest pain

DIAGNOSIS AND INVESTIGATION

- Chest x-ray shows a pleural mass with effusion. Asbestosis of the lung may be evident
- CT scan is better in defining the pleural mass and assessing local invasion
- Pleural fluid cytology: the fluid is often bloody with a high protein level and high level (>50 ng/L) of hyaluronic acid. Malignant mesothelial cells may be found in 40% of cases
- Pleural biopsy is more reliable than fluid cytology to establish the diagnosis. It is done by ultrasound or CT-guided needle biopsy. There is a high incidence of false negative biopsies, and if this is not successful, an open biopsy at thoracoscopy is required

TREATMENT

Surgery

The usual treatment for mesothelioma is drainage of the pleural effusion, chest tube pleurodesis or thoracoscopic pleurodesis. Because of the restrictive nature of the disease,

control of the effusion may be difficult.

Pleurectomy or pleural decortication is a debulking procedure with minimal morbidity for control of pleural effusion. A radical resection by pleuro-pneumonectomy (excision of lung, pleura, hemi-diaphragm and ipsilateral half of the pericardium) may be appropriate treatment for a few select patients; there is a high morbidity and mortality rate with this procedure.

Radiation therapy

The target volume of the tumor and toxicity of the surrounding tissues restricts the use of radiation. Radiation therapy is used primarily for palliation of chest pain.

Chemotherapy

A few drugs have limited activity. They include cisplatin, pemetrexed, gemcitabine and raltitrexed which produce partial tumor responses in about 15% of patients. Epithelial mesotheliomas are more responsive to chemotherapy, but even so responses are of short duration, usually a few months. Combination chemotherapy (cisplatin with pemetrexed or raltitrexed) increases response rates to 25-40% with a small survival benefit of about 3 months.

Intracavity therapy with chemotherapeutic agents (e.g. mitomycin C, cisplatin or Ara-C) or cytokines (interferon) or radioisotopes is of limited value.

OUTCOME

Mesotheliomas can have a variable natural history. The median survival is 9 months and the 2-year survival is 15%. In the presence of three or more adverse prognostic factors, the median survival is <6 months. A minority of patients have indolent disease and they can live for a few years.

Chapter 10

UROLOGICAL ONCOLOGY

PROSTATE CANCER

INCIDENCE

Cancer of the prostate is a relatively common cancer in elderly men, and the chance of a man developing invasive prostate cancer during his lifetime is 1 in 8. It is uncommon below the age of 50. Prostate cancer is the second leading cause of cancer-related deaths in men after lung cancer in the US, and the third after lung and colorectal cancers in Canada.

RISK FACTORS

• Age
About 70% of men over the age of 80 years have some histological evidence of cancer in their prostate. However, the finding of histological changes does not imply that the cancer is clinically relevant.
• Race
Prostate cancer is more common in men of African descent and less common in Asian men compared with Caucasians.
• Diet
High intake of dietary fats, particularly the fatty acid, α-linoleic acid, in red meats and butter, is believed to increase the risk 2- to 3-fold. In contrast, the isoflavinoid genistein, a component of soy, may reduce the risk, presumably by inhibiting 5α-reductase, the enzyme that converts testosterone to its active metabolite, α-dihydrotestosterone.
• Genetic predisposition
A family history of prostate cancer is present in about 5-10% of patients, but if the disease occurs at an early age, 40% of patients will have a positive family history. The relative risk for a man with a first-degree relative with prostate cancer is 1.76. The risk increases with the number of relatives affected and with younger age of onset. A dominantly inherited gene is suggested in kindred studies, but it has not yet been identified. Inheritance of the mutated BRCA-2 gene, which is implicated in breast and ovarian cancers, increases the risk of prostate cancer in men 3-fold.

PATHOLOGY

Macroscopic

The normal prostate has two lobes with a firm rubbery consistency, similar to the thenar eminence of the palm. Cancer of the prostate usually develops in the peripheral part of the prostate, and it is often multifocal. The cancer appears as an infiltrating hard, pale yellow area.

Microscopic

In situ cancer, or prostate intraepithelial neoplasia (PIN), is the precursor to invasive disease. Adenocarcinoma is the most common histological subtype, accounting for almost 95% of prostate cancer. Other uncommon cancers include transitional cell carcinoma, carcinosarcoma, basal cell carcinoma, lymphoma and stromal sarcoma.

Grading

The differentiation or grade of prostate cancer is a major prognostic factor. The Gleason system is the most commonly used histological grading system. This is a 5-part scheme with a grade of 1 to 5 being assigned to the growth pattern of the cancer (Figure 10.1). Pattern 1 tumors are the most differentiated with discrete glandular formation, and pattern 5 tumors are poorly differentiated with complete loss of the glandular architecture. A modification of the Gleason system is the Gleason score, which is the sum of the two most prevalent grades; the score ranges from 2 to 10. For example, a tumor with a mixture of a moderately well-differentiated (Grade 2) and poorly differentiated (Grade 5) cancers would be scored 2 + 5 or 7/10. The higher the score, the greater is the chance of extra-capsular spread and nodal metastases. Sums of 2 to 4 are regarded as well-differentiated tumors; 5 to 7 are moderately differentiated tumors; and 8 to 10 are poorly differentiated tumors.

Figure 10.1 Gleason grades and scores

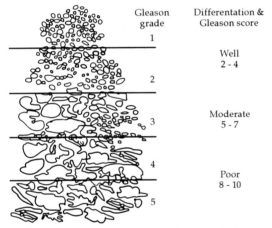

Combined score of the two most prevalent areas is the Gleason score, range 2 to 10.

Spread

Local extension occurs through the prostatic capsule with invasion of adjacent organs, i.e. base of the bladder and seminal vesicles, or, less commonly, the urethra or rectum.
Lymphatic to the obturator lymph nodes, followed by the presacral, presciatic and iliac nodes.
Blood-borne to bone by retrograde venous spread through the vertebral plexus of veins. Up to 80% of patients who die with metastatic prostate cancer have sclerotic bone metastases, most commonly to the spine, followed by femur, pelvis, ribs, skull and humerus. Metastases to lungs or liver are less common.

CLINICAL FEATURES

There are two common conditions of the prostate that require clinical attention: benign prostatic enlargement or hypertrophy (BPH) and carcinoma. Some degree of enlargement of the prostate is common after age 45. Often, this causes little or no symptoms in the early stages, but over time the enlargement can lead to elongation and tortuosity of the prostatic urethra, and the median lobe may compress the internal urinary meatus, resulting in outflow obstruction. Early symptoms of BPH are urinary frequency, decreased flow, nocturia, post-void dribbling and repeated urinary tract infections.

As a result of Prostate Specific Antigen (PSA) screening, an increasing number of patients are diagnosed at an asymptomatic stage. *Symptoms from local growth* are not unlike those of BPH: difficulty in passing urine and poor, intermittent stream with post-void dribbling.
Blood-borne metastasis to the spine causes back pain. *Generalized effects* include fatigue, which is common in men with metastatic disease.
Digital rectal examination reveals a hard area of induration or a hard nodule in one lobe of the prostate, usually in the periphery. As the primary cancer enlarges, it forms a craggy mass, replacing the prostate and abolishing the normal sulcus between the two lobes. Eventually, there is infiltration of the tissues on either side of the prostate. A uniformly enlarged gland with normal consistency is more likely due to BPH. *Blood-borne* metastasis to the axial skeleton causes tenderness on palpation of the spine. Metastatic involvement of the vertebral bodies may result in spinal cord compression.

DIAGNOSTIC AND STAGING TESTS

• Complete blood count

- Biochemistry: urea, creatinine, alkaline phosphatase and calcium
- Trans-rectal ultrasound (TRUS) is the most sensitive means to assess the prostate, and it permits biopsy of any suspicious area. Systematic biopsy strategies have been developed. Traditionally, 6 biopsies are taken along the parasaggital line between the edge and the midline of the gland at the apex, mid-gland and base. Additional samples of the peripheral zones more laterally with a total of 8 biopsies are now taken (Figure 10.2)
- Prostate Specific Antigen (PSA) is a normal glycoprotein found in the prostate and seminal vesicles, where it maintains the semen in a liquid state to ensure fertility. The normal PSA level is related to age and prostate volume (Table 10.1). The prostate gland enlarges with age, and inflammation is more common in older men. The increase in tissue to produce PSA and its increased leakage into the blood due to inflammation lead to higher levels of serum PSA with advancing age
- CT scan or MRI to assess regional nodes
- A bone scan should be done if there is bone pain or if the PSA is >20 ng/mL

Figure 10.2 Octant biopsy technique of the prostate gland

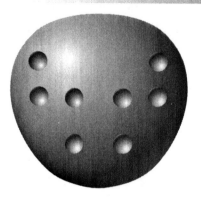

Table 10.1 Age-specific reference ranges for PSA

Age range (years)	Serum PSA range (ng/mL)
40 – 50	0 – 2.5
51 – 60	0 – 3.5
61 – 70	0 – 5.5
>70	0 – 6.5

STAGING

The TNM system is used. The important distinction to be made is whether the cancer is localized, locally advanced or metastatic.

TNM Criteria

T1 Asymptomatic incidental finding
T2 Palpable, confined within the capsule
T3 Extends beyond the capsule
T4 Fixed or invades structures other than seminal vesicles
N0 No regional nodes
N1 Regional node metastases
M0 No distant metastases
M1 Distant metastasis present

EARLY DETECTION AND SCREENING

The standard method of early detection of prostate cancer is a digital rectal examination (DRE), which should be done yearly in fit men between 50 and 70 years of age or if obstructive or other urinary symptoms are present. The American Cancer Society, the American Urological Association, and the American College of Radiology recommend that all men above the age of 50, who have a life expectancy of more than 10 years, undergo an annual DRE and serum PSA measurement. In African-American men or those with a positive family history of prostate cancer, screening should begin at age 40 years. These recommendations are not endorsed by the Canadian Task Force on Periodic Health Examination or the United States Preventive Services Task Force.

In men who are ultimately diagnosed with prostate cancer, the serum PSA rises 5-10 years prior to diagnosis. This implies that a 5- to 10-year lead-time on clinical diagnosis can be achieved by screening asymptomatic men by PSA measurements. However, PSA screening is not universally accepted because there are no data to prove that prostate cancer-specific mortality is reduced through screening, while morbidity of treatment can be significant. The high incidence of prostate cancer in autopsy series also suggests that not all prostate cancers become clinically significant.

Until the debate of the benefits of PSA as a population screening test is settled by clinical trials, it is prudent that fit men between 50-70 years with a life expectancy of at least 10 years be made aware of the availability of PSA as a detection test for prostate cancer and its potential benefits and risks.

APPROACH TO THE PATIENT WITH ELEVATED SERUM PSA

The present widespread use of PSA in general clinical practice leads to the discovery of an elevated PSA in men who do not have symptoms of prostate disease. An elevated serum PSA is not by itself confirmatory for cancer. Men with BPH, prostatitis, prostatic infarction, urological manipulation (including digital rectal examination, trans-rectal ultrasound or biopsy), and those who exercise strenuously can also have elevated PSA. Rarely, undifferentiated cancers at other sites can cause serum PSA to increase. Nonetheless, an isolated elevation of PSA level in a man with no other manifestation of disease (benign or malignant) requires a systematic approach to diagnosis.

The major decision is whether a biopsy is required. PSA cut-off levels at 4 and 10 ng/mL provide the best levels of sensitivity and specificity. Men with levels <4 ng/mL are at very low risk for prostate cancer, and follow-up monitoring is appropriate. On the other hand, those with levels >10 ng/mL are at sufficiently high risk to justify a biopsy. For levels between 4 and 10 ng/mL, several strategies have been developed.

- Age-specific reference ranges (see Table 10.1)

Patients with PSA values above the age-specific ranges may benefit from TRUS-guided biopsy even though there is no palpable abnormality on DRE.

- Free and protein-bound PSA

PSA circulates in both free (30%) and protein-bound (70%) forms. Patients with cancer have a lower percentage of the free PSA compared with men with BPH.

- PSA density and velocity

PSA density is a measure of PSA production per unit volume of prostate gland. When the ratio between serum PSA level and prostate volume is >0.15, there is a higher probability of cancer. However, the difficulty in assessing prostate volume in clinical practice limits this approach. PSA velocity refers to the rate of rise of PSA level over time. Men with prostate cancer have a faster rise (approximately 0.5 ng/mL/year) than do those with BPH (approximately 0.18 ng/mL/year). The variability in PSA assays, however, makes this strategy unreliable.

Table 10.2 shows the risk of prostate cancer in relation to the findings at DRE and PSA levels.

Table 10.2 Detection of early prostate cancer

DRE	PSA level*	Risk assessment/evaluation
Negative	Normal	Very low
Negative	Elevated	High. TRUS-guided biopsies
Positive	Any	Very high. TRUS biopsy of lesion and octant biopsies

*age specific
DRE: digital rectal examination   TRUS: Trans-rectal ultrasound

TREATMENT

Many prostate cancers may be clinically insig-
nificant and may not cause symptoms during a
man's lifetime. Therefore, several factors should
be taken into consideration when planning treatment; these include:

- Patient factors
  - age (younger patients are more likely to
    develop problems)
  - general health
  - personal preference
- Tumor factors
  - stage of cancer
  - Gleason score
  - pre-treatment PSA

A plan of active surveillance or deferred
therapy may be appropriate in an elderly man
with asymptomatic low-risk prostate cancer,
who also has other co-morbid medical problems.
Likewise, a radical prostatectomy is not advised
for a cancer not localized to the gland or if the
PSA is very high (>50 ng/mL), since a PSA in
this range almost always indicates metastatic
disease.

Cancer confined to the prostate

Low-risk disease
Low-risk disease is defined by a PSA <10 ng/mL
and Gleason score <6. In a fit individual with a
life expectancy over 10 years, radical prostatectomy or radiation is an option. Potential
complications include erectile dysfunction, incontinence, and rectal/bladder irritation and
minor bleeding from radiation.

Because patients with low risk cancer have
high 10-year cancer-specific survival rates, another option is active surveillance with institution of treatment if there is disease progression. Active surveillance of patients with
low risk prostate cancer includes:

- PSA every 3 months for 2 years, then 6
  monthly
- DRE every 6 months for 2 years, then 6
  monthly
- Re-biopsy every 3 years

Intermediate-risk cancer
Intermediate risk cancer includes those with a
PSA of 10-19ng/mL and Gleason score of 7. In a
fit individual with a life expectancy over 10
years, radical prostatectomy or radiation
(external beam radiation or brachytherapy
[implantation of radioactive gold seeds in the
prostate gland]) should be considered. In
general, radical surgery is reserved for patients
<70 years of age who are in excellent health. A
nerve sparing procedure should be done to
preserve potency, although this may be un-
avoidable on the side of the lesion or with significant apical disease. Neo-adjuvant anti-
androgen therapy can reduce the risk of positive
margins by 50%, but the effect on recurrence
rates is unclear.

High-risk disease
High-risk disease is defined by a PSA >20 ng/
mL, Gleason score >8 or Stage T3. External
beam radiation therapy combined with hormone
therapy is the standard treatment. Neo-adjuvant
anti-androgen therapy for several months prior
to radiation is usually recommended. Improved
overall survival and local tumor control can be
achieved with external beam radiation therapy
combined with concurrent and adjuvant anti-
androgen therapy of up to three years duration
compared with radiation therapy alone.

T4 disease

Treatment is individualized and may involve
radical or palliative radiotherapy and/or early
or delayed hormone therapy. It is questionable
whether patients with locally extensive disease

are curable with radiation therapy alone and, therefore, combination therapy with neo-adjuvant or adjuvant anti-androgen therapy is appropriate. The main intent is to achieve local control, i.e. to relieve symptoms and prevent or relieve ureteric or bladder outlet obstruction.

Node-positive disease

Hormone therapy is the mainstay of treatment. The general trend is towards immediate androgen ablation therapy at the time of diagnosis of metastatic disease rather than waiting for symptomatic progression. However, some delay of treatment in sexually active, asymptomatic men is a reasonable alternative, and the potentially adverse effect on quality of life should be taken into account.

Distant metastatic disease

• Hormone therapy
The median survival for men with metastatic prostate cancer is 4 years, but the natural history is variable and a small proportion of men with bone metastases can live >5 years. About 80% of men with prostate cancer will respond to androgen ablation therapy and this is the first choice for treatment of metastatic disease. Androgen ablation is achieved through surgical orchiectomy or "medical" castration by lu-teinizing hormone-releasing hormone (LHRH) agonists, such as leuprolide, buserelin or gos-erelin. These agents cause an initial surge, followed by suppression of LH release from the pituitary gland. LH is responsible for stimulating release of testosterone from the testis. To avoid an initial flare of the disease or symptoms with the LHRH agonists, a non-steroidal anti-an-drogen, such as flutamide, nilutamide or bica-lutamide, is given for one week prior to treatment and during the initial two weeks of treatment.

A common clinical issue is the treatment of asymptomatic patients with a rising PSA. One approach is to offer early hormone treatment, since this reduces later complications. This must be weighed against the side effects of treatment, such as loss of libido, erectile dysfunction and hot flashes.

In general, patients receiving initial hormonal therapy will develop hormone resistance after about 18 months. The addition of an anti-androgen, like bicalutamide, on progression of their disease may result in further response in about one-third of patients, although this response is usually short, about 3 months.

Unfortunately, all patients with metastatic prostate cancer will become hormone resistant unless they succumb to their disease or other illness. In addition, about 20% are hormone-resistant at the outset. For these patients, a few options are available:

• Other hormone therapy
Conventional androgen deprivation therapy removes 90% of circulating androgens produced in the testes. As much as 10% of circulating testosterone remains, in part, due to peripheral conversion of adrenal steroids to testosterone. Abiraterone, an inhibitor of 17-α-hydroxylase/$C_{17,20}$ lyase which is important in adrenal androgen synthesis, may be a useful second-line hormone treatment.

• Chemotherapy
Docetaxel is the drug of choice for patients with hormone-refractory prostate cancer. There is no standard chemotherapy for patients whose cancer progresses after docetaxel, but one option is mitoxantrone and prednisone. A number of drugs are under investigations, of which sat-raplatin appears to be the most promising. Satraplatin is an oral platinum compound which in combination with prednisone produces an improvement in progression-free survival when used as second-line treatment.

- Radiation therapy
Thus can relieve pain from bone metastases.
- Treatment with radioisotopes
Strontium-89 resembles calcium and radioactive Strontium is taken up by sclerotic bone metastases. Another radioisotope is Samarium-153, which is also taken up into bone.
- Supportive measures
Regular narcotic analgesics and other measures may be an appropriate treatment choices for some patients, especially those who are elderly or infirm.

FOLLOW-UP EVALUATION

The main goal of follow-up evaluation is early detection of recurrence where salvage therapy can be curative or can prolong life. A rising PSA is indicative of recurrent disease, but it does not distinguish local from metastatic relapse. Two situations can arise:

After radical prostatectomy: Two successive increases in the PSA to a level >0.3 ng/mL are indicative of recurrent disease.

After radical radiation therapy: PSA level reaches a nadir, which typically takes 12-24 months. Three consecutive rises from the nadir with a minimum of 0.5 ng/mL suggest recurrent disease.

Follow-up recommendations

Post-radical prostatectomy: DRE and PSA are recommended every 3 months for one year, then every 6 months. Elevation of PSA or a palpable nodule suggests disease recurrence and local radiation or hormone therapy may be considered.

Post-radical radiation: Young (<70 years) fit men who had primary radiation for early stage prostate cancer may be candidates for salvage surgery. A rising PSA or development of a palpable nodule is indication for local therapy.

PSA every 6 months for three years, then yearly is recommended for follow-up evaluation.

Older or unfit men with recurrent disease may be considered for hormone therapy. It is, however, unclear whether early treatment of asymptomatic men improves quality of life or overall survival and, therefore, routine follow-up examinations or tests are controversial in this group of patients.

TESTICULAR CANCER

INCIDENCE

Testicular cancer is the most common solid tumor in men between the ages of 20 and 40 years. There are three peaks of occurrence: infancy, ages 20 to 40, and at about age 60. Testicular tumors in older men are more likely to be lymphoma. The lifetime probability of developing testicular cancer is 0.2%. Over the past 20 years, the incidence of testicular cancer has doubled, and the reason for this is not clear.

RISK FACTORS

- Cryptorchidism
The only definite condition associated with testicular cancer is maldescent of the testis. It is suggested that exposure of the germinal epithelium *in utero* to high levels of free maternal estrogens could lead to cryptorchidism, but this hypothesis has not been conclusively proven. Cryptorchidism increases the risk of testicular cancer 3- to 14-fold, resulting in a 3-5% chance of developing cancer in either testis. Cancer is more likely in an abdominal cryptorchid testis compared with an inguinal cryptorchid testis. Orchioplexy seems to reduce the risk, especially if done before puberty. Interestingly, men with a history of cryptorchidism can develop cancer in the normally descended testis, suggesting that the underlying

mechanism of oncogenesis is intrinsic, and not due to the maldescent *per se*.

- Race

Testicular cancer is four times more frequent in Caucasians compared with African-Americans.

- Genetic

Testicular cancer has been reported in siblings and twins, but the risk is unclear.

- Klinefelter's syndrome (47, XXY karyotype)

This is associated with an increased risk of mediastinal germ cell tumors. Affected individuals also have testicular atrophy, absence of spermatogenesis, eunuchoid habitus and gynecomastia.

PATHOLOGY

Macroscopic

The testis is oval, smooth and sensitive to pressure. The epididymis lies above and posterior to the testis and it is separated from it by a thin groove. Testicular cancer starts in the testis itself, forming a mass. The cancers are bilateral in 1-2% of cases.

Microscopic

The vast majority of cancers of the testis are germ cell tumors, which are classified into three major subgroups:

- Seminoma – 45%
- Non-seminoma – 40%
  - Embryonal carcinoma
  - Teratoma
  - Choriocarcinoma
  - Yolk sac tumor
- Mixed tumors – 15%

Biology

Germ cell tumors have the unique ability for totipotential differentiation, and tumors with a mixture of embryonal carcinoma, seminoma, yolk sac tumor, choriocarcinoma and teratoma may be evident. α-Fetoprotein, a product of the normal yolk sac, and hCG (human chorionic gonadotropin), a product of trophoblastic tissues, are elevated in yolk sac tumors and choriocarcinomas, respectively. Elevations of these proteins may, however, be present in mixed tumors or even when there is no distinct histological component of these observed within the tumor.

Certain cytogenetic abnormalities are consistent in germ cell tumors:

- They are almost always hyperploid
- They have at least one X and one Y chromosome
- An isochromosome of the short arm of chromosome 12 is present. This suggests that a gene on chromosome 12p is central to malignant transformation of the cell
- There is widespread gene loss from virtually all chromosome arms, even in the very early stages of the disease. This contrasts with the gradual allelic loss during progression from dysplasia to invasive carcinoma observed in other cancers

Spread

Local growth leads to progressive destruction of the testis. Invasion into the tunica vaginalis and along the spermatic cord may occur. Involvement of the scrotum is a relatively late event.

Lymphatic spread is the most common route of metastatic spread. This occurs directly to the para-aortic nodes via the lymphatics accompanying the testicular veins. In more advanced stages of the disease, the left supraclavicular nodes can be involved. Pelvic and inguinal node involvement is rare.

Blood-borne spread tends to occur late in seminoma, but non-seminomatous tumors spread commonly to the lungs and liver. In the late stages, bone, brain, kidney and gastrointestinal tract are involved.

CLINICAL FEATURES

Local growth commonly causes a painless testicular mass, varying in size from a few millimeters to several centimeters. About 45% of patients can experience diffuse testicular discomfort or pain associated with a swelling or hardness. Acute testicular pain may be due to intra-tumor bleed. A scrotal mass of acute onset, accompanied by severe pain, is more likely epididymitis or testicular torsion.

Lymphatic spread to retroperitoneal nodes causes back pain.

Blood-borne metastasis causes dyspnea or cough (lung metastasis), neurological symptoms (brain metastasis) or hepatic dysfunction (liver metastasis).

Generalized effects include weight loss and gynecomastia (due to hCG production).

Examination reveals a palpable mass in the testis. A mass separate from the testis is more likely due to epididymitis. Trans-illumination of the mass is helpful to distinguish a cyst (readily trans-illuminates) from a solid mass (does not trans-illuminate). A mass that cannot be separated from the testis and does not trans-illuminate is a neoplasm until proven otherwise.

Lymphatic spread to the retroperitoneal nodes may be palpable as a para-aortic mass. In late stages of the disease, a left supraclavicular node may be palpable. Inguinal node involvement is uncommon.

Blood-borne metastasis to distant organs leads to respiratory signs, neurological signs or hepatomegaly.

APPROACH TO THE PATIENT WITH A TESTICULAR MASS

The major distinction that needs to be made in a patient with a testicular mass is whether it is arising from the testis itself (neoplasm) or adjacent structure (epididymis), and whether it is cystic (benign) or solid (malignant). The main differential diagnosis is epididymitis. The differentiation between these two possibilities can be difficult as the epididymis may be thick and tense, and since it sits over the testis, the normal groove between the two structures can be obscured.

If the diagnosis is uncertain, a trial of antibiotics is justified. If there is no resolution of the symptoms within 2-4 weeks, a cancer is more likely. This requires urgent attention, since testicular cancer can be rapidly progressive, and a delay in diagnosis must, therefore, be avoided.

DIAGNOSIS

A radical inguinal orchiectomy, using an inguinal incision is the only acceptable therapeutic and diagnostic procedure when a tumor is detected on clinical examination and verified by ultrasound. A trans-scrotal biopsy must not be done as this violates the lymphatic drainage of the testis and, consequently, permits the spread of the cancer to inguinal and pelvic nodes.

STAGING TESTS

- Complete blood count
- Biochemistry: creatinine, liver function tests
- Tumor markers: α-fetoprotein, hCG and LDH. These should be done before surgery and weekly after treatment until they return to normal levels. LDH is a useful marker in seminoma. About 90% of patients with non-seminomatous germ cell tumors have elevated α-fetoprotein or hCG, and in half of these, both are raised

- Testicular ultrasound
- Chest x-ray
- CT scan of abdomen and pelvis
- Brain CT scan if there are neurological symptoms
- Sperm count (with or without sperm banking)

TNM STAGING SYSTEM

Tis   Intra-tubular germ cell neoplasia (carcinoma *in situ*)

T1   Tumor limited to the testis and epididymis without vascular/lymphatic invasion; tumor may invade into the tunica albuginea but not the tunica vaginalis

T2   Tumor limited to the testis and epididymis with vascular/lymphatic invasion, or tumor extending through the tunica albuginea with involvement of the tunica vaginalis

T3   Tumor invades the spermatic cord with or without vascular/lymphatic invasion

T4   Tumor invades the scrotum with or without vascular/lymphatic invasion

N0   No regional lymph node metastases

N1   Metastases with a lymph node mass <2 cm in greatest dimension; or multiple lymph nodes, none >2 cm in greatest dimension

N2   Metastases with a lymph node mass >2 cm but <5 cm in greatest dimension; or multiple lymph nodes, any one mass >2 cm but <5 cm in greatest dimension

N3   Metastases with a lymph node mass >5 cm in greatest dimension

M0   No distant metastasis

M1   Distant metastasis

M1a   Non-regional nodal or pulmonary metastasis

M1b   Distant metastasis other than to nonregional lymph nodes and lungs

Stage groupings

Stage I   T1-4 N0 M0
Stage II   Any T N1-3 M0
Stage III   Any T Any N M1

Because patients with advanced germ cell tumors are curable with chemotherapy, it is helpful to stratify patients according to the likelihood of cure. This depends on several prognostic factors (International Germ Cell Collaborative Group criteria) (Table 10.3):

- pre-treatment levels of α-fetoprotein, hCG and LDH
- site of primary (testis, mediastinum or retroperitoneum)
- presence of non-pulmonary visceral metastases (e.g. liver, brain, bone)

TREATMENT

Radical inguinal orchiectomy is performed as a diagnostic and therapeutic measure. (A scrotal approach must be avoided, since this leads to tumor implantation in the scrotal wound and subsequent relapse.) Postoperative treatment is determined by the clinical stage.

Seminoma

Stage I disease (T1-4 N0 M0)
There is a 20% risk of occult retroperitoneal metastases. Nevertheless, a very high cure rate can be achieved by three strategies: adjuvant radiation treatment, surveillance strategy with administration of irradiation or chemotherapy in the event of relapse, or adjuvant chemotherapy with carboplatin.

Adjuvant radiation (20-25 Gy) to the para-aortic is the most frequently used adjuvant treatment, resulting in a relapse rate of 3-4%.

Surveillance strategy may be used as an alternative to adjuvant irradiation. The potential advantage of surveillance is that patients

Table 10.3 Germ cell tumor risk classification: International Consensus Classification

	Seminoma	Non-seminoma
Good risk	- any hCG any LDH no non-pulmonary visceral metastases any primary site	αFP <1000 ng/ml hCG <5000 IU/L LDH <1.5 ULN no non-pulmonary visceral metastases gonadal or retroperitoneal site
Intermediate Risk	- any hCG any LDH non-pulmonary visceral metastases any primary site	α-FP 1,000-10,000 hCG 5,000-50,000 LDH 1.5-10 ULN no non-pulmonary visceral metastases present gonadal or retroperitoneal site
Poor Risk	-	α-FP >10, 000 hCG >50,000 LDH >10 ULN non-pulmonary visceral metastases present (e.g. liver, brain) mediastinal site

ULN: upper limit of normal

are spared acute and late radiation toxicity and possibly an associated increased risk of secondary malignancies. Relapse rate on surveillance are approximately 20%. However, almost all relapses can be cured with further therapy.

Adjuvant chemotherapy with carboplatin is an alternative to radiation therapy or surveillance; relapse rates are low, about 3-4%.

Stage II disease (Any T N1-3 M0)
Radiation treatment to the para-aortic and ipsilateral pelvic area is the standard treatment option. Chemotherapy with cisplatin, etoposide and bleomycin (BEP), or etopside and cisplatin (EP) is an alternative treatment for patients, in particular those with larger retroperitoneal disease where radiation may not be possible due to inclusion of the kidney in the radiation field. Cure rates are 90-95%.

Stage III disease
These patients are treated with BEP chemo-

therapy and may require subsequent resection of residual masses. Cure rates are >90%.

Non-seminomatous germ cell tumor

Stage I disease (T1-4 N0 M0)
The cure rate is 99%. Vascular invasion by the primary tumor is the most important prognostic indicator for relapse with a 48% risk of developing metastatic disease, whereas only 14–22% of patients without vascular invasion suffer a relapse. Three treatment options are available:
- Surveillance is the preferred treatment option and should be considered only if all staging is unequivocally normal
- Retroperitoneal lymph node dissection (nerve-sparing)
- Adjuvant chemotherapy with 2 cycles of BEP chemotherapy may be considered in selected high risk patients. With this approach, the risk of relapse is reduced to 4-5%

Stage II "good prognosis" disease
(Any T N1-2 M0)

Two treatment approaches are available, producing cures in up to 98% of patients.

- Primary chemotherapy is recommended for a retroperitoneal mass or an abnormal/equivocal scan and persistent elevation of tumor markers. Residual post-chemotherapy masses should be resected
- For patients with minor (<3 cm) lymphadenopathy and negative markers, two options can be considered: First, radical bilateral retroperitoneal lymph node dissection with postoperative adjuvant chemotherapy if the resected tumor is >2 cm, or >5 nodes are involved, or there is extra-nodal extension; otherwise close follow-up for early detection of relapse with institution of chemotherapy may be undertaken. Second, observation for patients willing to undergo close observation with repeat CT scans

Stage II "intermediate" or "poor" prognosis disease and Stage III disease (Any T Any N M1)

BEP or EP chemotherapy is the standard approach for these patients. If after chemotherapy, the tumor markers are normal, but there is a residual mass, it should be resected. Histologically, about 35% of these residual masses will reveal necrosis, 50% will contain mature teratoma with a risk of late relapse due to malignant change over years, and 15% will have residual active cancer. If residual cancer is evident in the resected specimen, two further cycles of intensive chemotherapy are given.

Patients with brain metastases at initial presentation are potentially curable and should be treated with chemotherapy. If brain metastases persist after an otherwise complete systemic response to chemotherapy, they should be resected, if possible, and cranial radiation given afterwards.

FOLLOW-UP EVALUATION

Follow-up of patients with testicular cancer is important. Patients with early stage disease (Clinical Stage I), who had orchiectomy and are on a surveillance program, require careful follow-up to detect relapse. The patterns of failure are well defined, and follow-up investigations with tumor markers, chest x-ray and CT scans can detect recurrent disease. Recurrences are less likely after 2 years.

OUTCOME

Testicular cancer is a highly curable disease. Almost all patients with Stage I cancer are cured. Even for the more advanced stages, the cure rate is about 85%. Unfortunately, a small minority relapse and the outlook for them is not as good. Patients who relapse are increasingly being treated with high-dose chemotherapy with peripheral stem cell or autologous bone marrow transplantation. About 20-30% of these will have long-term remission of their disease.

RENAL TUMORS

Cancers of the kidney are divided into those arising from the kidney itself and those arising from the renal pelvis. The latter are similar pathologically to those arising from the ureter and bladder.

CLASSIFICATION

Renal Tumors

Benign

- Adenoma
- Hemangioma
- Oncocytoma

Malignant

Primary
- Nephroblastoma
- Renal cell carcinoma

Secondary

The kidney is an uncommon site for secondary metastases, but melanoma, breast and lung cancers can rarely metastasize to it. The kidney may also may be involved in the late stages of lymphoma and leukemia.

Renal Pelvis Tumor

Benign

- Papilloma

Malignant

- Transitional cell carcinoma
- Squamous cell carcinoma

RENAL CARCINOMA

INCIDENCE

Renal carcinoma accounts for 3% of adult cancers, and it is more common in the age group 50-70 years. The male:female ratio is 2:1.

RISK FACTORS

- Cigarette smoking increases the risk of renal cancer and it is associated with 30% of cases
- Occupational factors: there is an increased incidence of renal cancer among leather tanners, shoe workers, and those exposed to asbestos, cadmium, thorium (a radioactive agent), and petroleum products
- Abuse of phenacetin-containing compounds with analgesic nephropathy
- Adult polycystic disease of the kidney and horseshoe kidneys
- Hereditary renal carcinoma (2%)

- von Hippel-Lindau disease, which occurs in 1 of 36,000 live births, with a predisposition to develop cancer in several organs (kidney, brain, spine, eye, adrenal gland, endocrine pancreas, inner ear and epididymis)
- Hereditary papillary renal carcinoma, an autosomal dominant disease, in which individuals develop bilateral, multifocal renal cancers
- Familial renal carcinoma is associated with HLA-BW44 and HLA-DR8
- Familial renal oncocytoma

PATHOLOGY

Macroscopic

Renal carcinoma arises from the epithelium of the proximal convoluted tubule. It tends to be a large, spherical, vascular, golden-yellow mass, usually in one or other pole of the kidney. A pseudo-capsule forms due to compression of surrounding tissues by the tumor. Hemorrhage or a central area of necrosis may be present.

Microscopic

They are adenocarcinomas and five main cellular subtypes are recognized:
- Clear cell (75%)
- Papillary (12%)
- Chromophobe (4%)
- Collecting duct carcinoma
- Renal cell carcinoma, unclassified

The degree of differentiation can vary from well-differentiated tumors to anaplastic tumors. While the majority of renal cancers in adults are renal cell carcinomas, it is important not to overlook the possibility of a more treatable histology in the younger patients or where atypical clinical features are present, e.g. transitional cell carcinoma of the renal pelvis, sarcoma, lymphoma or adult Wilms' tumor.

Molecular genetics

A large proportion of clear cell renal cancers have a loss of a portion of chromosome 3p, the likely site of a tumor suppressor gene. Papillary renal cancers have trisomies and tetrasomies of chromosomes 7 and 17.

Spread

Locally throughout the renal substance with invasion of the perinephric tissues. Invasion of the renal vein is common and, thence, to the inferior vena cava (IVC).

By lymphatics to renal hilar nodes and then to the para-aortic nodes.

Blood-borne to lungs and bone. Other sites of metastasis include the brain, liver and skin.

CLINICAL FEATURES

With the increasing use of imaging studies, especially ultrasound, for investigations of abdominal complaints, an increasing proportion of renal cancers are found incidentally.

Symptoms from local disease include hematuria, abdominal mass and pain, each of which may be present in 60% of patients. The classic triad of hematuria, abnormal mass and pain occurs in less than 10% of patients. Venous extension of the disease with growth along the renal vein to the IVC causes sudden onset of left-sided varicocele in 2% of patients with renal cancer.

Blood-borne metastasis is present in about 25% of patients at presentation, manifesting as bone pain or pathological fracture (bone metastasis), neurological symptoms (brain metastasis), or cough with or without hemoptysis (lung metastasis). Of patients with metastasis, about 2% have a solitary metastatic deposit, which may be amenable to surgical resection with good long-term results.

Generalized symptoms of malignancy are relatively common: weight loss (30%), anemia (30%) due to hematuria or hemolysis, and fever (20%).

A number of paraneoplastic syndromes are also associated with renal carcinoma, including hypercalcemia (parathyroid hormone-related protein), hypoglycemia (insulin), diabetes mellitus (glucagon), Stauffer's syndrome (abnormal liver function tests without liver metastases), polycythemia (erythropoietin), and polyneuropathy. Secondary amyloidosis occurs in 5% of patients.

Prognostic factors

Six features associated with a poor outcome, known as the modified Motzer criteria, are:

- low Karnofsky performance status (<80%)
- high LDH (>1.5 x normal)
- low hemoglobin
- high serum calcium
- absence of nephrectomy
- >1 metastatic site

0 risk factor = favorable risk
1-2 risk factors = intermediate risk
>3 risk factors = poor risk

STAGING INVESTIGATIONS

- Complete blood count
- Biochemistry: electrolytes, urea, creatinine, and liver function tests
- Chest x-ray
- IVP
- CT or MRI of abdomen
- Skeletal x-ray survey is done if bone metastasis is suspected. (Because bone metastasis from renal cancer is typically lytic, isotope bone scan can give false negative results.)
- Inferior venacavography (if the tumor is large or there is uncertainty about tumor involvement of the vena cava)
- CT brain scan (if neurological symptoms are present)

TNM STAGING

T0   No evidence of primary tumor

T1   Tumor <7 cm in diameter and limited to the kidney

T2   Tumor >7 cm in greatest dimension limited to the kidney

T3   Tumor extends into major veins or invades the adrenal gland or perinephric tissues, but not beyond Gerota's fascia

T4   Tumor invades beyond Gerota's fascia

N0   No regional lymph node metastases

N1   Metastasis in a single regional lymph node

N2   Metastasies in more than one regional lymph node

M0   No distant metastasis

M1   Distant metastasis

Stage Grouping

I   T1 N0 M0

II   T2 N0 M0

III   T1-2 N1 M0 T3 N0-1 M0

IV   T4 N0-1M0

       Any T N2 M0 Any T Any M1

TREATMENT

Surgery

Radical nephrectomy is the main curative treatment and it is suitable for patients with localized or locally advanced disease. This involves the *en bloc* resection of the kidney, perirenal fat, perirenal fascia, adrenal gland and regional nodes. Cancer invading the renal vein can be removed and, thus, this is not a contraindication to radical treatment. Direct infiltration of the vena cava is associated with a poor prognosis.

The occasional patient may develop a solitary metastasis to brain, lung or liver, which can be resected with good long-term survival.

Radiation therapy

The benefit of adjuvant radiation after nephrectomy is inconclusive. Radiation may be useful for palliation of symptoms due to metastasis to bone, brain or soft tissues. It is also used to control bleeding and pain from the primary cancer.

Chemotherapy

Renal carcinoma is a relatively resistant to chemotherapy and this is seldom used.

Immunotherapy

Interferon-alpha and interleukerin provide a modest survival benefit, although the occasional patient may have long-term survival. Clinical use of these agents is, however, limited by their side effects, and they have been supplanted by targeted agents.

Targeted therapy

Tyrosine kinase inhibitors

Two tyrosine kinase inhibitors have demonstrated clinical activity in advanced renal cell cancer and are considered the new standard of care. Sunitinib is a tyrosine kinase inhibitor with activity against VEGFR, PDGFR, kit and FLT-3. In patients with good or intermediate Motzer risk factors, sunitinib improved progression-free survival (11 vs. 5 months) compared with interferon. As a result of this, sunitinib is the standard first-line therapy in patients with metastatic renal cell cancer. Sorafenib is another tyrosine kinase inhibitor with activity against Raf kinases, VEGFR-2, and PDGFR. It significantly improves progression-free survival as second-line therapy in patients with metastatic renal cell cancer after cytokine treatment.

Bevacizumab

Bevacizumab, a monoclonal antibody directed against VEGF, in combination with interferon significantly improves response rates and prolongs disease-free survival compared with interferon alone.

mTOR inhibitors
Temsirolimus, an inhibitor of the mammalian target of rapamycin (mTOR), significantly improves both progression-free and overall survival compared with interferon in patients with poor prognosis metastatic renal cell cancer. Everolimus, another mTOR inhibitor, is also an active drug.

OUTCOME

The risk of recurrence is related to the stage of the disease and the completeness of surgical resection. The lung is the most common site of distant relapse, occurring in 50-60% of patients. Some patients with metastatic disease may have an indolent course, and 5-10% with unresectable lung metastases can live for 5 or more years.

Stage	5-year survival (%)
I	65-85
II	45-80
III	15-35
IV	0-10

Regular follow-up with abdominal ultrasound may detect the development of a contralateral primary kidney cancer.

BLADDER TUMORS

CLASSIFICATION

Benign

• Transitional cell papilloma

Malignant

Primary
• Transitional cell carcinoma (90%)
• Squamous cell carcinoma – arising in an area of metaplasia (8%)
• Adenocarcinoma (2%)
• Small cell carcinoma – uncommon
• Sarcoma – rare

Secondary
Invasion from cancers of adjacent organs: rectum, colon, prostate, uterus and ovary

CANCER OF THE BLADDER

INCIDENCE

Bladder cancer is the fourth most common cancer in men and the ninth in women. It is rare below age 40, and the median age of patients at diagnosis is 65 years. It is more common among Caucasians than among African-Americans, Asians or Native Indians.

RISK FACTORS

• Tobacco smoking
Tobacco smoking is associated with up to one-half of bladder cancer cases.
• Environmental or occupational carcinogens
Occupational exposure to carcinogens, e.g. aromatic amines and alinine dyes, accounts for about one-quarter of cases. These carcinogens and their metabolites are excreted in the urine where they come in contact with the bladder mucosa. There is a long lag period between exposure and the development of cancer. Individuals at increased risk include painters and aluminum, textile, rubber and cable workers. Persons whose sole source of drinking water for most of their lifetime is chlorinated surface water appear to be at increased risk.
• Drugs
  ◆ Phenacetin-containing analgesics
  ◆ Cyclophosphamide (used for cancer

treatment)

- Infections

Exposure to *Schistosoma hematobium*, a parasite found in many developing countries increases the risk for both transitional cell and squamous cell bladder cancer. Chronic urinary tract infections, e.g. in those with paraplegia or indwelling Foley catheters, increase the risk for squamous cell cancer, presumably due to nitrate production by bacteria.

PATHOLOGY

Macroscopic

About 70% of bladder tumors appear as an exophytic papillary growth, usually located on the lateral wall or base of the bladder. They form fine fronds, which are friable and bleed easily. The more malignant tumors are sessile, solid growths, which infiltrate the bladder wall with ulceration. Often, there is surrounding cystitis.

Microscopic

Papillomas resemble the normal urothelium. In more than half of bladders with multiple papillomas, dysplasia or carcinoma *in-situ* is present. This indicates that the uroepithelium is unstable, and the typical pattern is for multiple tumors to develop within the bladder as well as the rest of the urinary tract (ureter and renal pelvis).

Transitional cell carcinoma makes up 90% of bladder carcinomas. In countries where *S. hematobium* infestation is endemic, squamous cell carcinoma is more common, accounting for up to 30% of bladder cancers.

Grading

Bladder cancers are graded as low (G1), intermediate (G2) or high (G3) grade. For non-invasive tumors, grading is an important prognostic factor. It is less important for invasive cancers, which are almost all high grade, and tumor stage is more important in this setting.

Spread

Local invasion occurs into the bladder wall and perivesical tissues. Later, the cancer infiltrates into the prostate, urethra, ureter, sigmoid colon and rectum or anterior vaginal wall. Hydronephrosis and renal failure ultimately occur.

By lymphatic spread to the iliac and para-aortic nodes.

Blood-borne spread occurs late to the lungs, bone and liver.

Implantation may take place to other parts of the bladder wall or in surgical scars.

CLINICAL FEATURES

Bladder cancer usually presents with gross or microscopic hematuria. This is intermittent and the degree of hematuria is not necessarily related to the seriousness of the underlying cause. Painless hematuria in a person over 40 years should prompt further investigations for a possible bladder cancer. Malignant tumors ulcerate, causing dysuria, frequency and urgency. Occasionally, ureteral obstruction leads to hydronephrosis with flank pain, and local invasion into pelvic structures causes pelvic pain. Metastasis is uncommon at presentation, but cough and hemoptysis (lung metastasis) or bone pain (bone metastasis) may occur. Generalized symptoms include anorexia, weight loss and malaise.

Examination is negative in benign papillomas, but a malignant tumor may be palpable on bimanual examination.

INVESTIGATIONS

- Complete blood count
- Serum biochemistry: electrolytes, urea,

creatinine, liver enzymes
- Tumor markers: CEA
- Urinalysis
- Urine cytology is more likely to be diagnostic in high-grade tumors, and it is done in conjunction with IVP and cystoscopy
- Chest x-ray
- IVP or retrograde pyelogram may show a filling defect in the bladder and renal tract obstruction. Also, a concomitant tumor elsewhere in the urinary tract may be detected
- CT scan or MRI provides information about extravesical extension of the cancer and lymph node enlargement
- Cystoscopy is the definitive investigation to assess the cancer and obtain a biopsy. Biopsy provides important staging and grading information

STAGING

Clinical staging is based on the depth of invasion of the bladder wall by tumor (Figure 10.3). Bimanual examination under anesthesia and cystoscopy with biopsy are important to assess the size and mobility of the cancer, degree of involvement of the bladder wall and extravesical extension.

Figure 10.3 TNM classification of bladder cancer

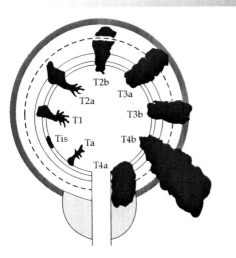

Stage

Superficial tumor
Ta Non-invasive papillary carcinoma
Tis Carcinoma *in situ*: flat tumor
T1 Superficial invasive cancer confined to the sub-epithelial connective tissue
Invasive tumor
T2 Invasion of bladder wall
    T2a Invasion of superficial muscle
    T2b Invasion of deep muscle
T3 Invasion through muscle wall
    T3a Microscopic invasion of perivesical fat
    T3b Macroscopic invasion of perivesical fat
T4 Disease beyond the bladder
    T4a Invasion of surrounding pelvic structures
    T4b Invasion of pelvic wall or abdominal wall
Lymph node
N0 No regional node
N1 Single regional node <2cm
N2 Single regional node 2-5cm
N3 Node >5cm
Distant metastasis
M1 No distant metastasis
M1 Distant metastasis

TREATMENT

Treatment depends on the extent of local invasion into the bladder, tumor differentiation and distant spread.

Superficial tumors

- Low grade Ta, T1 tumors
Most bladder tumors are superficial papillary tumors. They are frequently solitary, but in about one-third of cases, they are multiple. The standard treatment is complete endoscopic resection. Careful follow-up by cystoscopy and urine cytology is mandatory to detect the emergence of new cancers. Factors associated with

increased risk of recurrence include:

- Tumor grade (G1 vs. G2-3)
- Stage (Ta vs. T1)
- Large size
- Multicentricity
- History of prior recurrence

Intra-vesical instillations of chemotherapeutic drugs (mitomycin C, thiotepa, doxorubicin), immunotherapy agents (BCG) or cytokines (interferon) can reduce the rate of development of new bladder tumors. Uncommonly, intra-vesical treatment may be used to treat residual disease despite attempts at complete resection, but it is unclear whether this is of any benefit, as the instilled agents do not penetrate beyond the superficial few cellular layers of the bladder wall.

- Tis and high grade Ta, T1 tumors

Carcinoma *in-situ* of the uroepithelium of the high-grade, flat type is distinct from papillary *in-situ* disease as it tends to behave more aggressively. There is a high risk (40-80%) of progression to muscle-invasive disease and subsequent metastases. Standard treatment is cystectomy. Tis does not respond reliably to radiation therapy. For selected patients with focal disease, consideration may be given to intravesical therapy with BCG or mitomycin C. This decreases the risk of invasive disease in patients with high grade Ta, T1 and selected cases of Tis. Careful follow-up is required to detect progression to more deeply invasive cancer.

Superficial muscle invasion (T2a)

Definitive single modality treatment with either cystectomy, or radiation (with or without concurrent chemotherapy) are curative treatment options. Patients treated with radiotherapy must be followed closely cystoscopically, since they may be candidates for salvage cystectomy.

Invasive tumors

(T2b - deep muscle invasion), (T3 - perivesical fat), (T4a - prostate)

Radical Cystectomy

Radical cystectomy is the most frequent curative treatment option in North America with a 5-year survival range from 35% for patients with node-positive disease to 89% for T2 muscle-invasive disease.

External Beam Radiation Therapy

An alternative to cystectomy is external beam radiation therapy, which is a potentially curative treatment with the possibility of bladder preservation. However, careful follow-up is essential, since 15-25% of patients require salvage cystectomy for either recurrence or bladder contracture. External beam radiation therapy is also an option for patients who are unsuitable for surgery because of advanced age or concurrent medical problems. Five-year survival after external beam radiation therapy alone is 20-40%.

Combined Modality Therapy with Chemotherapy

- Neo-adjuvant chemotherapy

The rationale for giving chemotherapy before definitive treatment is to treat micro-metastatic disease that may be present at diagnosis. In addition, chemotherapy is often better tolerated given before surgery or radical radiation. Neo-adjuvant platinum-based combination chemotherapy followed by surgery improves survival at 5 years (from 45% to 50%) compared with surgery alone.

- Concurrent chemotherapy and radiation

The role of concurrent chemo-radiation is uncertain, but this approach may improve local control.

- Postoperative adjuvant chemotherapy

Postoperative adjuvant chemotherapy is not a widely accepted standard of care and randomized trials are underway to address this issue.

However, selected high risk patients (e.g. extra-vesical extension, node-positive) can be considered for treatment.

• Tri-modality Therapy

Bladder-sparing by means of "tri-modality" therapy comprises aggressive trans-urethral resection of tumors and induction chemo-radiation, followed by cystoscopic reassessment with cystectomy for those not in complete remission, or further chemo-radiation for those in remission. Several non-randomized studies demonstrate survival rates with tri-modality therapy similar to those achieved with radical cystectomy.

Locally advanced disease (T4b)

Initial treatment with combination chemo-therapy followed by reassessment and further local measures (surgery or radiation) is the usual approach. For elderly or unfit patients, a course of palliative radiation may be appropriate.

Metastatic disease

About 5-10% of patients have metastatic disease at presentation, and most with metastatic disease develop this after initial treatment. Chemotherapy is the standard treatment with gemcitabine plus cisplatin or carboplatin. Chemotherapy extends median survival from 3-6 months to 12 months. The addition of paclitaxel to cisplatin and gemcitabine can improve the results with higher response rates and a trend toward longer survival.

OUTCOME

Superficial bladder cancer tends to recur within the bladder and regular follow-up by cystoscopy and urine cytology is, therefore, important.

The prognosis depends on the stage of the cancer. For T1 bladder cancer, the 5-year survival rate is 70%, but for T3 and T4 cancers, the 5-year survival rates are 20% and <5%, respectively.

Chapter 11

GASTROINTESTINAL ONCOLOGY

CANCER OF THE ESOPHAGUS

ANATOMY

The esophagus extends from the hypopharynx to the stomach. It is divided into three regions: the upper third spans the interval from the lower border of cricoid cartilage (level of 6th cervical vertebra) to the superior portion of the aortic arch; the middle third from the superior portion of the aortic arch to the inferior pulmonary vein; and the lower third from the inferior pulmonary vein to the gastro-eso-phageal junction. About 10% of esophageal cancers occur in the upper third; 40% in the middle third; and 50% in the lower third.

CLASSIFICATION

Benign

• Leiomyoma

Malignant

Primary
• Carcinoma (most common)
• Small cell carcinoma (2%)
• Lymphoma (1%)
• Leiomyosarcoma (rare)
Secondary – Invasion from cancer of lung or stomach

ESOPHAGEAL CARCINOMA

INCIDENCE

Esophageal carcinoma has a wide variability in incidence globally. It is highest in China, Russia, Turkey, Iran and southern Africa, while it is uncommon in Canada and the US. Most patients with esophageal cancer are between 55 and 70 years of age. It is more common in men than women (3:1).

RISK FACTORS

• Smoking and alcohol
Individually, smoking and alcohol increase the risk of cancer of the esophagus, but together the risk is substantial due to chronic irritation of the mucosa.

• Barrett's esophagus
This is a pre-malignant condition characterized by glandular metaplasia of the squamous epithelium of lower esophagus, usually related to gastro-esophageal reflux disease (GERD). About 10% of patients with GERD and 1-2% of patients who undergo upper GI endoscopy for other reasons are found to have Barrett's esophagus. There is a high risk of adeno-carcinoma in these persons, with an incidence of about 0.5% per year.

• Tylosis
This is a rare autosomally dominant inherited condition, characterized by hyperkeratosis of the palm and soles, and papillomas of the esophagus.

• Achalasia
This causes food and secretions to pool in the dilated esophagus, leading to increased contact between the mucosa and any carcinogens in the food or produced by bacterial action.

• Caustic injury
Squamous cell cancer arising from strictures due to lye accounts for 1-4% of esophageal cancers.

• Esophageal diverticula

• Esophageal web
This occurs in Plummer-Vinson or Paterson-Kelly syndrome (upper esophageal webs, iron-deficiency anemia, glossitis and splenomegaly). About 10% of affected persons develop cancers

of the esophagus or hypopharynx.

- Infectious agent

Human papillomavirus is associated with squamous cell cancer in Japan and China.

- Vitamin-deficient diet
- Second primary tumors

Esophageal cancer may develop as a second primary cancer in individuals with other primary cancers of the upper aero-digestive tract. The underlying factor is exposure to the carcinogens in tobacco smoke, which is responsible for the development of these multiple tumors; this phenomenon is called "field cancerization."

PATHOLOGY

Macroscopic

The cancer starts as a nodule, which then develops into an ulcer, an exophytic mass or an annular constriction.

Microscopic

The major histological types of esophageal cancer are squamous cell carcinoma and adenocarcinoma. In the past, squamous cell cancer made up the majority, but the incidence of adenocarcinoma is rapidly increasing in North America and parts of Western Europe, especially in men. Squamous cell cancer arises in the upper two-thirds of the esophagus and its incidence is stable. Adenocarcinoma is more common in the lower third; its incidence is increasing and it now accounts for about one-half of all esophageal cancers.

Spread

Local growth occurs longitudinally and circumferentially with obstruction of the esophagus. Submucosal spread can cause "skip" lesions some distance from the primary cancer.

Invasion through the esophagus leads to involvement of the mediastinal structures: trachea, mediastinal pleura, main stem bronchus, vertebra and major vessels.

By lymphatic spread to the regional lymph nodes. Cancers in the upper third drain to the cervical and supraclavicular areas; those in the middle third to the mediastinal nodes; and those in the lower third to lesser curvature, left gastric and celiac axis areas.

Blood stream spread to liver, lungs, pleura and bone.

SCREENING

In endemic areas, such as South-East Asia, screening is practised. Swallowing an inflatable balloon is used to obtain cytological samples. Early cancers detected by this method are more curable by surgery. Endoscopic surveillance has been suggested for persons with chronic GERD symptoms, who are most likely to have Barrett's esophagus. However, the effectiveness of this has not been verified by clinical studies.

CLINICAL FEATURES

Local symptoms include dysphagia or odynophagia. Dysphagia is the most frequent presenting symptom; this symptom invariably has a pathological cause and must always be investigated. Dysphagia starts as a sensation of food sticking, usually for solids such as meat, but progressively worsens to softer foods and liquids. Retrosternal discomfort may accompany the dysphagia, and later there is regurgitation of food. Unlike gastro-esophageal reflux, there is not a sour or acid taste. Recurrent aspirations occur when the obstruction is severe, and these cause repeated lung infections.

Lymphatic spread to the neck and supraclavicular nodes leads to nodal enlargement.

Blood-borne spread may result in upper abdominal discomfort or pain due to hepatomegaly, shortness of breath or cough due to metastases to the pleura or lung, or bone pain due to bone metastasis.

Systemic symptoms include anorexia, weight loss, fatigue (anemia).

INVESTIGATIONS

- Complete blood count: microcytic anemia may be present
- Biochemistry: liver enzymes, bilirubin
- Tumor markers: CEA, CA19-9
- Barium swallow provides an initial assessment of the tumor length
- Endoscopy is required for histological confirmation and documentation of the location of the primary cancer. Endoscopic ultrasound permits evaluation of the depth of invasion of the cancer and possible involvement of the paraesophageal lymph nodes
- Chest x-ray
- CT scan of the chest and upper abdomen is required preoperatively to evaluate the thorax, mediastinum and upper abdominal organs (liver and adrenal glands) for metastases
- Bronchoscopy is recommended in middle or upper third cancers to exclude invasion of the trachea or main-stem bronchus
- Positron emission tomography (PET) scanning is used increasingly to detect nodal or distant metastases in operable patients

STAGING

The TMN staging system is used.

Tis - carcinoma *in situ*
T0 - no evidence of primary tumor
Tx - primary cannot be assessed
T1 - invasion of the lamina propria (T1a) or submucosa (T1b)
T2 - invasion of the muscularis propria
T3 - invasion of adventitial tissues

T4 - invasion of surrounding structures
N0 - no nodal involvement
N1 - regional nodes involved
    N1a - 1-3 nodes involved
    N1b - 4-7 nodes involved
    N1c - >7 nodes involved
M0 - no distant metastasis
M1 - distant metastasis present
    M1a – metastasis in distant nodes (celiac, supraclavicular)
    M1b – other distant metastases

Staging groups

Stage 0	TisN0M0	
Stage 1	T1N0M0	
Stage IIA	T2N0M0	T3N0M0
Stage IIB	T1N1M0	T2N1M0
Stage III	T3N1M0	T4 any N M0
Stage IVA	any T any N M1a	
Stage IVB	any T any N M1b	

TREATMENT

Resectable disease

Surgery is the only potentially curative modality, and patients with resectable disease have better outcome than those whose disease is unresectable. Surgery remains the treatment of choice for localized lesions, especially those in the lower third, which is the most surgically accessible part of the esophagus. For cancers in the upper third, radiation therapy is favored as surgery is technically difficult. (Also see Cancer of the Stomach below for adjuvant therapy for gastro-esophageal adenocarcinoma.)

Locally advanced disease

For locally advanced cancers, radiation therapy is favored. However, because of the low survival rates, combined modality treatment with surgery, radiation and chemotherapy is increasingly being used to improve local control, and this may also confer a small survival benefit. The usual chemotherapy is cisplatin with infusional 5-fluorouracil (5FU), which gives a response rate of 30-60%. There is also an increased use of concurrent chemotherapy (cisplatin-5FU) with radiation, particularly for patients with squamous cell carcinoma or inoperable tumors. This may lead to down-staging of the cancer to facilitate surgery or provide a longer period of disease control for those whose cancer remains unresectable. Chemo-radiation is also used with radical intent for patients who are not fit candidates for surgery.

Metastatic disease

Palliation is the primary goal for patients with inoperable or metastatic disease. Relief of dysphagia is the chief aim. This can be achieved by radiation therapy, simple dilation, esophageal intubation or laser ablation of the obstructive lesion.

Chemotherapy with 5FU and cisplatin may be useful in relieving dysphagia in patients fit for chemotherapy. For squamous cell carcinoma, this produces a response rate of about 50%. Adenocarcinoma of the gastro-esophageal junction has a 50% response rate to ECF (epirubicin-cisplatin-5FU). An alternative combination is docetaxel-cisplatin-5FU, which produces response rates similar to ECF, but has more side effects.

Many patients with esophageal cancer are in poor nutritional state. Liquid dietary supplements to maintain adequate caloric intake or enteral feeding, via a nasogastric or percutaneous gastrostomy tube, may be advised.

OUTCOME

The overall 5-year survival for all patients is 10%. For patients with resectable disease, the 5-year survival rate is about 20%; for the subgroup with node-negative disease, it is 40-50%, while for node-positive disease it is 10-20%.

CANCER OF THE STOMACH

CLASSIFICATION

Benign

- Epithelial – adenoma
- Connective tissue – leiomyoma, fibroma, neurofibroma

Malignant

Primary
- Adenocarcinoma (95%)
- Lymphoma (3%)
- Stromal tumors (uncommon)
- Carcinoid tumor (uncommon)

Secondary: Invasion from cancer of adjacent organs, such as pancreas or transverse colon

GASTRIC CARCINOMA

INCIDENCE

Gastric cancer was a common cancer in Canada and the US in the early 1900s, but its incidence has decreased dramatically in the past 60 years. However, the number of new cases of cancer of the proximal stomach (cardia) and gastro-esophageal junction has risen faster than other GI cancers over the past 25 years. Stomach cancer remains a common cancer in Asian countries, like Japan and Korea, in Latin American countries, like Chile and Costa Rica, and in Eastern Europe. Men are affected more commonly than women (2:1), and the peak incidence occurs in the seventh decade of life in men and slightly later in women.

RISK FACTORS

- Nutritional factors

The stomach is exposed to various carcinogens both ingested with food and produced from food by bacterial action in the stomach. Factors associated with an increased risk include:

  - salted meat or fish
  - certain types of food preparation, such as smoking
  - high nitrate intake (converted to nitroso-amines by bacteria)
  - low dietary vitamins A and C (antioxidants)
- Environmental factors
  - lack of refrigeration
  - poor drinking well-water
  - *Helicobacter pylori* infection
- Social factors

Persons of low social class have an increased incidence. This may be related to above factors, e.g. poor food preparation or storage.

- Medical factors
  - prior gastric surgery for benign diseases, such as gastric ulcer
  - gastric atrophy and gastritis
  - achlorhydria
  - history of pernicious anemia
- Genetic factors

Persons with blood group A have an increased risk of stomach cancer, whereas those with blood group O seem at less risk.

SCREENING

Population screening for gastric cancer in Japan was introduced in the 1960s as part of screening programs for several cancers, including uterus, breast, lung, and colon, in individuals older than 40. Barium studies were done with an upper GI endoscopy if any abnormality was detected. This has resulted in a greater proportion of early cancers being found and an overall decline in gastric cancer mortality. In general, screening for gastric cancer is not recommended outside of a few countries with a high incidence of gastric cancer.

Eradication of *H. pylori* has the potential to reduce the burden of gastric cancer, but the ideal means to implement a screening program and the settings in which it would be appropriate remain unclear.

PATHOLOGY

Macroscopic

The cancer forms an ulcerating, nodular or polypoid lesion, but occasionally may be diffuse, infiltrating. About 50% occur in the pylorus, and of those arising in the body of the stomach, most are located along the lesser curvature.

Microscopic

The majority of stomach cancer is adeno-carcinoma. There are two distinct types:

- *Intestinal type* is associated with precancerous conditions, such as gastric atrophy or intestinal metaplasia. This type is more common in men, and occurs with a higher frequency in high incidence areas, suggesting an environmental cause
- *Diffuse type*, characterized as signet ring carcinoma, is slightly more frequent in women and younger patients, and has a higher association with blood group type A, suggesting a genetic etiology

Spread

Local growth within the stomach causes narrowing of the lumen and rigidity of the wall (linitis plastica). Invasion through the stomach wall leads to infiltration of adjacent structures: omentum, pancreas, transverse colon, spleen, kidney or adrenal gland. Extension of proximal cancers to the lower end of the esophagus can cause dysphagia.

Lymphatic spread occurs to the nodes along the gastric vessels and to the celiac axis. Splenic hilar nodes and those around the pancreas are also frequently involved. Spread through the thoracic duct leads to involvement of the left supraclavicular node (Virchow's node).

Blood-borne dissemination is to the liver (via the portal vein) as well as to the lungs and bone. Bone marrow infiltration occurs infrequently. Brain metastasis is a late, uncommon event.

Transcelomic spread produces seeding on the peritoneal surface or implantation on the ovaries (Krukenberg tumors).

CLINICAL FEATURES

Local symptoms include early satiety and anorexia, and their onset can be insidious. Later, dyspepsia and nausea/vomiting (due to gastric outlet obstruction) occur. These symptoms can be mistaken for more common benign conditions, such as gastritis or peptic ulcer disease. Antacids, H2 blockers or proton pump inhibitors may sometimes temporarily relieve the symptoms, and this leads to further delay in diagnosis. As the disease progresses, back pain (due to infiltration of retroperitoneal structures), or dysphagia (due to obstruction of the gastroesophageal junction by proximal cancers) can be present. Occasionally, hematemesis may occur or there may be melena. A few patients present with iron-deficiency anemia due to chronic blood loss.

Secondaries may lead to jaundice (due to biliary obstruction by enlarged porta hepatis nodes) or abdominal distension from ascites.

Systemic manifestations include anorexia (common), fatigue (due to anemia), or weight loss.

Examination may disclose an emaciated, pale or icteric patient with an epigastric mass. There may be hepatomegaly, ascites, Virchow's node, or a rectal shelf due to deposits in the pouch of Douglas. Infrequently, dermatomyositis or ancanthosis nigricans may be seen.

INVESTIGATIONS

- Complete blood count: microcytic anemia may be present
- Biochemistry: liver enzymes and bilirubin
- Tumor markers: CEA, CA19-9
- Upper GI barium may demonstrate mucosal abnormalities although in some cases these cannot be distinguished from peptic ulcer disease
- Upper GI endoscopy allows accurate anatomic assessment of the lesion and permits biopsy for histological confirmation. An endoscopic ultrasound allows assessment of the depth of invasion and lymph node involvement
- Chest x-ray
- CT scan of abdomen and pelvis provides information about the extent of the cancer beyond the stomach, involvement of the celiac nodes or presence of liver metastasis

STAGING

The TNM staging system is used.

Tis - carcinoma in situ

T0 - no evidence of primary tumor

Tx - primary cannot be assessed

T1 - invasion of lamina propria or submucosa

T2 - invasion of muscularis propria (T2a) or subserosa (T2b)

T3 - penetration of serosa

T4 - invasion of adjacent structures

N0 - no nodal involvement

N1 - 1-6 nodes involved

N2 - 7-15 nodes involved

N3 - more than 15 nodes involved

M0 - no distant metastasis

M1 - distant metastasis present

Staging groups

Stage 0	Tis N0M0		
Stage 1A	T1N0M0		
Stage 1B	T1N1M0	T2a/bN0M0	
Stage II	T1N2M0	T2a/bN1M0	T3N0M0
Stage IIIA	T2a/bN2M0	T3N1M0	T4N0M0
Stage IIIB	T3N2M0		
Stage IV	T1-3N3M0	T4N1-3M0	
	Any T Any N M1		

TREATMENT

Resectable disease

Surgery by partial or total gastrectomy, depending on the location and extent of the cancer, is the only potentially curative modality. About two-thirds of patients are candidates for an operation after staging investigations, and of these, one-third will be deemed resectable at laparotomy. The traditional approach in North America is removal of the stomach and the first echelon nodes (perigastric nodes), referred to as a D1 node dissection. There is some evidence in favor of a more extensive node dissection (D2 dissection) with removal of the second echelon nodes. This is associated with higher operative morbidity and mortality, but it may improve the surgical cure rates.

Adjuvant therapy for gastric and gastro-esophageal cancers

Following surgery, many patients remain at high risk for local recurrence and distant metastases, and they are candidates for postoperative adjuvant therapy. Postoperative adjuvant therapy with 5FU chemotherapy and radiation to the upper abdomen improves overall survival in patients with high-risk gastric cancers extending through the stomach wall or with regional lymph node metastasis. Fit patients, who are able to maintain a daily caloric intake of more than 1500 calories postoperatively, are suitable for postoperative adjuvant chemo-radiation. This strategy increases the 3-year disease-free (48% vs. 31%) and overall survival rates (50% vs. 41%) compared with surgery alone. The median survival is significantly longer (36 vs. 27 months) in favor of the combined modality therapy.

Another approach is preoperative chemotherapy to downsize the primary tumor and enhance the probability of an R0 resection as well as eliminate microscopic metastases. Two regimens have been evaluated for preoperative chemotherapy. Two cycles of epirubicin-cisplatin-5FU (ECF) followed by surgery and then two more cycles of ECF improved R0 resection rates compared with surgery alone (79% vs. 70%) and 5-year survival rates (36% vs. 23%). Another regimen is cisplatin-5FU with two cycles before surgery followed by four cycles postoperatively. The R0 resection rate is better for the chemotherapy arm compared with surgery alone (84% vs. 73%), and the 5-year disease-free survival rates are 34% vs. 17%.

Locally advanced or metastatic disease

Palliative surgery with a gastro-enterostomy may be performed to relieve the symptoms of obstruction by a distal cancer. Surgery may occasionally be advised to control bleeding.

Radiation therapy can be useful for palliation of obstruction caused by gastro-esophageal or cardia tumors. It may also reduce bleeding from an inoperable gastric cancer and relieve pain due to bone metastasis or tumor infiltration into the celiac plexus.

Advanced or metastatic disease

Chemotherapy can produce partial responses in locally advanced or metastatic gastric cancer with consequent palliative benefit. The commonly used drugs are 5FU and cisplatin with or without epirubicin. Newer active chemotherapy drugs include oxaliplatin, irinotecan, docetaxel and paclitaxel, and these are being now incorporated in chemotherapy regimens.

Endoscopic procedures, such as stenting or laser coagulation, can be helpful for obstruction.

OUTCOME

Early gastric cancer confined to the mucosa has a 5-year survival rate of 90%. Unfortunately, only a small minority of patients are diagnosed at this stage. Patients who undergo complete surgical resection have an overall 5-year survival of 20%. With adjuvant therapy, the 5-year survival rate is 35%. The outlook for patients with unresectable or metastatic disease remains poor with a median survival of 6 months.

COLORECTAL CANCER

ANATOMY

The large bowel is divided into the colon and rectum. For treatment purposes, the rectum is considered in terms of its extra-peritoneal location, and the portion below the peritoneal reflection is regarded as the rectum. The colon and upper rectum drain into the portal circulation. The distal 5-7 cm of the rectum has a dual drainage. The superior hemorrhoidal vein drains into the portal circulation whereas the middle and inferior hemorrhoidal veins drain into the inferior vena cava. The lymphatics begin as a plexus beneath the muscularis propria and drain to the extramural lymphatics, which converge along the vascular trunks. The paracolic chains of lymph nodes along the vascular arcades are the most important sites of metastasis from colorectal cancer.

CLASSIFICATION

Benign

- Adenomatous polyp
- Lipoma
- Neurofibroma
- Hemangioma

Malignant

Primary
- Carcinoma
- Carcinoid tumor (uncommon)
- Sarcoma (rare)
- Lymphoma (rare)

Secondary: Invasion from adjacent organs, e.g. stomach, prostate, ovary or bladder.

COLORECTAL CARCINOMA

INCIDENCE

Colorectal cancer is the third most common cancer that affects approximately 1 in 15 persons in industrialized countries. Ninety percent of cases occur in persons over 50 years of age with an almost equal distribution between men and women, although rectal cancer is slightly more common in men, and colon cancer is slightly more common in women. In North America and some Western European countries, there has been a steady decline in mortality over the past 25 years, although the incidence is fairly constant. This is probably due to improved treatment and earlier diagnosis. In some South-East Asian countries, like Taiwan, there is an increasing incidence of colorectal cancer, possibly due to a change to a more western-style diet. Colorectal cancer is uncommon in Africa and Asia.

RISK FACTORS

- Nutritional factors

These may explain the large geographic differences in incidence. The important factors are:
  - increased meat consumption
  - high fat diet
  - low fibre diet; thus results in slower transit bowel time, which allows a longer period of contact between the bowel mucosa and any carcinogenic substance (e.g. fecal pentenes or 3-ketosteroids) in the stool
- Genetic factors
  - family history of colorectal cancer (20%)
  - genetic syndromes (3-5%)
    ▷ familial adenomatous polyposis (FAP) (1%)
    ▷ hereditary nonpolyposis colorectal

cancer (HNPCC) (2-4%)
    ▷ Gardner's, Turcot's, Oldfield's syndromes (rare)
- Pre-existing diseases
  - inflammatory bowel disease (e.g. ulcerative colitis or Crohn's colitis)
  - colorectal polyps
  - previous colorectal cancer
- Others
  - ureteric diversion to sigmoid colon
  - previous cholecystectomy

FAP and HNPCC are two important heritable syndromes associated with a high risk for colorectal cancer. The most important features of these are shown in Table 11.1

Table 11.1 Features of FAP and HNPCC

Feature	FAP	HNPCC
Inheritance pattern	Autosomal dominant	Autosomal dominant
Penetrance	100%	80%
Genetic defect	Mutation in APC gene	Mismatch repair gene defect
Age of onset	Adolescence	4th-5th decade
Number of adenomas	>100	<10
Site of adenomas	Left or total	Mainly right side
Site of cancer	Random	Mainly right side
Other cancers	Duodenum, gastric, thyroid, CNS, liver	Endometrium, ovary, ureter, small bowel, pancreas, stomach, hepatobiliary, possibly prostate

PATHOLOGY

Macroscopic

The rectum (30%) and sigmoid colon (25%) are the most common sites for cancers of the large bowel. Colorectal cancers arise from precursor polyps (tubular or villous adenomas), and progress in a stepwise sequence from adenoma to invasive carcinoma (see Chapter 2, Figure 2.5). Five percent of cancers of the large bowel are multiple.

The cancer may be ulcerating, nodular or polypoid in appearance.

Microscopic

Adenocarcinoma is the most common histological type, representing 95% of colorectal cancers. Other uncommon cancers are carcinoid tumors and sarcomas.

Important prognostic pathological features

Tumor features
- Depth of invasion through the layers of the bowel wall
- Involvement of the circumferential wall, especially for rectal cancers
- Mucinous cell type
- Venous invasion
- Perineural invasion

Lymph node features
- Total number of nodes removed (12-14 recommended)
- Number of nodes involved
- Lymphatic invasion

Spread

Locally with the encircling and infiltration of the muscle layers of the bowel wall. Occasionally, there is extension to adjacent organs or structures, such as small bowel, stomach, vagina, sacrum, sacral plexus and lateral pelvic wall.

Lymphatic spread to the paracolic nodes and regional mesenteric nodes; in later stages, the left supraclavicular node is involved.

Blood-borne spread – colon: via the portal vein to liver and later to lungs; rectum: via the middle or inferior hemorrhoidal veins to the inferior vena cava and, thence, to the lungs; or via the superior hemorrhoidal vein to the portal system and, thence, to the liver.

Transcelomic spread with malignant deposits throughout the peritoneal cavity may also occur.

SCREENING

There is good evidence that fecal occult blood testing of asymptomatic individuals above age 50 years on an annual or biennial basis reduces the mortality from colorectal cancer. The incidence of positive tests is between 1-4%, of which 10-20% are due to adenomatous polyps, and 5-10% to colorectal cancer. Fecal occult blood test allows the diagnosis of early cancers with an increase in the proportion of Stages I and II cancers in the screened population. This results in an increase in surgical cure rates.

Because of the low specificity and sensitivity of FOBT, other options for screening have been advocated (see also Chapter 1). An immuno-chemical fecal occult blood test, which detects intact human haemoglobin, potentially increases the specificity of the fecal occult testing. Alternative options include endoscopic screening by flexible sigmoidoscopy (with or without annual occult blood tests) at 5-year intervals , or colonoscopy at 10 year-intervals.

High-risk individuals require regular colonoscopic surveillance. These include those with familial adenomatous polyposis, HNPCC, inflammatory bowel disease, family history of colorectal cancer or adenomas in a first-degree relative before age 60 years, or a personal history of colorectal adenomatous polyps or cancer.

PREVENTION

Because of the links to dietary factors, dietary changes with an increase in fibre and reduction of fat or meat may be an effective preventive strategy. There is some suggestion for the chemopreventive effects of aspirin or NSAIDs in reducing the incidence of colorectal cancer (see also Chapter 1.)

STAGING

The TNM staging system is used.
Tx   primary tumor cannot be assessed
T0   no evidence of primary tumor
Tis carcinoma *in situ*

T1   tumor invades submucosa

T2   tumor invades muscularis propria

T3   tumor invades through muscularis propria

T4   tumor invades other organs or structures or perforates visceral peritoneum

Nx   regional nodes cannot be assessed

N0   no regional nodes metastasis

N1   metastasis in 1-3 regional lymph nodes

N2   metastasis in 4 or more regional lymph nodes

Mx   distant metastasis cannot be assessed

M0   no distant metastasis

M1   distant metastasis

Stage Grouping

Stage 0	Tis N0 M0
Stage I	T1-T2 N0 M0
Stage IIA	T3 N0 M0
Stage IIB	T4 N0 M0
Stage IIIA	T1-T2 N1 M0
Stage IIIB	T3-T4 N1 M0
Stage IIIC	Any T N2 M0
Stage IV	Any T Any N M1

INVESTIGATIONS

- Complete blood count: microcytic, hypochromic anemia is commonly present due to chronic blood loss
- Biochemistry: liver enzymes and bilirubin (if jaundice is present)
- Tumor markers: CEA, CA19-9
- Colonoscopy is the most important diagnostic investigation. In addition, it permits detection of any synchronous primary cancer and removal of any polyps. (Double-contrast barium enema also allows visualization of the entire bowel, but is used less frequently now)
- Chest x-ray
- Imaging study of the abdomen and pelvis by CT scan
- Endorectal ultrasound and pelvic MRI are recommended for mid or low rectal cancers to determine the lateral extent of the cancer within the pelvis

CLINICAL FEATURES

Local symptoms most commonly include a persistent change in bowel habits with constipation or diarrhea or the two alternating. Bleeding, which may be bright red, melena or occult, is common. For cancers arising in the left colon where the stool is more solid, obstructive symptoms (intermittent, colicky abdominal pains) due to a constricting cancer predominate, whereas in the right colon, the stool is more liquid and obstructive symptoms are less common. Cecal cancers can bleed slowly with significant anemia. Uncommonly, acute peritonitis results from perforation of the cancer. Rectal cancer causes rectal pain or tenesmus.

Blood-borne metastases may be present in up to 20% of patients at diagnosis. The most common site of distant metastases is the liver, which can cause upper abdominal discomfort. Metastases to the lung may occur later in colon cancer patients, but can be present in rectal cancer patients without liver metastases. However, dyspnea is an uncommon symptom at presentation.

Transcolemic spread results in ascites.

General effects include anorexia, weight loss or fatigue (anemia).

Examination may reveal a rectal mass with heaped-up margins and a friable ulcer that bleeds easily. A rectal shelf may be palpable due to metastases in the Pouch of Douglas and is an indication of peritoneal spread. Large cecal cancers may occasionally be palpable in the right lower quadrant of the abdomen. Metastasis to the left supraclavicular node (Virchow's node) may be evident, and liver metastases cause hepatomegaly. In later stages, ascites may be present due to liver dysfunction; another cause of ascites is peritoneal carcinomatosis.

Differential diagnosis

- The differential diagnosis is from diseases producing local symptoms – diverticular disease, ulcerative colitis or infectious diarrhea
- A palpable rectal mass may be due to:
  - benign tumors
  - secondary deposits in the pelvis (rectal shelf)
  - ovarian or uterine tumors
  - invasion from cancer of the prostate or cervix
  - endometriosis
  - diverticular disease
  - feces
  - the cervix can be palpated through the anterior rectal wall and should not be confused with an abnormal mass

TREATMENT

Curative treatment

Surgery
Surgical resection is the mainstay of therapy. Colon cancers are treated by segmental resection of the colon with re-anastomosis. Rectal cancer surgery is more difficult due to the technical challenges of its location within the confines of the pelvis. Local pelvic recurrence rates can be high, historically up to 25-30%. However, the adoption of the specialized technique of total mesorectal excision (TME), with meticulous circumferential resection down the avascular plane between the mesorectum and the pelvic sidewall, has brought about a remarkable re-duction of local recurrence rates which are now less than 10%. Mid or high rectal cancers are resected by an anterior resection of the rectum with primary end-to-end anastomosis. For low rectal cancers, an abdominoperineal resection of the rectum with a permanent colostomy is performed.

Radiation therapy
Because of the high risk for local recurrent disease within the pelvis, postoperative radiation to the pelvis is routinely given to patients with Stages II or III rectal cancers. The typical dose of radiation is 45-50 Gy over 5 weeks. This is usually combined with 5FU chemotherapy. There is good evidence that a short course of preoperative radiation (25 Gy in 5 days) followed by TME within 7 days can reduce pelvic recurrences from mid to low rectal cancers. Similar results can be achieved with long course radiation (45-50 Gy over 5 weeks) followed by surgery in 6 weeks. Adjuvant pelvic radiation is now routinely offered to patients with high risk rectal cancers and preoperative radiation is being increasingly favored. For locally advanced rectal cancer that is unresectable, radiation with or without 5FU chemotherapy, may be used to down-stage the cancer to render it resectable.

In colon cancer, radiation therapy has little role, since local recurrence is not a problem, and delivery of high doses of radiation is limited by the toxicity to the abdominal organs, especially the small bowel.

Chemotherapy
Postoperative adjuvant chemotherapy with the combination of 5FU, folinic acid and oxaliplatin (FOLFOX) for 6 months is recommended for patients with Stage III colon cancer. Adjuvant chemotherapy can improve the overall 5-year survival rates from 50% for surgery alone to 70% with postoperative chemotherapy. Patients

not fit for FOLFOX chemotherapy may be treated with 5FU or oral capecitabine although the magnitude of benefit is smaller. There is some controversy over the need for postoperative adjuvant chemotherapy for Stage II colon cancer patients, but it may be considered if there are adverse features, such as T4 (invasion of adjacent structure or perforation) or poorly differentiated tumors. The value of the addition of targeted therapies, such as bevacizumab or cetuximab, to FOLFOX chemotherapy as adjuvant treatment for colon cancer is being examined in clinical trials.

For both Stages II and III rectal cancer patients, adjuvant chemotherapy is recommended in addition to pelvic radiation. The common regimen is folinic acid and 5FU for 6-8 months, and studies of adjuvant FOLFOX chemotherapy are in progress.

Palliative treatment

Surgery
Palliative surgery is indicated for an obstructing primary cancer or when there is obstruction of the small bowel due to peritoneal implants. Even in the presence of metastatic disease, a surgical bypass procedure may be beneficial. Multiple levels of obstruction of the bowel, however, cannot be effectively managed by surgery.

In patients with a limited number of liver metastasis and no evidence of extra-hepatic metastatic disease, partial hepatic resection can lead to 5-year survival of 25-40%. Preoperative chemotherapy (oxaliplatin-5FU or irinotecan-5FU) can decrease the risk of progression for patients with resectable liver metastases, but it is associated with more complications (liver failure or biliary fistulas). Patients with liver metastases that are considered borderline for R0 resection can be down-staged by che-

motherapy to render them resectable.

Radiofrequency ablation of a few, small liver metastases also provide good long-term control of liver metastases when surgery is not feasible. This is usually used when there are few (<5), small (<5 cm) lesions.

Radiation therapy
Palliative radiation therapy can be useful to reduce bleeding or mucus discharge from unresectable rectal cancer, and relieve pain due to infiltration of the sacral nerve plexus.

Chemotherapy
Chemotherapy can be beneficial to patients with metastatic disease in reducing tumor-related symptoms and extending survival. Active drugs include 5FU (or capecitabine), irinotecan and oxaliplatin. For fit patients with good performance status (ECOG 0-1), the combination of folinic acid and 5FU with irinotecan (FOLFIRI) or oxaliplatin (FOLFOX) is recommended. Combination chemotherapy with sequential FOLFIRI and FOLFOX can extend median patient survival from 9 months to about 18 months. Not all patients are fit for combination chemotherapy, and capecitabine is a suitable choice for elderly or sicker patients with metastatic colorectal cancer.

Targeted therapy
Bevacizumab, a monoclonal antibody directed to VEGF (vascular endothelial growth factor), increases response rates and prolong patient survival when combined with chemotherapy in patients with advanced colorectal cancer in the first- or second-line setting. Similarly, monoclonal antibodies directed to the extracellular domain of epidermal growth factor receptor (EGFR) can exert several biological effects, including reversal of drug resistance to irinotecan. It also delays tumor progression in advanced cases. Two anti-EGFR drugs available for the treatment of colorectal cancer are cet-

uximab and panitumumab. A third anti-EGFR drug, nimotuzumab, which has fewer side effects, also looks promising.

Other treatment modalities
Laser therapy can occasionally be helpful to relieve the symptoms of obstruction or reduce bleeding or mucus discharge from unresectable rectal cancers. For constricting rectal lesions, an endorectal stent may be placed.

OUTCOME

Stage	5-year survival
Stage I (T1-2N0)	93%
Stage IIA (T3N0)	85%
Stage IIB (T4N0)	72%
Stage IIIA (T1-2N1)	83%
Stage IIIB (T3-4 N1)	64%
Stage IIIC (N2)	44%
Stage IV	<5%

The stage of the cancer and its resectability are the two most important determinants of patient survival. Patients with metastatic disease (Stage IV) are generally incurable, except for a small proportion with limited resectable liver or lung metastases. Untreated, the average life expectancy of patients is 9 months, but those fit for chemotherapy have a median survival of about 11 months with single-agent 5FU chemotherapy, and about 18 months with combination chemotherapy regimens.

CANCER OF THE PANCREAS

CLASSIFICATION

Benign

- Serous cystadenoma
- Neuroendocrine neoplasm

Uncertain malignant potential

- Mucinous cystadenoma
- Papillary cystic neoplasm

Malignant

Primary
- Ductal adenocarcinoma (most common)
- Mucinous cystadenocarcinoma
- Acinar cell carcinoma
- Malignant neuroendocrine tumors
- Pancreatoblastoma
- Small cell carcinoma

Secondary
Invasion from carcinoma of the stomach, duodenum or ampulla of Vater

PANCREATIC ADENOCARCINOMA

INCIDENCE

The incidence of pancreatic cancer has decreased slightly since the 1970s in North America, but has increased in Japan. Most patients are between the ages of 65 and 80 years at diagnosis. The male:female ratio is about 1.3:1. Pancreatic adenocarcinoma accounts for 5% of all cancer deaths.

RISK FACTORS

- Cigarette smoking is the most firmly established risk factor. Carcinogens in cigarette smoke, especially nitrosoamines, cause mutation in the K-ras oncogene
- Diet: high intake of fat or meat and low consumption of fruits and vegetables
- Long-standing diabetes is associated with an increased risk for pancreatic cancer. Pancreatic cancer should be considered when there is the recent onset of diabetes

with no obvious predisposition, such as a family history
- Chronic pancreatitis is associated with about 5% of pancreatic cancer cases
- Previous abdominal surgery: peptic ulcer surgery may increase the risk, but previous cholecystectomy as a risk factor is controversial
- Exposure to chemicals, e.g. 2-naphthylamine, benzene, gasoline derivatives or DDT
- Occupations, e.g. stone miners, cement workers, gardeners and textile workers
- Familial cancer syndromes: Lynch syndrome type II and familial atypical multiple mole melanoma (FAMM) syndrome

PATHOLOGY

Macroscopic

The cancer forms a circumscribed mass or a diffuse infiltration of the pancreas.

Seventy-five percent are located in the head of the pancreas, 15% in the body, and 10% in the tail.

Microscopic

Ductal adenocarcinoma accounts for 95% of pancreatic cancers.

Spread

Locally with diffuse infiltration of the gland or along the pancreatic ducts to the common bile duct. Breaching of the capsule leads to invasion of the celiac and mesenteric plexus, duodenum or distal stomach and portal vein.
Lymphatic spread to adjacent nodes and nodes in the porta hepatis and celiac axis.
Blood-borne to liver and lungs.
Transcelomic spread with malignant peritoneal implants.

CLINICAL FEATURES

Because of the deep-seated location and the nonspecific symptoms, pancreatic cancers are difficult to diagnose, especially in the early stages of the disease. Cancers of the pancreatic body and tail do not cause obstruction of the intrapancreatic portion of the common bile duct and early diagnosis is uncommon.
Local symptoms include pain, which tends to be dull and constant. Pain is present in over 50% of patients at diagnosis, and in 90% during the course of the disease. It is due to invasion of the celiac and mesenteric plexus, and it is usually experienced in the epigastrium or upper abdomen. Back pain may be associated with the abdominal pain, and in some patients back pain occurs independently. Cancer arising in the head of the pancreas often causes obstructive jaundice. As the cancer progresses, gastric outlet obstruction may occur. Malabsorption and steatorrhea due to pancreatic enzyme insufficiency may result from obstruction of the pancreatic duct or destruction of the organ by the cancer. Changes in stool frequency are common, but diarrhea is uncommon.
General effects
- Diabetes is present in 80% of patients
- Cancer cachexia due to cytokines produced in response to the growing tumor
- Depression is a common symptom
- Paraneoplastic syndromes: migratory thrombophlebitis and hypercoaguable syndrome, e.g. deep venous thrombosis, pulmonary embolism
Examination typically reveals an underweight person, who is icteric. There may be evidence of scratch marks on the trunk due to pruritis caused by bile salts retention. A palpable gall bladder may be present (Courvoisier's Law). In the late stages, a fixed epigastric mass may be

palpable, and the liver is enlarged. Ascites may be present. Metastasis to the left supraclavicular node is common. In advanced stages, purpura and bruising due to DIC can occur, and thrombophlebitis is not uncommon.

Differential diagnosis

The differential diagnosis is from other causes of obstructive jaundice and from other causes of upper abdominal pain. Causes of obstructive jaundice include:

- Gallstones
- Benign biliary tract strictures, e.g. following surgical trauma
- Lymph node metastases at the porta hepatis
- Sclerosing cholangitis
- Cholangiocarcinoma

   Three other important malignant conditions must be distinguished from pancreatic carcinoma.

- Malignant neuroendocrine tumors of the pancreas (see also Chapter 15)

These arise from the clusters of islet cells within the pancreas. About one-half are functioning tumors that give rise to specific syndromes due to hypersecretion of hormones (insulin, gastrin, vasoactive intestinal polypeptide, glucagon or somatostatin). The other one-half are nonfunctioning, and they come to attention incidentally or due to their "mass" effect. The histology of these cancers is distinct from pancreatic adenocarcinoma, and serum chromogranin A level is often elevated. Islet cell cancers are indolent, and patients can live for years despite metastasis to the liver.

- Periampullary cancer

Periampullary cancers often present earlier than pancreatic cancers and they have a more favorable prognosis after resection.

- Duodenal cancer

Invasion into the head of the pancreas by a duodenal cancer can sometimes be difficult to distinguish from a primary pancreatic cancer.

INVESTIGATIONS

- Complete blood count
- Biochemistry: liver enzymes and bilirubin. (Serum amylase is rarely elevated)
- Clotting profile: INR may be prolonged due to impaired production of vitamin K-dependent clotting factors
- Tumor markers (CA19-9 and CEA). CA19.9 is elevated in most pancreatic cancers, but it is not specific enough to be diagnostic
- Chest x-ray
- Ultrasound or CT scan of the upper abdomen. A fine needle aspirate of the pancreatic mass or metastatic deposits, e.g. in the supraclavicular node, is the procedure of choice to establish the histological diagnosis
- If a mass is not evident on abdominal CT scan, an endoscopic retrograde cholangiopancreatogram (ERCP) should be performed. Endoscopic ultrasound provides higher diagnostic accuracy
- MRI can delineate the cancer, ducts and vessels

STAGING

A practical staging system is guided by surgical resectability.

Localized (20%)

- no encasement of the celiac axis or superior mesenteric artery (SMA)
- patent superior mesenteric-portal vein (SMPV) confluence
- no extrapancreatic disease

Locally advanced (40%)

- extensive peripancreatic lymph node disease
- encasement or occlusion of the superior mesenteric vein or SMPV confluence
- direct involvement of SMA, inferior vena cava, aorta or celiac axis

Metastatic disease (40%)
- presence of liver, peritoneum or lung metastases

TREATMENT

Surgery

Only patients with localized disease are suitable for surgical resection. Pancreaticoduodenectomy or Whipple's resection is the surgical procedure for resectable pancreatic adenocarcinoma. The 5-year survival after Whipple's resection is 20%. Patients with unresectable cancer are candidates for palliative surgical bypass procedures for decompression of the biliary tree (choledochojejunostomy) or gastric outlet obstruction (gastrojejunostomy).

Radiation therapy

External beam radiation may be used for locally advanced pancreatic cancer, but no definite survival benefit has been documented. In some centres, intra-operative radiation is used with possibly improved local control of the disease. Radiation therapy may also relieve pain due to infiltration of the nerve plexus. Combined modality treatment with radiation and 5-FU has not been consistently successful in prolonging disease remission or patient survival.

Chemotherapy

Adjuvant chemotherapy
Because of the high rate of relapse after complete surgical removal of pancreatic cancer, adjuvant chemotherapy has been investigated. A study by European investigators suggests that 5FU chemotherapy after surgical resection may confer a small survival advantage, but this requires confirmation. A different approach in North America is to offer chemo-radiation with infusional 5FU chemotherapy during radiation.

Postoperative adjuvant gemcitabine also produces a significant improvement in patient survival. The 3-year survival rate is 37% for patients receiving gemcitabine compared with 20% for those who had no additional postoperative treatment.

Chemotherapy for metastatic or advanced disease
Metastatic pancreatic cancer has a poor prognosis with a median survival of about 5-6 months. Gemcitabine chemotherapy improves the 1-year survival from 2% to 18% compared with 5FU, and about one-third of treated patients experience clinical improvement of their symptoms (reduced pain, weight gain and improved performance status). The combination of capecitabine and gemcitabine prolongs patient survival, but only by a small amount. Also, the addition of erlotinib, a tyrosine kinase inhibitor of EGFR, to gemcitabine produces a small but statistically significant improvement in overall survival.

Other palliative measures
Obstruction of the common bile duct is common and can be relieved by the placement of a biliary stent or by percutaneous trans-hepatic cannulation of the intra-hepatic bile ducts. Patients with pancreatic cancer may also experience symptoms from several coexisting conditions that can be relieved by appropriate measures; e.g. insulin for diabetes, enzyme supplements for pancreatic insufficiency, opioids for pain, enteric nutrition for malnutrition, and antidepressants for clinical depression.

OUTCOME

The prognosis for patients with pancreatic cancer is poor. The overall 5-year survival is <5%. Even among those who undergo surgical resection, the 5-year survival is only 20%.

HEPATOCELLULAR TUMORS

CLASSIFICATION

Benign

- Benign epithelial tumors (adenoma, regenerative nodule)
- Benign mesenchymal tumors (cavernous hemangioma, hamartoma, leiomyoma, myxoma, fibroma, lipoma)
- Cysts

Malignant

Primary
- Hepatocellular carcinoma (80%)
- Cholangiocarcinoma (20%)
- Sarcoma (uncommon)

Secondary
The liver is the most common site of metastatic disease from cancers of other organs.
- Portal spread from the colon, stomach or pancreas
- Systemic blood spread, especially from lung, breast or melanoma
- Direct spread from gallbladder, stomach or hepatic flexure of colon

HEPATOCELLULAR CARCINOMA

INCIDENCE

Hepatocellular carcinoma is uncommon in North America, but it is one of the most common malignancies globally, especially in China, Korea and sub-Saharan Africa. In areas of high incidence of the disease, such as Asia and Africa, there is an association with endemic hepatitis B or aflatoxin contamination of stored grains (peanuts and corn). In endemic areas, the peak incidence is 20-40 years, whereas elsewhere it is 40-60 years. Men are affected twice as frequently as women.

RISK FACTORS

- Cirrhosis due to chronic hepatitis B or C virus infection, or alcohol
- Aflatoxin exposure
- Metabolic factors
  - genetic hemochromatosis
  - hereditary tyrosinemia
  - alpha-1 antitrypsin deficiency
- Environmental factors
  - thorotrast (which contains thorium, a radioisotope)
  - androgenic anabolic steroid use

Hepatitis and hepatocellular carcinoma

There is a strong association between chronic hepatitis B virus (HBV) infection and hepatocellular carcinoma. Also, chronic infection by hepatitis C virus (HCV), usually acquired through contaminated blood transfusion, substantially increases the risk for hepatocellular carcinoma. The role of HBV or HCV as direct carcinogens is unclear as the HCV genome is not integrated in the host genome, and HBV is integrated in a random fashion. One hypothesis is that repeated rounds of liver damage, followed by replicative repair, lead to accumulation of mutations associated with cancer development.

PATHOLOGY

Macroscopic

About 80% of patients with hepatocellular carcinoma have underlying cirrhosis. In South-East Asia, the cirrhosis is usually of the macro-nodular variety, whereas in Europe and North America, micro-nodular cirrhosis is also seen. The cancer grows rapidly and it may be solitary or multifocal.

Microscopic

Most are epithelial malignancies, and only a

small minority are primary sarcomas. Fibro-lamellar hepatocellular carcinoma is a distinct variant, which is more common in the West. It is often encapsulated with abundant fibrous stroma arranged in parallel lamellae. It occurs in young patients without underlying cirrhosis.

Spread

Local growth leads to destruction of the liver parenchyma. Spread occurs along the intra-hepatic ducts and hepatic veins. Infiltration through the liver capsule leads to invasion of the hepatic veins, portal vein and IVC as well as adjacent structures, such as the diaphragm, right kidney, stomach and transverse colon.
Lymphatic spread occurs to the hilar nodes at the base of the liver and portal nodes.
Blood-borne metastasis is to lungs, bone, skin and brain.
Transcelomic spread with peritoneal metastases.

PREVENTION/SCREENING

In endemic areas certain preventive strategies have been introduced:
- HBV vaccination of newborns to protect them from persistent infection. This has brought about a significant decrease in the incidence of hepatocellular cancer (see Chapter 1)
- Change of drinking water from pond or ditches to deep well or tap water to avoid contamination
- Change of food from corn to rice in rural areas to minimize exposure to aflatoxin
  Secondary prevention by screening has also been advocated, but remains controversial. In China, screening of high-risk populations by alpha-fetoprotein and/or liver ultrasonography to detect small, resectable cancers is practised. A prospective study in Shanghai suggests that screening HBV carriers permits early detection of resectable hepatocellular cancer and increases patient survival at an acceptable cost. A similar outcome was reported in an Alaskan Native study that used ultrasonography as a screening method. In North America, screening/sur-veillance by liver ultrasonography and alpha-fetoprotein every 6-12 months should be considered for certain high-risk groups: patients with cirrhosis from any cause, chronic hepatitis C patients with significant fibrosis and/or cirrhosis, and chronic HBV infected patients.

CLINICAL FEATURES

Patients with hepatocellular cancer often have a known diagnosis of cirrhosis and related problems. *Local growth* of the cancer can cause discomfort or pain due to stretching of the liver capsule from hepatomegaly. Occasionally, bleeding into the tumor leads to rapid expansion with acute upper abdominal pain. Obstruction of the bile ducts produces jaundice. Invasion of the portal vein results in portal hypertension with splenomegaly and ascites.
Blood-borne spread may cause bone pain (bone metastasis) or, uncommonly, respiratory symp-toms (lung metastasis).
Generalized effects include anorexia with weight loss. These may be present in the early stage of the disease. Weakness and fever may also occur.
Paraneoplastic syndromes
A number of paraneoplastic syndromes have been associated with hepatocellular carcinoma, although these are seldom of clinical signi-ficance: hypoglycemia, erythrocytosis, hyper-calcemia, hypercholesterolemia, dysfibrino-genemia, carcinoid syndrome, increased thyroxine-binding globulin, sexual changes from estrogen (gynecomastia, testicular at-rophy, precocious puberty), and porphyria cutanea tarda.

Examination reveals stigmata of chronic liver disease. Hepatomegaly is frequently present, and in more advanced cases, there is ascites from impairment of liver function or peritoneal implants. An arterial bruit and hepatic rub may be heard over the cancer. Compression of the inferior vena cava leads to leg edema. If portal vein thrombosis occurs, splenomegaly may develop.

DIAGNOSIS

• Serological Assay

Serum alpha-fetoprotein is elevated in 80% of Asian patients with hepatocellular carcinoma, and about 65% of North American patients.

• Fine needle aspiration

Biopsy of hepatocellular cancer carries a risk of bleeding due to thrombocytopenia, elevated INR, as well as the hypervascular nature of the cancer. However, fine needle aspirate (FNA) can be carried out safely under ultrasonic guidance. In conjunction with the serum alpha-fetoprotein, FNA confirms the diagnosis and distinguishes it from metastatic adenocarcinoma. There is a small risk of spillage of the tumor or implants of tumor cells along the needle track. Hence, for potential liver transplant patients, an FNA is contraindicated.

INVESTIGATIONS

• Complete blood count: thrombocytopenia is frequently present due to hypersplenism
• Biochemistry: bilirubin, liver enzymes and serum albumin. (Liver function tests are needed for diagnosis and selection of the appropriate treatment modality)
• Coagulation studies: INR, PTT
• Alpha-fetoprotein
• Imaging studies: ultrasound of the liver is a good screening test, but a CT scan is required to determine the local extent of the cancer. For operable patients, a CT arteriogram is advised to define the tumor size, location and vascular supply as a prerequisite to surgical resection

TREATMENT

The only curative treatment is surgical resection of the cancer. Unfortunately, this is possible only in a minority of patients with small cancers, typically less than 5 cm. Adverse prognostic features include vascular invasion, tumor size (>50% of liver involvement), and poor liver function. The Pugh-Child's grading of cirrhosis is helpful in determining liver function as a guide to resectability. It takes into account a combination of clinical and biochemical parameters (Table 11.2).

Table 11.2 Pugh-Child Grading of Cirrhosis

Measurement	1 Point	2 Points	3 points
Bilirubin (micromol/L)	<34	34-51	>51
INR (International Normalized Ratio)	<1.7	1.7-2.3	>2.3
Albumin (g/L)	>35	30-35	<30
Ascites	None	Mild	Moderate-severe
Encephalopathy	None	Minimal	Advanced coma

Class A: 5 to 6 points (well-compensated cirrhosis)
Class B: 7 to 9 points (decompensating cirrhosis)
Class C: 10 to 15 points (decompensated cirrhosis)

Generally, partial hepatectomy is offered only to patients with Pugh-Child Class A and selected Class B patients. Class C patients are not candidates for surgery or any aggressive non-surgical treatment, and they should be considered for supportive care.

Good results are obtained in patients with fibrolamellar hepatocellular carcinoma, likely due to the well-circumscribed nature of the cancer without associated cirrhosis. The resectability rates are 50-75%. Orthotopic liver transplantation may be considered in highly selected cases.

Because hepatocellular cancer receives its blood supply through the hepatic artery, hepatic artery chemoembolization is an option. This produces tumor responses in up to 50% of patients with symptomatic improvement. In addition, other options for patients with few (<5), small lesions (<5 cm) are percutaneous intralesional ethanol injection and radio-frequency ablation.

Chemotherapy has a limited role for hepatocellular cancer. Doxorubicin is the usual drug prescribed, but tumor response rates are low.

Sorafenib, a multi-targeted receptor tyrosine kinase inhibitor with anti-angiogenic and pro-apoptotic properties, improves patient survival compared with best supportive care in patients with advanced hepatocellular cancer.

OUTCOME

Surgery is the only potentially curative modality, but <20% of patients are long-term survivors. Survival for patients with unresectable hepatocellular carcinoma is poor with a median time of 3 months for those with cirrhosis, and 12 months for those without cirrhosis. The overall 5-year survival rate is 7%.

CHOLANGIOCARCINOMA

INCIDENCE

Cholangiocarcinoma is rare in developed countries with an incidence of 1-2/100,000. It is more common in South-east Asia, where liver flukes are endemic. The peak age incidence is 50-70 years, and is slightly more common in women.

RISK FACTORS

- Liver flukes *(Clonorchis sinensis and Opisthorchis viverrini)* in endemic area, such as South-east Asia
- Primary sclerosing cholangitis, a rare complication of chronic ulcerative colitis, carries a 9-40% risk
- Chronic cholangitis due to gallstones
- Congenital biliary abnormalities, such as choledochal cysts
- Environmental toxins: dioxins, asbestos, nitrosoamines and Thorotrast

PATHOLOGY

Macroscopic

Cholangiocarcinomas are divided into three groups: intrahepatic (20%), perihilar (50%) and extrahepatic (20%); in 10% of cases the cancer is multifocal. Perihilar cancers are defined as arising between the cystic duct-common duct junction and the confluence of the hepatic ducts (Klatskin tumors). The cancers may be diffusely sclerosing, nodular or papillary.

Microscopic

They are usually well-differentiated, mucin-secreting adenocarcinomas.

Spread

The cancer spreads locally into the liver (proximal cancers), or duodenum and pancreas (distal cancers). Lymphatic metastases occur to the hepatic hilar, superior mesenteric and celiac nodes. Blood-borne spread is most common to the liver, but may also occur to the lungs or bone.

CLINICAL FEATURES

The most common symptom is obstructive jaundice with scleral icterus, dark urine, pale stools and pruritis. The gallbladder may be palpable. Hepatomegaly may be present.

INVESTIGATIONS

- ERCP allows accurate anatomical localization and brushing or aspirates can confirm the diagnosis
- Percutaneous transhepatic cholangiogram may be done if ERCP is unsuccessful
- CT scan of the abdomen can detect enlarged nodes or liver metastases

TREATMENT

Surgery

Surgery is the only curative modality, but only about 30% of patients with intrahepatic or perihilar cancers, and 40% with distal cancers are candidates for curative surgery. Intrahepatic cancers are resected by partial hepatectomy; perihilar cancers require biliary resection and major hepatic resection; and more distal cancers are resected by pancreaticoduodenectomy. For unresectable disease, a biliary stent is placed to relieve the obstruction. A palliative choledochojejunostomy is required when biliary stenting is not possible.

Radiation

Brachytherapy with iridium-192 to deliver radiation to the site of an extrahepatic bile duct cancer can be offered when there is an indwelling percutaneous biliary catheter. If there is extraductal extension of the cancer, this is combined with external beam radiation.

Chemotherapy

Chemotherapy is not extensively studied. Palliative chemotherapy for advanced disease includes 5FU and cisplatin; gemcitabine is an alternative choice.

OUTCOME

Cholangiocarcinomas tend to grow more slowly than other hepatobiliary cancers. The median survival about 24 months and the overall 5-year survival is 14-40%.

GALLBLADDER CANCER

INCIDENCE

Gallbladder cancers are rare, accounting for <5% of all cancers. It occurs more frequently in women (female:male ratio 3:1) in the age group 60-80 years. It is more common in southwestern Native Americans and Hispanic Americans. Caucasians are affected more often than African-Americans.

RISK FACTORS

- Gallstones are the main risk factor, present in 75% of cases
- Gallbladder polyps
- Calcification of the gallbladder wall (porcelain gallbladder) is associated with a 10-20% risk of cancer
- Choledochal cysts and other biliary tract anatomical anomalies

- Chronic *Salmonella typhi* carriage
- Rubber plant workers
- Medications: methyldopa, oral contraceptives, isoniazid

PATHOLOGY

Most cancers arise in the fundus or neck of the gallbladder. Ninety percent are adenocarcinomas; uncommon histologies include small cell carcinoma, squamous cell carcinoma, sarcoma and lymphoma. The cancer spreads locally into the adjacent liver or by lymphatic spread to the hilar nodes around the base of the liver. Blood-borne spread occurs to the liver and lungs. Transcelomic spread with peritoneal carcinomatosis is common.

CLINICAL FEATURES

Many patients with early invasive gallbladder cancer are asymptomatic or have symptoms that mimic or are due to gallstones or cholecystitis. Some cancers are diagnosed incidentally at laparoscopic cholecystecomy; cancer is discovered in 0.2% of gallbladders removed for gallstones. The symptoms of more advanced cancer are pain, anorexia, nausea and vomiting. Weight loss, obstructive jaundice and duodenal obstruction occur later. Examination may reveal a mass in the right upper quadrant of the abdomen. Ascites is present when there are peritoneal metastases.

INVESTIGATIONS

- Liver function tests
- Endoscopic ultrasound is an accurate imaging study
- CT scan of the abdomen

TREATMENT

About 10% of patients have disease confined to the gallbladder wall at diagnosis, and fewer than 30% have potentially resectable disease. Surgery comprises cholecystectomy with a wedge resection of the surrounding liver, excision of the extrahepatic bile duct and regional node dissection. When the cancer is discovered incidentally in the resection specimen of laparoscopic cholecystectomy, patients may be cured if there is only superficial involvement of the mucosa. However, if the cancer extends beyond the muscular layer of the gallbladder wall, a laparotomy is required for wider margins of excision and regional node dissection. Chemotherapy is not well studied. 5FU is a reasonable choice for advanced disease, and gemcitabine, with or without cisplatin, is an alternative. Radiation may be used for palliation of pain due to local infiltration. Stenting of the bile ducts or other drainage procedures may relieve biliary obstruction.

OUTCOME

Gallbladder cancer is an aggressive malignancy. When there is liver, lung or peritoneal metastases, the median survival is 3 months, and <5% of patients are alive at one year.

ANAL CANCER

INCIDENCE

Anal cancer is an uncommon malignancy, comprising about 1.5% of GI cancers. It affects persons in the age group 50-70 with a slight preponderance of women over men.

RISK FACTORS

- Infection with human papillomavirus (HPV) types 16 and 18 is evident in 50% of cases; this is more common in homosexual men

- Genital condyloma acuminatum
- The incidence is high in homosexual males regardless of HIV status. However, the incidence is not higher in HIV-positive patients who do not practice anal receptive intercourse
- Immune suppression (HIV infection and post-transplantation immunosuppressive therapy) facilitates activation of HPV and is, therefore, associated with an increased risk
- Women with a history of cervix cancer, which is also strongly associated with HPV infection, are at slightly increased risk for anal cancer
- Cigarette smokers have an increased risk of anal cancer in smokers. (Of note, cigarette smoking is also highly associated with cervical neoplasia and is thought to act as a co-carcinogen)

PATHOLOGY

Macroscopic

The cancer forms a nodule, polyp or ulcer in the anal canal.

Microscopic

The vast majority (90%) are squamous cell cancers. Keratinizing squamous cancers generally arise in the lower anal canal, and non-keratinizing cancers, which are also called cloacogenic, basaloid, or transitional cell anal cancers, predominate in the transitional zone between the dentate line and the junction with the rectal mucosa. The behavior of keratinizing and non-keratinizing squamous anal cancers is similar, and they are treated the same way. Adenocarcinoma can rarely arise from the mucus glands in the anal canal. Other anal malignant histologies, including Bowen's or Paget's disease (high-grade intraepithelial neoplasia), occur rarely.

Spread

Local spread occurs to the perianal skin, the anal sphincter muscle, vagina, urethra and ischiorectal fossae.

Lymphatic spread is to the inguinal nodes and femoral nodes, and thence to the iliac nodes for cancers below the dentate line. Cancers arising above the dentate line spread to the perirectal and paravertebral nodes.

Blood borne spread is uncommon at presentation, but may occur later to the liver, lungs and bone.

SCREENING/PREVENTION

Homosexual and bisexual men may have asymptomatic anal intraepithelial neoplasia (AIN) comparable to cervical intraepithelial neoplasia (CIN). Screening high-risk individuals allows detection of AIN, which is managed by laser therapy.

"Safe sex" practice among homosexual men can prevent the transmission of HPV. A decrease in the incidence of HPV 16 after vaccination offers hope that immunization may decrease the risk of HPV-related diseases, including anal canal cancer in high-risk individuals.

CLINICAL FEATURES

Local growth causes pain and discomfort, bleeding, tenesmus and discharge from the anus. In the early stages, the symptoms are mild and may be attributed to hemorrhoids.

Examination reveals an indurated ulcer on digital examination. Enlarged inguinal nodes may be present.

Differential diagnosis

- Genital condyloma acuminatum or warts
- Basal cell cancer of the perianal skin
- Crohn's disease of the anus
- Melanoma (uncommon)

INVESTIGATIONS

- An HIV test should be considered in all patients who may be at high risk of contracting HIV. A positive test may have implications in terms of treatment, such as opportunistic infections and increased treatment-related toxicities
- Proctoscopy is the main investigation that permits visualization of the cancer and biopsy of the lesion
- Fine needle aspirate of enlarged inguinal lymph nodes can distinguish between metastasis and reactive changes due to concomitant infection
- Chest x-ray to rule out lung metastases (uncommon at presentation)
- CT scan or MRI of pelvis to assess the depth of invasion of the primary cancer and possible involvement of the iliac nodes

TREATMENT

Small cancers at the anal margin, including carcinoma *in situ* and early invasive carcinoma, is treated by local excision, providing adequate margins can be obtained without endangering sphincter function. More extensive tumours should be considered for combined radiation and chemotherapy, which is the standard of care. Radiation is delivered to the pelvis and inguinal regions with concurrent chemotherapy (5FU and mitomycin C). This brings about a complete remission is up to 80% of cases and also allows anal sphincter preservation. Most local recurrences occur within the first year and can be salvaged by an abdominoperineal resection.

OUTCOME

The overall 5-year survival is 70%. Adverse prognostic factors include:

- Location in anal canal vs. anal margin
- Poor tumor differentiation
- Higher stage of disease at presentation

Chapter 12

GYNECOLOGICAL ONCOLOGY

OVARIAN CANCER

CLASSIFICATION

Epithelial tumors

- Serous tumor
- Endometroid tumor
- Mucinous tumor
- Clear cell tumor

Germ line tumors

- Germ cell tumor
- Gonadoblastoma

Sex cord-stromal tumors

- Granulosa-stromal tumor
- Androblastoma (Sertoli-Leydig tumor)

OVARIAN EPITHELIAL CARCINOMA

INCIDENCE

Ovarian cancers account for 5% of all cancers in women with the majority occurring in post-menopausal women. The median age at diagnosis is 66 years. The incidence has remained stable over the past 30 years with the lifetime risk of a woman developing ovarian cancer in the general population being 1.5%.

RISK FACTORS

- Hormonal factors

The risk of ovarian cancer increases in situations where there is incessant ovulation, and the higher the number of ovulatory cycles in a woman's life span, the greater the risk of ovarian cancer. With each ovulatory cycle the surface epithelium of the ovary undergoes proliferation and repair. Therefore, the factors that reduce the number of ovulatory cycles also reduce the risk of ovarian cancer. These include pregnancy and use of oral contraceptive. Likewise, factors that increase the risk are infertility and nulliparity. Drugs like clomiphene used to stimulate ovulation in infertile women also increase the risk.

- Environmental factors

An association between the use of talcum powder and ovarian cancer has been suggested. There is some evidence that exposure to asbestos increases the risk of ovarian cancer.

- Genetic factors

About 5% of cases are hereditary. Three genotypes are identified:

  - Breast-ovarian cancer syndrome - linked to inheritance of a BRCA-1 gene mutation
  - Ovarian cancer syndrome
  - Lynch type II familial cancer syndrome - hereditary nonpolyposis colorectal cancer, endometrial cancer and ovarian cancer

PATHOLOGY

Macroscopic

The cancer appears as a cystic enlargement of the uterus. Two types are common:

- Serous cyst with clear fluid within a thin-walled cyst containing papillary structures
- Pseudo-mucinous cyst with large, multi-loculated masses containing mucinous material

Microscopic

Ovarian epithelial neoplasms display a range of malignant potential. Serous or mucinous tumors of low malignant potential have a good prognosis compared with their invasive counterparts. The distinction between these tumors is based on the presence of an infiltrating, destructive growth pattern with malignant cells invading the stromal spaces. Epithelial ovarian cancers account for 90% of ovarian malignancies; the remaining 10% of tumors arise from the germ cells or stromal cells. There are four subtypes of epithelial adenocarcinomas:

- Serous carcinoma (40-50%)
- Endometroid carcinoma (15-30%)
- Mucinous carcinoma (10-15%)
- Clear cell carcinoma (10-15%)

Spread

Transcelomic spread by exfoliation of malignant cells from the ovarian epithelial surface through the peritoneal cavity is the most common form of dissemination of ovarian cancer. The omentum is a frequent site of metastases.

Lymphatic spread occurs in about 10% of patients. This is primarily through the infundibulopelvic ligament to lymph nodes around the aorta and vena cava. In addition, lymphatic drainage through the broad ligaments and parametrial channels or retrograde lymphatic spread leads to involvement of the external iliac, obturator and hypogastric nodes.

Direct spread to the bladder, rectosigmoid colon and pelvic peritoneum is possible.

Blood stream dissemination to extra-abdominal sites is uncommon.

SCREENING

The impact of routine screening for ovarian cancer is unproven. A National Institutes of Health Consensus Conference on Ovarian Cancer recommended taking a careful family history and performing an annual pelvic examination in all women; other screening procedures, such as CA 125 testing and ultrasonography, are recommended only for women with a presumed hereditary cancer syndrome.

CLINICAL FEATURES

In the early stages of the disease, women have little or no symptoms. About 70% of patients present with advanced stages of cancer. Abdominal discomfort and bloating are common symptoms, followed by vaginal bleeding, gastrointestinal symptoms, such as altered bowel habits, and urinary tract symptoms.

Examination may reveal a palpable ovarian or adnexal mass as well as ascites. A pleural effusion may be detectable, and in advanced cases, a left supraclavicular node may be present.

APPROACH TO THE PATIENT WITH AN ADNEXAL MASS

The adnexum refers to the ovaries, fallopian tubes, broad ligament and structures in it. An adnexal mass typically comes to attention as an incidental finding on routine pelvic examination. Occasionally, pelvic or abdominal pain leads to its discovery. Adnexal masses originate in gynecologic organs, but they may also arise from the intestine, urinary tract, abdominal wall or retroperitoneum (Table 12.1).

During the reproductive years, the most common adnexal mass is an ovarian cyst. Endometriosis is also frequent with ectopic endometrial tissue on the peritoneal surfaces of the pelvis. Pelvic inflammatory disease, resulting from tubo-ovarian abscess, hydrosalpinx or chronic adhesions, commonly presents as a tender adnexal mass. The major concern is that the adnexal mass is a cancer. Ovarian neoplasms represent the most common adnexal tumors, and they may be either benign or malignant.

Table 12.1 Causes of an adnexal mass

Gynecologic causes

Organ/structure	Mass
ovary	cyst, endometrioma, inflammation (subacute or chronic infection), infection (ovarian or tubo-ovarian abscess), neoplasm
fallopian tube	ectopic pregnancy, hydrosalpinx, infection (pyosalpinx or abscess), neoplasm
broad ligament	cyst, neoplasm
uterus	leiomyoma, pregnancy (in bicornuate uterus)

Non-gynecologic causes

Organ/structure	Mass
intestine	feces, diverticula, pelvic appendicitis, colon cancer
urinary tract	distended bladder, ectopic pelvic kidney, neoplasm
abdominal wall	hematoma, abscess, desmoid tumor
retroperitoneum	neoplasm

INVESTIGATIONS

- Complete blood count
- Serum biochemistry: creatinine, electrolytes
- Serum tumor markers: CA 125 is elevated in about 80% of women with advanced ovarian cancer, but it is not specific for a malignant tumor. In patients under age 40 years, hCG and α-fetoprotein should be done to rule out a germ cell tumor
- Chest x-ray
- Ultrasound of pelvis
- CT scan of abdomen and pelvis is useful to assess the extent of disease when a pelvic mass is identified on physical examination or by ultrasound
- Ascitic fluid cytology can be helpful. (Note: Pap smear is inadequate to identify ovarian cancer)

STAGING

Ovarian cancer is a surgically staged disease. The International Federation of Obstetrics and Gynecology or FIGO system is widely used.

Stage I
Tumor confined to the ovary
  Ia - one ovary involved
  Ib - both ovaries involved
  Ic - Ia or Ib tumor but with tumor on surface of one or both ovaries; or with capsule ruptured; or with malignant ascites or peritoneal washings

Stage II
Tumor spread to the pelvis
  IIa extension and/or implants on uterus and/or tubes
  IIb extension to other pelvic tissues
  IIc pelvic extension with malignant cells in ascites or peritoneal washings

Stage III
Tumor spread to the abdominal cavity (peritoneal implants outside the pelvis or positive retroperitoneal or inguinal nodes or superficial liver implants; tumor limited to the true pelvis, but with histologically verified malignant extension to small bowel)
  IIIa - microscopic peritoneal metastasis beyond pelvis

IIIb - macroscopic peritoneal metastasis beyond pelvis 2 cm or less
IIIc - peritoneal metastasis beyond pelvis 2 cm or greater and/or lymph node metastasis

Stage IV
Distant metastasis; if pleural effusion is present, it must be cytologically positive

TREATMENT

Early stage ovarian cancer (Stages I and II)

Early stage disease is managed surgically by total abdominal hysterectomy (TAH), bilateral salpingo-oophorectomy (BSO) and omentectomy.

Advanced stage ovarian cancer (Stages III and IV)

Surgery is recommended to surgically stage all patients and to reduce or remove all gross intra-abdominal disease. The bulk of disease preoperatively and the amount left postoperatively determine the patient's overall survival. Patients, who have undergone optimal de-bulking surgery with no remaining tumor >1 cm in diameter, fare best. Surgery is followed by chemotherapy with carboplatin and paclitaxel. In selected cases, primary chemotherapy may be used prior to surgery to facilitate complete resection.

Stage IV patients with liver metastases, extra-abdominal metastases or enlarged retrocrural nodes are not candidates for de-bulking surgery, and they are treated primarily by chemotherapy.

Intraperitoneal chemotherapy
For women with stage III cancer who have low-bulk residual (<1 cm) cancer, intraperitoneal chemotherapy (carboplatin and paclitaxel) can improve progression-free survival and overall survival in the short and medium term compared with standard intravenous chemotherapy. The long-term disease-free survival rate at 8 years is, however, unchanged.

Treatment at relapse

The majority of patients who relapse after first-line treatment are incurable. A second de-bulking surgery can be carried out, but its value is uncertain. Chemotherapy is usually used. If the relapse occurs >6 months after completion of a platinum-based therapy, patients are usually retreated with a platinum-based chemotherapy regimen. However, if the relapse is <6 months, re-challenge with a platinum-based regimen is unlikely to produce a response. Second-line chemotherapy, such as topotecan or liposomal doxorubicin, may be used.

OUTCOME

The prognosis for patients with Stage I ovarian cancer is good with a 10-year survival of 80%. For women with Stages II and III disease, the 5-year survival is 45% and 25%, respectively. Patients with Stage IV disease have a median survival of a few months.

CERVICAL CANCER

INCIDENCE

Although cervical cancer is common, death from the disease is unusual in developed countries. The adoption of routine screening with pelvic examination and cervical cytology by the Papanicolaou or Pap smear is largely responsible for this.

RISK FACTORS

• Human papillomavirus
There is a strong association between human

papillomavirus (HPV) and cervical neoplasia. More than 80 subtypes of HPV have been identified, but the subtypes 16 and 18 are the most commonly associated with cervical cancers in North America. Parts of the viral genome become integrated into the cellular genome in high-grade neoplasms and invasive cancers of the cervix.

• Sexual habits

Squamous cell cervical cancer and its precursor lesions occur commonly in prostitutes and in women who have sexual intercourse starting at a young age, multiple sex partners, sexually transmitted diseases or who have children at a young age. Many of these associations may be explained by HPV infection.

• Cigarette smoke

Nicotine metabolites are detectable in cervical mucus which may explain the association. However, the effect of smoking disappears when HPV infection is taken into account.

• Immune suppression (e.g. AIDS)
• Oral contraceptive use (controversial)

PREVENTION/SCREENING

The early detection of precancerous lesions through cervical cytology smears, or Pap tests, can prevent invasive squamous cell cancer of the cervix. About three years after onset of vaginal intercourse, but no later than age 21 years, women should begin screening. Until age 30 years, annual screening with conventional Pap tests or biennial screening using liquid-based Pap tests should be done. At or after age 30 years, women who have had three consecutive normal Pap tests may undergo screening every 2-3 years by either conventional or liquid-based cytology, or alternatively, by the combination of HPV DNA testing and conventional or liquid-based cytology. Women over age 70 years who have had three or more normal Pap tests and no abnormal tests in the last 10 years, and women who have had a total hysterectomy may choose to stop screening (see also Chapter 1.)

Squamous cell cervical cancer is associated with human papillomavirus (HPV). Prevention of HPV transmission does not appear feasible at present. Condom use does not completely prevent the spread of HPV genital infections. While HPV infection is common, only a small percentage of infected women will develop cervical cancer. Of note is that the HPV subtypes associated with visible genital warts do not predispose to invasive cancer. At present, the role of HPV testing for cervical cancer prevention is being evaluated.

An HPV vaccine protecting against the most common HPV subtypes associated with cervical cancer is now available. This could prevent the infection and likely bring about a further reduction in the incidence of cervical cancer. The American Cancer Society recommends routine vaccination principally for girls aged 11-12 years, as well as girls 13-18 years to "catch up" those who missed the opportunity to be vaccinated. There is insufficient data to recommend for or against universal vaccination of women aged 19-26 years. At present, standard screening is recommended for both vaccinated and unvaccinated women.

PATHOLOGY

Macroscopic

The cancer arises at the junction between the squamous epithelium of the ectocervix and the columnar epithelium of the endocervix. Metaplastic cells at the squamo-columnar junction are probably particularly sensitive to HPV-induced changes, and they can progress to cervical intraepithelial neoplasm (CIN).

Invasive tumors develop as an exophytic

growth protruding from the cervix into the vagina or as an endocervical lesion that distends the cervix.

Microscopic

Cervical intraepithelial neoplasia
CIN is characterized by the presence of cellular disorganization, cellular immaturity and increased mitotic activity. It is graded from CIN I to CIN III. CIN I may undergo spontaneous regression in 60% of cases, whereas CIN II and III lesions precede micro-invasive and invasive carcinoma.

Micro-invasive carcinoma
There is extension of cells from the epithelium into the underlying stroma with multiple foci of protrusion evident as the cancer progresses.

Invasive carcinoma
• Squamous cell carcinoma (90%)
• Adenocarcinoma (10%)
Adenocarcinoma of the cervix is far less common than squamous cell carcinoma, but it is increasing in incidence, especially in young women in their 20s and 30s.
• Anaplastic small cell carcinoma
This is uncommon and runs a more aggressive course.

Spread

Local spread occurs to the lower uterus, upper vagina or into paracervical spaces via the broad or uterosacral ligaments. The cancer later becomes fixed to the pelvic sidewall or invades the bladder or rectum.

Lymphatic spread occurs through a rich lymphatic supply to the nodes in the pelvis (internal and external iliac, presacral and obturator nodes), and then to the para-aortic nodes. The disease can extend from involved para-aortic nodes to the lumbar spine.

Blood-borne metastasis is rare at initial diagnosis. In the late stages of the disease, distant metastasis may be evident in lungs, liver and bone.

CLINICAL FEATURES

CIN is detected during routine cervical cytology screening of asymptomatic women, although patients with early invasive disease may also be asymptomatic. In general, the presenting symptoms are caused by local growth of the cancer. The first symptom is vaginal bleeding, usually following coitus. Occasionally, there is foul-smelling vaginal discharge. Extension of the cancer to adjacent structure causes pelvic pain, and obstruction of the ureter leads to flank pain. Direct extension of the cancer to the bladder results in hematuria, or a vesicovaginal fistula causes incontinence. A large tumor may compress the rectum with obstructive symptoms, but invasion of the rectal mucosa is rare. Sciatic pain and leg edema can also occur.
Bimanual examination reveals a hard cervix and mobility is reduced in advanced cases.

APPROACH TO THE PATIENT WITH AN ABNORMAL PAP SMEAR

Cervical Pap smear is the most effective method of identifying the patient with pre-invasive cervical cancer. The finding of a cytological abnormality requires specific management according to the type of finding. Two broad classes of abnormalities are recognized according to the Bethesda system.

Benign cellular changes

• Infections, such as *Candida* species, herpesvirus, *Trichomonas vaginalis* or *Actinomyces* species
• Reactive changes associated with atrophy, inflammation, post-radiation changes or the

presence of an intrauterine device (IUD)

Epithelial cell abnormalities

Epithelial cell abnormalities are more serious, and they may be of three types.

(i) Squamous cell

- atypical squamous cells (ASC)
  - of undetermined significance (ASC-US)
  - cannot exclude high grade squamous intraepithelial lesion (ASC-H)
- low-grade squamous intraepithelial lesion (LSIL) consistent with HPV infection or mild dysplasia, CIN I
- high-grade squamous intraepithelial lesions (HSIL): moderate/severe dysplasia, CIN II, CIN III
- squamous cell carcinoma

(ii) Glandular cell

- atypical endocervical cells, endometrial cells or glandular cells, not otherwise specified
- atypical endocervial cells glandular cells, favour neoplastic
- endocervical adenocarcinoma *in situ* (AIS)
- adenocarcinoma (endocervical, endometrial, extra-uterine)

(iii) Other malignant neoplasms

Management of patients with abnormal PAP smears

Patients with infections require appropriate antibiotics, while those with reactive changes, such as from previous radiation or IUD use, are treated expectantly. Atrophic changes can be managed with hormones. A repeat smear in 4-6 months is advised.

When epithelial cell abnormalities are found on Pap smear, a firm diagnosis is required. This includes repeat Pap smear, inspection of the lower genital tract and colposcopy. A colposcope is a stereoscopic, binocular microscope that allows examination of the visible cervix to de-tect and biopsy abnormal areas. Endocervical curettage is also performed at the time of colposcopy if the lesion extends into the cervical canal or if the squamo-columnar junction is not seen.

Atypical squamous cells (ASC) are a common finding during cervix cancer screening. The cells display cellular abnormalities more marked than simple reactive changes, but not meeting the criteria for squamous intraepithelial neoplasia. Two categories are defined: ASC-US, which is qualified as "of undetermined significance", and ASC-H, in which a high grade squamous intraepithelial lesion cannot be excluded. While the risk of invasive cancer in patients with ASC is low (0.1-0.2%), there is a higher risk of precancerous lesions (5-17% with ASC-US, and 24-94% with ASC-H). Hence, further investigation is required.

The options for ASC-US are:

- HPV typing: Women who test positive for high-risk HPV types should undergo colposcopy. Women who test negative for high risk HPV types are followed with repeat cervical cytology in 12 months
- Repeat cytological evaluation in 6 and 12 months, and if normal, routine screening may be resumed. A second abnormal smear is evaluated by colposcopy
- Immediate colposcopy

For women with ASC-H, colposcopy and endocervical sampling should be done. If no lesion or CIN I is found, follow-up with either cytology in 6 and 12 months or HPV testing in 12 months is acceptable. If CIN II or CIN III is identified, additional treatment is needed. This may be either procedures to ablate the abnormal tissue (e.g. cryotherapy or laser ablation), or procedures to excise the area of abnormality to allow further histological study.

If colposcopic biopsy demonstrates early

invasive cancer (micro-invasion) or if there is a disparity between the Pap smear cytology and colposcopic biopsy, a cervical cone biopsy is required, especially in the setting of high grade cytology.

Evaluation of an abnormal Pap smear done during pregnancy can be difficult. Pregnancy causes hyperplastic changes that may appear atypical. If the changes are mild, observation is appropriate until the postpartum period. If, however, an invasive lesion is suspected, appropriate sampling is required to confirm the diagnosis.

INVESTIGATIONS

- Complete blood count: anemia may be present or the white cell count elevated if there is chronic infection
- Serum creatinine
- Chest x-ray
- CT scan of pelvis and abdomen to assess the local extension of the cancer and enlargement of the regional nodes
- MRI can define soft tissues around the cervix better than CT scan
- Cystoscopy and proctoscopy in patients with bulky cancers

STAGING

Stage 0   CIN
Stage I   Micro-invasive disease limited to the cervix (IA) or confined to the cervix with invasion >5 mm depth from the surface or >7 mm spread in horizontal direction (IB)
Stage II   Tumor involvement of the upper two-thirds of the vagina (IIA); extension to parametrium, but not to the pelvic wall (IIB)
Stage III Tumor involvement of the lower third of the vagina (IIIA); extension

to the pelvic sidewall (IIIB)
Stage IV   Tumor involvement of the bladder or rectal mucosa (IVA) or distant metastasis present (IVB)

TREATMENT

Pre-invasive disease (Stage 0)
Non-invasive squamous cervical lesions are treated by superficial ablative therapy, such as cryotherapy, CO_2 laser therapy, loop electrosurgical excision or cone biopsy. (A cone biopsy involves the removal of the ectocervix and most of the endocervix.)

Micro-invasive carcinoma (Stage 1A)
Treatment is simple hysterectomy. Selected patients who wish to maintain fertility may be offered a cervical conization if negative resection margins can be achieved.

Early stage disease (Stages IB and IIA)
Early stage disease is treated with combined external beam radiation and brachytherapy or by radical hysterectomy. Chemo-radiation may be indicated for patients with bulky cancers.

Locally advanced disease (Stages IIB, III and IVA)
Radical radiation therapy combined with platinum-based chemotherapy is the standard treatment for patients with locally advanced cervical cancer.

Metastatic disease (Stage IVB)
For patients with metastatic disease, pelvic radiation may be useful to relieve local symptoms, such as bleeding. Chemotherapy produces responses in about 20-30% of patients. The active drugs include cisplatin, ifosfamide and paclitaxel.

OUTCOME

Stage	Cure rates
Stage 0	Local recurrence rate is 10-15%, and progression to invasive disease is rare (2%) after local therapy
Stage I	85%
Stage II	55-60%
Stage III	25-30%
Stage IV	5-10%

ENDOMETRIAL CANCER

INCIDENCE

Endometrial cancer is the most common gynecological malignancy. It occurs in post-menopausal women with the average age at diagnosis being 60 years. It is rare before the age of 40.

RISK FACTORS

- Hormones

The endometrium is a hormonally regulated organ with the stimulatory action of estrogen balanced by the maturating effect of progesterone. Chronic estrogen exposure, therefore, predisposes a woman to endometrial cancer. This arises in the following situations:

  - oral intake of estrogen without progestin
  - low parity
  - extended periods of anovulation (e.g. polycystic ovarian disease)
  - obesity (obese women convert androstenedione from adrenal and ovaries to estrone in their adipose tissues)
  - granulosa-theca tumor (a rare estrogen-secreting tumor associated with endometrial cancer)
- Genetic factors
  - family history of endometrial, ovarian or colorectal cancer
- Coexisting conditions
  - white race
  - high socioeconomic status
  - prior pelvic radiation therapy
  - long-term use of tamoxifen (for treatment of breast cancer), which has a pro-estrogenic effect on endometrial tissues

PATHOLOGY

Macroscopic

The cancer arises in the inner epithelial lining and forms a polypoid mass within the uterine cavity. The lesion is friable and tends to bleed easily.

Microscopic

About 90% of endometrial tumors are adenocarcinomas.

- Grade 1 cancers have identifiable endometrial glands and are well-differentiated (50%)
- Grade 2 cancers are intermediate cancers which are moderately well-differentiated (30%)
- Grade 3 cancers show solid growth patterns and are poorly differentiated (20%)

The remaining 10% include papillary serous carcinoma, clear cell carcinoma, papillary endometroid carcinoma and mucinous carcinoma. These tend to occur in older women and have a worse prognosis.

Spread

Local growth produces a mass within the uterine cavity, which eventually extends to the lower end of the uterus and cervix. Invasion of the wall of the uterus occurs at the same time. Growth through the endometrium leads to direct invasion of bladder, colon or adnexal structures.

Lymphatic drainage occurs through the rich lymphatic network to the para-aortic nodes in the upper abdomen or via broad ligaments to the pelvic nodes.

Blood-borne spread is uncommon, but metastasis to lungs, liver and bone can occur.

CLINICAL FEATURES

The most common symptom is vaginal bleeding in a postmenopausal woman or heavy and prolonged bleeding in a perimenopausal woman. There may be associated vaginal discharge. The diagnosis should be considered in premenopausal women with abnormal bleeding, especially if they are oligo-ovulatory or obese.

Examination reveals a bulky uterus, and bleeding from the os may be evident. The adnexa should also be assessed as there is a 5% incidence of concomitant ovarian tumors.

DIAGNOSIS

Patients with postmenopausal bleeding should have a vaginal ultrasound to assess the endometrial wall thickness, which, after the menopause, is <4 mm. The main diagnostic test is hysteroscopy and biopsy, which is done under local or general anesthesia. This also allows determination of the site of the cancer as well as the presence of other uterine pathology.

INVESTIGATIONS

- Complete blood count
- Serum creatinine
- Chest x-ray
- CT scan or MRI of abdomen and pelvis to assess the extent of the tumor and lymph node enlargement
- Cystoscopy or sigmoidscopy, if the cancer is at an advanced stage

STAGING

Endometrial cancer is surgically staged.

Stage I   Tumor confined to the uterine fundus
    Ia – tumor limited to endometrium
    Ib – invasion to less than half the myometrium
    Ic – invasion to more than half the myometrium

Stage II   Tumor invades the cervix, but does not extend beyond the uterus

Stage III   Regional spread to uterine serosa, adnexa, vagina, or pelvic or para-aortic nodes

Stage IV   Bulky pelvic disease with invasion of bladder or bowel mucosa (IVA); or distant spread, including intra-abdominal or inguinal nodes (IVB)

TREATMENT

Surgery is the mainstay of treatment. Fortunately, most patients are diagnosed with early stage cancer and are amenable to surgical resection. Treatment depends on the stage of the cancer and its histological grade.

Stage I "low risk"

Patients are considered to be at "low risk" for recurrence if the following are present:

- Stage 1A grade 1-2
- Stage 1B grade 1
- No lymphatic or vascular invasion

Total abdominal hysterectomy and bilateral salpingo-oophorectomy (TAH-BSO) is the standard treatment. For patients who are medically unfit for surgery, radiation therapy may be considered.

Stage I "intermediate risk"

Women with Stage 1B grade 2 are treated by TAH/BSO, followed by radiation therapy to the vaginal vault. Overall prognosis is still good even without radiation treatment.

Stage I "high risk"

This comprises patients with one or more of the following features:

- Stage 1C disease
- Lymphatic or vascular invasion identified
- Grade 3 disease

There is a higher risk of local or regional relapse, and women with this stage of disease are treated by TAH/BSO followed by external beam radiation to the pelvic lymph nodes and a vaginal vault brachytherapy.

Stage II

Patients with endometrial cancer which involves the cervix are treated with preoperative radiation, followed by hysterectomy.

Stage III

Stage III endometrial cancers are usually treated with a multimodal approach and their treatment is individualized as follows:

- Resectable disease

Surgical resection (TAH/BSO) is performed. Additional treatment is determined as follows:

   ◆ Women with no macroscopic residual disease, Grade 1 and 2, and only adnexal involvement receive postoperative pelvic radiation therapy
   ◆ Women with Grade 3 disease, or more than adnexal involvement, or macroscopic residual disease receive chemotherapy with carboplatin-paclitaxel, followed by radical radiation therapy to the pelvis and site of bulk disease

- Unresectable disease

Women with advanced disease unsuitable for TAH/BSO are treated with initial chemotherapy with or without radiation therapy. Responding patients may be considered for surgery.

Stage IV

Chemotherapy with carboplatin and a taxane (docetaxel or paclitaxel) is given to suitable patients. Radiation therapy may be useful for local control of pain or bleeding.

SPECIAL SITUATION

Papillary Serous Adenocarcinoma of the Endometrium

Carcinoma with a papillary serous component is an aggressive variant of endometrial adenocarcinoma. It tends to present with more advanced disease and survival rates are lower. Since the pattern of spread appears to mimic that of ovarian epithelial cancer, the initial laparotomy should include peritoneal cytology, lymph node evaluation, total hysterectomy and bilateral salpingo-oophorectomy, and omentectomy. For Stage I and fully de-bulked Stage II patients, postoperative radiation is given to the pelvis and abdomen, followed by vaginal vault brachytherapy.

Women with Stage II cancer who have residual disease after surgery, and those with Stage III or Stage IV cancer, are treated with chemotherapy (carboplatin-paclitaxel). Depending on the clinical response, radiation may also be given to the original site of bulk disease.

OUTCOME

Stage of disease	5-year survival
Stage I	85-90%
Stage II	80%
Stage III	25%
Stage IV	<10%

Chapter 13

DERMATOLOGICAL ONCOLOGY

CLASSIFICATION OF SKIN CANCER

- Non-melanomatous skin cancers
  - Basal cell carcinoma
  - Squamous cell carcinoma
  - Merkel cell carcinoma (rare)
- Melanoma

BASAL AND SQUAMOUS CELL CARCINOMA

INCIDENCE

Basal cell carcinoma (BCC) is the most common skin cancer. Squamous cell carcinoma (SCC) is less common than BCC. Both are diseases of fair skin people, and the incidence rises from the poles to the equator. The median age of onset of these cancers is 68 years with a preponderance of men (4:1).

RISK FACTORS

- Sun exposure accounts for 90% of skin cancers, which commonly occur in the sun exposed areas of the body, such as the head, neck, arms and legs
- Other less common factors include the following:
  - atrophic skin changes resulting from skin damage
  - genetic syndromes, e.g. xeroderma pigmentosum or Gorlin's syndrome
  - prolonged immune suppression, e.g. in organ transplant or lymphoma
  - chemical exposure to arsenic, tar, nitrogen mustard
  - ionizing radiation
  - sites of trauma, such as burns

SCREENING/PREVENTION

Because of the increased risk from sun exposure, Caucasians living in sunny regions should avoid excessive sun exposure. Covering parts of the body by light clothing or a hat, limiting outdoor activities during the period of intense sunlight (from 11 am to 3 pm), and using protective sunscreens with a minimum Sun Protection Factor of 15 in all exposed areas are prudent measures.

PATHOLOGY

Macroscopic

BCC is slow growing and forms a well-defined papule with a "pearly" appearance and surface telangiectases. As the lesion enlarges, the central portion may become ulcerated. SCC has a variety of appearances - hyperkeratosis, an ulcer or a scaly patch that bleeds. Some may be mistaken for benign proliferative lesions, such as keratoacanthoma.

Microscopic

BCC forms nests of palisading, small basal type cells with relatively large basophilic nuclei.
SCC arises from the epidermal keratinocytes and is distinguished by keratinization and horny pearl formation.

Spread

BCC grows *locally*, forming a painless nodule that later ulcerates and bleeds. The borders are rolled and shiny. *Lymphatic* or *blood-borne spread* is rare.
Local growth of SCC leads to an expanding, red, irregular lesion, which later ulcerates and forms

a crust. *Lymphatic spread* to the regional lymph nodes occurs in about 1-2% of cases. *Blood-borne* metastasis to distant organs, such as lung or liver, may occur, but is uncommon.

CLINICAL FEATURES

Both BCC and SCC usually remain asymptomatic for a long time, and the lesion may be noted on routine clinical examination. In other cases, the patient is aware of the skin lesion, which may cause local symptoms, such as discomfort, itchiness or bleeding on contact. Examination reveals a discrete skin lesion. When telangiectases are present, a BCC is more likely. SCC is associated with solar keratosis. In the advanced stages, deep invasion causes the cancer to be tethered to the underlying structures.

DIAGNOSIS

Any suspicious skin lesion should be biopsied for histological confirmation. This may be done by a shave biopsy or by a punch biopsy. (Lesions that are suspicious for melanoma should have a complete excision biopsy rather than a shave or punch biopsy.) Full inspection of the skin is important to rule out a synchronous, second primary skin cancer. For very large lesions on the face and scalp, further investigations by imaging studies (CT scan or MRI) may be necessary to rule out invasion of underlying structures, such as bone.

Differential diagnosis

The main lesions to be distinguished from BCC or SCC are:

- Keratoacanthoma: a benign hyperkeratotic lesion which grows rapidly and becomes cone-shaped with a central pit containing keratin. It occurs on sun-exposed areas, such as the face or hands and arms. It tends to resolve spontaneously within a few weeks or months
- Wart: a common lesion caused by viruses; it resolves spontaneously
- Seborrheic keratosis: a common lesion in older persons. It is a brown, round to oval lesion with a slightly irregular surface that appears "waxy"
- Solar keratosis: a benign lesion on sun-damaged skin on the dorsum of the hands, face, neck and nose. It appears as a flat or hyperkeratotic, red, scaling macule. It may progress to squamous cell carcinoma over time
- Bowen's disease: an erythematous patch, representing carcinoma *in situ* of the skin

TREATMENT

Surgery

Complete surgical excision is curative for the majority of BCCs and SCCs. For BCC, a 2- to 5-mm margin of clearance is adequate, but for SCC, a wider, 5- to 10-mm margin is required. Incomplete deep margins should be re-excised. In the unusual instance of regional lymph node metastases, a nodal dissection is recommended.

Curettage and electrocautery (C&E)

C&E is adequate for small BCCs (<1 cm). There is, however, a higher risk for local recurrence, since the margins may not be free of tumor.

Cryotherapy

Liquid nitrogen freezing can be effective for small, superficial lesions.

Radiation therapy

When surgery is not possible because of the location of the lesion (lip, nose, eyelid or ear) or for large primary skin cancers, radiation therapy can produce cure rates close to 100%. This allows good preservation of function and cosmesis. The disadvantages are the late effects of radiation on the tissues: atrophy and telangiectases. Because of this, radiation therapy is generally reserved for older patients.

Chemotherapy

Metastasis from BCC or SCC is uncommon. There is no standard chemotherapy, but fluorouracil (5FU) with cisplatin is a reasonable choice.

Topical 5FU is used for solar keratosis, Bowen's disease and small, flat BCC. One disadvantage of topical 5FU for BCC is that there may be superficial regression of the cancer while its deep portions progress.

MELANOMA

INCIDENCE

Cutaneous melanoma is an important health problem due to a marked increase in its incidence worldwide, particularly in Australia and New Zealand. The incidence and mortality rates have begun to level off, especially in younger individuals. The reason for the epidemic is likely the increased recreational exposure to sunlight, coupled with an increased amount of ultraviolet B (UVB) radiation from sunlight that reaches the earth's surface. Melanoma is primarily a disease of Caucasians.

RISK FACTORS

• Sun exposure
Intense, irregular exposure to UV radiation in recreational activities is the main hazard. Exposure to other sources of UV radiation, such as sun-beds, also increases the risk.
• Skin type

Individuals with fair complexion and light skin, who tan poorly and burn easily, are at greatest risk. Those with a tendency to freckling are also at increased risk.
• Number of moles
An increased number of moles >2mm increases the risk. Almost everyone has one or more moles; some have many although they may not become apparent until puberty.
• History of dysplastic nevi
• Past history of melanoma
The risk of developing a new melanoma is about 3-7%.
• Family history of melanoma
About 4-10% of patients have a family history of melanoma in a first-degree relative. The familial atypical multiple mole (FAMM) syndrome predisposes to melanoma. Patients with this disorder have 10-100 pigmented lesions, mainly on the trunk, buttocks or lower limbs. The pattern of inheritance is autosomal dominant with incomplete penetrance.

PATHOLOGY

Melanoma progresses in a stepwise fashion from dysplasia to melanoma *in situ* to invasive malignant melanoma. There is a superficial or radial growth phase during which the lesion expands horizontally at the basal lamina. This is followed by a deep or vertical growth phase with dermal invasion.

Lymphatic spread occurs to the regional nodes. Metastases that develop within the dermal and subdermal lymphatics prior to reaching the regional lymph nodes are referred to as in-transit metastases if there are >2 cm from the primary lesion. Skin or subcutaneous lesions within 2 cm of the primary tumor are satellite lesions, which are considered intra-lymphatic extensions of the primary mass. The tumor biology associated with satellite and in-transit metastases is similar.

Blood borne metastases may occur to almost any organ.

A convenient way to classify melanoma is by its pattern of growth. Four major patterns are recognized.

• Superficial spreading melanoma

This is the most common type of melanoma and makes up about 65% of all cases. It occurs at any age after puberty. Superficial spreading melanoma may arise either *de novo* or from a pre-existing dysplastic lesion. It usually undergoes a slow change over 1-5 years. As it grows, it becomes irregular, asymmetric with variation in color, sometimes with areas of depigmentation. The clinical characteristics include the ABCDE of early detection: *a*symmetry in the shape, *b*order irregularity, *c*olor variation, *d*iameter (>6 mm), and *e*volving (faster growth rate than other lesions, pruritis, pain, bleeding and crusting).

• Nodular melanoma

Nodular melanoma is the second most common type of melanoma, accounting for 25% of all cases. As the name suggests, it is raised or dome-shaped, and appears as if it is stuck to the skin. Nodular melanoma is more frequent on the trunk or head and neck area, and often there is no preceding history of a mole. While most are typically black or blue in color, about 5% may be amelanotic and have a fleshy appearance.

• Lentigo maligna melanoma

Lentigo maligna melanoma accounts for about 5% of melanomas. It occurs in the elderly, more often in women. The lesion tends to be large (>3 cm) and flat, and it is usually present on the face or neck, or occasionally on the back of the hands or lower legs. It is usually tan in color with occasional mottling and varying shades of brown. The border is irregular with notching and indentation. Often, the lesion is present for a long time, 5-15 years.

• Acral lentiginous melanoma

Acral lentiginous melanoma occurs on the palms, soles or under the nail beds. It makes up only 5% of melanoma cases in Caucasians, but it is more common in dark-skinned persons, such as African-Americans, Asians and Hispanics, where it accounts for 35-60% of cases. The lesion may grow rapidly. Subungual melanoma of this type appears as a brown or black streak under the nail bed, and may be misdiagnosed as a hematoma.

PREVENTION/SCREENING

Because exposure to UVB radiation of sunlight is the major risk factor for melanoma, prudent measures to avoid excessive sun exposure should be followed. As for BCC and SCC, these include wearing proper clothing, wearing of hats, avoidance of direct sun exposure, especially noon-day sun, and use of sunscreens with a high Sun Protection Factor.

Melanoma has a detectable phase of radial growth during which it is less likely to metastasize. The radial growth phase, which can last for years, allows early detection and removal of "atypical" pigmented lesions.

CLINICAL FEATURES

Melanomas can occur anywhere on the body, but are most common on the legs in women and on the back in men. Early lesions cause no symptoms, but the ABCDE features are typical. A common feature of a melanoma is its changing nature. Therefore, any pigmented lesion that shows a change in color, size or texture should be suspect.

Local growth causes the lesion to expand and eventually ulcerate or bleed. Ulceration is a poor prognostic sign. Patients may complain of local discomfort or itchiness.

Lymphatic spread produces satellite lesions, in-transit metastases or regional lymph node enlargement.

Blood-borne spread can be widespread, but the lungs, liver, brain and skin are common sites of metastasis. Splenic metastases may also occur, unlike most other cancers.

Generalized effect: Patients with extensive metastatic melanoma can occasionally have a slate-gray complexion due to circulating melanin released by the melanoma cells.

DIAGNOSIS

Any suspicious or atypical pigmented skin lesion should be biopsied. A mole that undergoes a change in shape or color, or one that causes symptoms of itching or burning should be assessed further. An excisional biopsy is preferred to an incisional biopsy if a melanoma is suspected, since this allows detailed histological analysis and measurement of the thickness of the lesion.

Differential diagnosis of pigmented skin lesions

• Junctional nevus

This occurs at the junction of the basal layer of the epidermis and the dermis. The lesion is pigmented, varying in shade from light brown to almost black. It is usually flat, smooth and hairless. It may be present anywhere on the body, including the palm, sole and genitalia. A small percentage can become malignant.

• Intradermal nevus

This is a common variety of benign mole. It may be skin-colored, light brown or dark in color, and may be flat or warty. A hairy mole is almost always intradermal. It is found on every part of the body, except the palm, sole or scrotal skin.

• Compound nevus

Clinically, it is indistinguishable from the intradermal nevi. It can become malignant.

• Congenital nevus

A small percentage of these can undergo malignant transformation; the risk of this increases with the size of the lesion.

• Spitz nevus

This is a benign lesion in children. It is usually under 1 cm in diameter and its importance lies in the difficulty in distinguishing it from melanoma.

INVESTIGATIONS

• Liver enzymes
• Chest x-ray
• CT scan of the abdomen in high-risk disease (3-mm or thicker lesions or positive lymph nodes)
• CT of the brain if neurological symptoms or signs are present

STAGING AND PROGNOSIS

Micro-staging

Micro-staging is an important part of the staging of melanoma. The Breslow method measures the thickness in millimeters of the melanoma using an ocular micrometer. A second method is Clark staging, which takes into account the increasing depth of penetration into the dermal layers and subcutaneous fat (Levels I to V). The Breslow method is favored because of its better accuracy. The presence of ulceration of the primary lesion is associated with a poorer prognosis (Table 13.1).

TREATMENT

Surgery

Surgery is the main modality of treatment.

Table 13.1 Breslow micro-staging and its relationship to patient survival

T stage	10-year survival (%)	
	No ulceration	Ulceration present
Tis – melanoma *in situ*	100	na*
T1 – melanoma <1.0 mm	88	83
T2 – melanoma >1.01-2.0 mm	79	64
T3 – melanoma >2.01-4 mm	64	51
T4 – melanoma >4 mm	54	32

*not applicable

Local control of primary melanoma requires local excision of the cancer or biopsy site with a wide margin of normal skin. A melanoma on a finger or toe often requires amputation at the proximal digit.

The recommendations for wide excision are shown below.

Melanoma thickness	Margins of excision
melanoma *in situ*	0.5 to 1 cm
<2 mm	1 cm
>2 mm	2 cm*

*A primary at a site where a 2-cm margin is difficult, e.g. on the face, can be managed by a narrower margin

Lymph node dissection
Regional lymph node dissection is recommended for clinically involved nodes. Prophylactic regional node dissection is not recommended. The technique of sentinel node mapping is increasingly being used for staging patients with moderate risk melanoma (>1 mm) with clinically negative lymph nodes. This identifies the first draining node, and its removal permits the detection of sub-clinical lymph node metastases. If a positive node is found by this technique, a full nodal dissection is carried out. While sentinel lymph node biopsy provides good prognostic information, there is presently no conclusive evidence that it leads to improved survival. Sentinel lymph node biopsy is indicated in the following situations:
- Melanoma >1 mm in thickness
- Clarke level IV melanoma (extension into reticular dermis)
- Presence of ulceration

Recurrent or metastatic disease
Local recurrence of melanoma can be surgically excised. Surgical excision is also indicated for satellite lesions or limited in-transit metastases. Solitary brain metastasis may sometimes occur and is treated by surgical excision followed by whole brain radiation in patients without systemic metastases.

Radiation therapy

Palliative radiation is used for painful bone metastasis. Patients with excised solitary brain metastasis or multiple brain metastases are treated with whole brain radiation.

Systemic therapy

Adjuvant therapy
A number of agents have been tested as adjuvant therapy for high risk melanoma, including cytotoxic drugs and several biological agents (BCG vaccination, levamisole, interferon), and vaccines prepared from cultured melanoma cells. Of these, only high-dose interferon given for one year after surgery for high-risk melan-

oma (>1.5 mm thick or lymph node metastasis) shows any benefit. This treatment improves disease-free survival, but its impact on overall patient survival is small, about 3% at 5 years.

Palliative chemotherapy

DTIC (dimethyl triazeno imidazole carboxamide) is the standard chemotherapy drug for metastatic melanoma. However, partial response rates are low, about 15%, and complete responses are infrequent. These responses are short-lived, often <6 months. Other active drugs include CCNU, vinblastine, cisplatin and paclitaxel. Combination chemotherapy with cisplatin, vinblastine and DTIC (CVD) is not better than DTIC alone. Temozolomide, an oral pro-drug of MTIC, produces similar results to DTIC, and its oral route makes it more convenient for patients. Temozolomide penetrates the blood-brain barrier and is preferred to DTIC for patients with brain metastases.

Biological Response Modifiers

Topical imiquimod cream may be considered for large, unresectable lentigo maligna when radiation is not feasible. Imiquimod is believed to induce local production of cytokines, such as interferon, which exert an anticancer effect. Intralesional BCG may be useful in the treatment of isolated cutaneous metastases.

Interleukin-2 (IL-2) produces modest response rates (16%) in metastatic disease, and a small proportion (29%) of responding patients live for 5 years, suggesting this regimen can benefit some patients, especially those with soft tissue metastases. Bio-chemotherapy, which combines DTIC-based chemotherapy regimes with IL-2 and interferon, yields higher response rates, but overall patient survival is not improved.

Anti-CTLA4 monoclonal antibodies directed against the CTLA4 receptor on T-lymphocytes have shown anti-tumor activity in some patients with metastatic melanoma. Although responses to these monoclonal antibodies develop slowly, some are relatively long-lasting.

A variety of tumor vaccines have been studied, but they have very limited efficacy.

OUTCOME

The prognosis of patients with melanoma is affected by the following factors:

- Stage of disease
- Depth or thickness (see Table 13.1)
- Regional lymph nodal metastases. This is a poor prognostic sign, and cure rate after surgery is 20-60%, depending on the size and number of nodes involved
- Patients with distant metastatic disease have a median survival of 6 months
- Ulceration of the primary lesion: this is a late development, but carries a poor prognosis, especially if bleeding occurs
- Gender: women have a better prognosis than men
- Age: men over 50 years fare worse than others
- Site: melanoma on the limbs has a better outcome than other sites, such as head, neck or trunk
- Type: nodular melanoma is more aggressive than the other types

Chapter 14

HEMATOLOGICAL ONCOLOGY

NON-HODGKIN'S LYMPHOMAS

INCIDENCE

Non-Hodgkin's lymphomas rank fifth in cancer incidence, and they are the sixth most common cause of cancer-related deaths. Over the past 30 years, the incidence of non-Hodgkin's lymphoma has been increasing. This is due, in part, to the development of lymphomas in persons with AIDS as well as an increasing incidence in patients over 65 years of age. While there is a steady increase in the incidence from childhood to old age, the average age of diagnosis of non-Hodgkin's lymphoma is 56 years, with the disease being more common in women. Certain types of lymphoma are more frequent in specific age groups. For example, in children, Burkitt's lymphoma and diffuse large cell lymphoma are more common, whereas the indolent lymphomas are infrequent. In addition, specific types occur more frequently in certain geographic areas: Burkitt's lymphoma in tropical Africa, and adult T-cell leukemia/lymphoma in the Caribbean and Japan.

RISK FACTORS

- Immune deficiency states
Congenital
  - Ataxia-telangiectasia
  - Wiskott-Aldrich syndrome
  - Severe combined immunodeficiency syndrome
  - X-linked lymphoproliferative syndrome, XLP
Acquired
  - Human immunodeficiency virus (HIV)
  - Post-transplantation
  Patients who receive immunosuppressive

therapy after organ transplantation have a high risk of developing a secondary lymphoid malignancy.
- Autoimmune disorders
Lymphomas are associated with some autoimmune disorders, such as Hashimoto's thyroiditis or Sjögren's syndrome.
- Infectious agents
  - *Helicobacter pylori* infection can cause chronic gastritis, which predisposes to the development of mucosa-associated lymphoid tissue (MALT) lymphoma
  - Epstein-Barr virus is linked to the development of Burkitt's lymphoma in Africa
  - Human T-cell lymphotrophic virus Type 1 (HTLV-1) is associated with a distinct type of adult T-cell lymphoma-leukemia (ATLL) in the Caribbean and Japan
  - Herpesvirus 8, which is associated with Kaposi's sarcoma, is linked with malignant lymphoma, especially of the pleura, pericardium and peritoneum
- Occupational exposures
Farmers have a higher risk of non-Hodgkin's lymphoma, likely due to exposure to herbicides. Forestry workers also appear to have an increased risk. A link has also been suggested with hair dyes.
- Chemical and physical agents
  - Solvents and chemicals: benzene, creosote, lead, formaldehyde, oils, arsenate, paint thinner and greases
  - Exposure to radioactive material
  - High nitrates in drinking water

CLASSIFICATION

Non-Hodgkin's lymphomas are a broad group of lymphoid neoplasms. There are several different classifications with a basic distinction being made between lymphomas of B- or T-cell lineage, as well as the degree of cellular differentiation. The recognition of specific chromosomal translocations has refined the classification. Many of these translocations result in insertion of an oncogene within a gene responsible for immunoglobulin or T-cell receptor, and they define the biological features of the lymphoma. The World Health Organization-Revised European American Lymphoma (WHO-REAL) is now widely accepted (Table 14.1).

Table 14.1 WHO-REAL classification of Non-Hodgkin's lymphoma

B-cell lymphoma

I Precursor B-cell lymphoma
   Precursor B-lymphoblastic-leukemia/lymphoma
II Mature B-cell lymphoma
   Small lymphocytic lymphoma/chronic lymphocytic lymphoma
   Lymphoplasmacytic lymphoma
   Mantle cell lymphoma
   Follicular lymphoma
   Marginal zone lymphoma, including MALT (mucosa-associated lymphoid tissue) lymphoma
   Splenic marginal zone lymphoma
   Diffuse large B-cell lymphoma
   Mediastinal (thymic) large cell lymphoma
   Intravascular large B-cell lymphoma
   Primary effusion lymphoma
   Burkitt's lymphoma

T/NK-cell lymphoma

I Precursor T-cell neoplasm
   Precursor T-lymphoblastic lymphoma/leukemia
   Blastic NK cell lymphoma
II Mature T-cell and natural killer (NK)-cell neoplasms
   Adult T-cell lymphoma/leukemia
   Extranodal NK/T cell lymphoma, nasal type
   Mycosis fungoides/Sézary syndrome
   Peripheral T-cell lymphoma, unspecified
   Angioimmunoblastic T-cell lymphoma
   Hepatosplenic T-cell lymphoma
   Enteropathy-type T-cell lymphoma
   Subcutaneos anaplastic large cell lymphoma
   Anaplastic large cell lymphoma
   Primary cutaneous anaplastic large cell lymphoma

A clinical schema has been developed, based on the clinical course of the disease and the outcome expected from available treatment (Table 14.2 [page 155]). In this, lymphomas can be divided into low-grade and high-grade diseases. Low-grade lymphomas are distinguished by the presence of well-differentiated, small lymphocytes and preservation of the follicular architecture of the node. High-grade lymphomas show diffuse infiltration of the lymph node by undifferentiated, large lymphoid cells.

Table 14.3 shows the frequency of the different subtypes of non-Hodgkin's lymphoma in adults and children.

Table 14.3. Relative frequency of specific lymphomas in adults and children

Lymphoma	Frequency
Adults	
B-cell lymphoma	
Diffuse large cell lymphoma	30%
Follicular lymphoma	25%
Others	30%
T-cell lymphoma	
Peripheral T-cell lymphoma	10%
Anaplastic large cell lymphoma	3%
Others	2%
Children	
B-cell lymphoma	
Burkitt's lymphoma	30%
Diffuse large cell lymphoma	5%
T-cell lymphoma	
Precursor lymphoblastic lymphoma	45%
Anaplastic large-cell lymphoma	15%
Peripheral T-cell lymphoma (unspecified)	5%

Table 14.2 Clinical grouping of non-Hodgkin's lymphomas

Grade	B-cell	T-cell
Indolent or low grade	Follicular lymphoma with any of the following cell types: - small cleaved cells - mixed small and large cleaved cells Well-differentiated diffuse small cell lymphocytic lymphoma MALTomas Mantle cell lymphoma	Mycosis fungoides/ Sézary syndrome
Aggressive or intermediate grade	Follicular lymphoma containing predominantly large cells Diffuse lymphoma containing any of the following cell types: - small cleaved cells - mixed small and large cells - predominantly large cells	Peripheral T-cell lymphoma Angioimmunoblastic lymphoma Anaplastic large cell (CD30-positive) lymphoma
Very aggressive or high grade	Precursor B-lymphoblastic lymphoma/leukemia Burkitt's lymphoma (small noncleaved cell lymphoma)	Precursor T-lymphoblastic lymphoma

CLINICAL FEATURES

The most common presentation is peripheral lymphadenopathy, which occurs in 70% of cases. The wide distribution of lymphoid tissues in the body results in a range of clinical presentations. Usually, the cervical nodes are affected, although the axillary or inguinal nodes can be involved. The presence of back pain may be a clue to enlargement of the retroperitoneal nodes (para-aortic nodes). Characteristic symptoms, called B symptoms, may be present; they include any of the following:

• recurrent fever over 38°C
• unexplained weight loss of >10% body weight in the preceding 6 months
• recurrent night sweats

Examination reveals palpable peripheral nodes, which are firm or rubbery, and not hard or craggy as in carcinoma. Hepatosplenomegaly may be present. Unlike Hodgkin's lymphoma, lymph node enlargement in non-Hodgkin's lymphoma is widespread, and this does not follow the pattern of spread to the adjacent regional node-bearing areas, e.g. from the neck to the supraclavicular region to the mediastinum. Hence, most patients with non-Hodgkin's lymphoma have generalized disease at presentation, but it is important to identify those with limited disease, which can be treated with radiation therapy. In addition to the stage and histological type of lymphoma, the bulk of lymphoma is an important prognostic indicator.

Assessment of the patient should include the anatomic extent of the disease by clinical examination with measurement of palpable nodes. Imaging studies, such as chest x-ray and CT scan, are useful to document the overall extent of the disease.

Since most patients with non-Hodgkin's lymphoma have peripheral lymph node enlargement, this provides a ready means to obtain adequate tissue for diagnosis.

GENERAL APPROACH TO THE PATIENT WITH ENLARGED LYMPH NODES

In a general clinical practice, evaluation of a patient with lymph node enlargement is common. The enlarged node may be found by the patient or discovered on routine physical examination. Important considerations in the evaluation of lymph node enlargement include the following:

- Patient's age

Young patients (<30 years) are more likely to have infections, especially viral infections of the upper respiratory tract, bacterial pharyngitis or infectious mononucleosis. Typically, there is cervical node enlargement, which is tender and associated with fever. In older patients, the probability of a benign cause is lower (40%). Older patients with generalized lymphadenopathy may have chronic infection, HIV, tuberculosis, disseminated fungal infections, sarcoidosis, drug reactions or immunological disorders. The presence of low-grade fever or sweats may not be helpful as these symptoms are not uncommon with lymphomas. When an obvious explanation for the lymphadenopathy cannot be identified, a malignancy must be considered.

Some general guidelines in assessing enlarged lymph nodes are as follows:

- Tender nodes usually indicate inflammation, e.g. infection
- Nodes that are stony hard are more likely due to metastatic cancer. Rubbery nodes may be due to lymphomas

- Matted nodes are likely due to cancer or lymphomas. Matted nodes refer to a group of nodes that are attached, and moving one moves the others as well
- Location of lymph node

The major nodal regions that are palpable include the cervical, supraclavicular, axillary, epitrochlear, inguinal and femoral nodes.

- The cervical nodes drain the head/neck region. Benign small (<1 cm), mobile nodes are common in the posterior cervical chain. Cervical node enlargement, especially if unilateral, in an older person with a history of cigarette smoking and alcohol abuse may be due to a cancer in the head/neck area. A palpable supraclavicular fossa node is almost always abnormal, and may represent a lymphoma or other malignancy of the head/neck region or thorax. Virchow's node is an enlarged medial left supraclavicular fossa node due to metastatic gastrointestinal cancer
- Axillary nodes drain the breast, arms, chest wall and intrathoracic organs. Small, soft or firm, mobile nodes are frequently palpable in the axilla; they are usually benign. Large, fixed or matted nodes indicate a malignancy, such as metastatic breast cancer. Infections of the breast, arm or chest wall or a recent history of vaccination may also be responsible for axillary node enlargement
- The epitrochlear nodes are located just proximal to the medial aspect of the elbow. Enlargement of these nodes is unusual, but may occur in lymphoma or some benign conditions, such as sarcoidosis or bacterial infections of the hand or arm
- Inguinal nodes, which lie along the inguinal ligament, drain the legs and genitalia. They are frequently enlarged, and nodes <1

cm may be palpable in most persons. Larger, fixed or matted nodes, or progressively enlarging nodes, or the appearance and enlargement of femoral or iliac nodes indicate a malignancy, such as lymphoma or metastatic genital or anal cancer. Inguinal nodes can be enlarged in sexually transmitted diseases, such as syphilis or lymphogranuloma venereum

- Distribution of lymph nodes

The distinction between local and generalized lymphadenopathy (>2 separate anatomic regions involved) is important in assessing the pathological significance of lymph node enlargement. It is not uncommon to palpate small nodes in the axilla or inguinal regions in normal persons, but generalized lymphadenopathy may be due to a number of causes. Table 14.4 lists some of these.

Laboratory studies

The work-up of a patient with lymphadenopathy is guided by the clinical setting and the impression obtained through the history and physical examination. A complete blood cell count is useful for those suspected of having an infection or hematologic malignancy. Serological tests may be helpful to rule out infectious causes, such as HIV, cytomegalovirus, toxoplasmosis, syphilis or lymphogranuloma venereum. A Monospot test can rule out infectious mononucleosis. Antinuclear antibody or rheumatoid factor is a useful screen for the collagen-vascular diseases.

Imaging studies are directed by the suspected diagnosis. A chest x-ray or imaging of the abdomen and pelvis can disclose enlargement of deeper nodes if a lymphoma is in the differential diagnosis.

Patients with persistent enlargement of the lymph nodes, especially when associated with systemic symptoms of fever, weight loss, night

Table 14.4 Some causes of lymphadenopathy

Infections

Acquired immunodeficiency syndrome (AIDS) and AIDS-related complex (ARC)
Measles
Infectious mononucleosis
Tuberculosis
Cytomegalovirus
Rubella
Cat-scratch disease
Rheumatic fever
Scarlet fever
Secondary syphilis
Toxoplasmosis
Brucellosis
Sporotrichosis

Collagen-vascular disease

Rheumatic arthritis
Systemic lupus erythematosus
Dermatomyositis
Still's disease

Neoplasms

Lymphoid leukemia
Lymphoma
Hodgkin's lymphoma

Metabolic diseases

Hyperthyroidism
Gaucher's disease
Nieman-Pick disease

Other causes

Intravenous drug abuse
Sarcoidosis
Phenytoin use
Amyloidosis
Scabies infestation
Serum sickness

sweats or pruritis, should have a lymph node biopsy. Excision biopsy of a whole node is advised to fully evaluate the nodal architecture and cytology, and rule out a reactive process. Usually, the largest and most accessible node is biopsied. Pathologic examination of the lymph node should include special stains and cultures for bacteria, fungi and mycobacterium. If a malignancy is suspected, standard histological examination and special immunohistochemical stains are needed. In the case of lymphoma, additional studies, such as immunotyping, cytogenetics, immunoglobulin and T-cell receptor gene rearrangement, are useful.

INVESTIGATIONS

- Complete blood count may show a mild anemia or pancytopenia if the bone marrow is involved. A high white cell count comprised mainly of lymphocytes is a poor prognostic sign
- Erythrocyte sedimentation rate is often elevated. Elevations of >40 mm/hr is a poor prognostic sign
- Biochemistry: serum creatinine, alkaline phosphatase, LDH, AST, bilirubin, calcium, protein electrophoresis, and β_2-microglobulin. Serum LDH is a useful marker of disease activity
- Bone marrow aspiration and biopsy
- Imaging studies
  - Chest x-ray can demonstrate any hilar or mediastinal node enlargement, lung infiltration or pleural effusion
  - CT scan of abdomen and pelvis is important to assess the abdominal and pelvic nodes
  - Positron emission tomography (PET) may be important in evaluating the effects of therapy

Certain tests are required for specific situations.

- Hepatitis B surface antigen and hepatitis C antibody
- HIV serology
- CSF cytology in primary lymphoma of brain, epidural lymphoma or any lymphoma if neurological abnormalities are present
- ENT examination in lymphoma involving the suprahyoid cervical lymph node or GI tract
- Upper GI series and follow-through contrast radiograph in lymphoma involving Waldeyer's ring
- Ophthalmologic examination in primary lymphoma of the brain

STAGING

The staging system in common use is based on the Ann-Arbor system with additional consideration of the bulk or size of individual tumors (Table 14.5).

Table 14.5. Ann-Arbor staging of lymphoid malignancies

Stage	Involvement
I	Single lymph node region (I) or one extranodal site (IE)
II	Two or more lymph node regions, on the same side of diaphragm (II) or local extranodal extension plus one or more lymph node regions on the same side of diaphragm (IIE)
III	Lymph node regions on both sides of diaphragm (III) which may be accompanied by local extranodal spread (IIIE)
IV	Diffuse involvement of one or more extra-lymphatic organs or sites

Bulk disease

Bulky   Any tumor with diameter >10cm
Nonbulky   All tumor <10 cm

Symptoms

A   No symptoms
B   Presence of at least one "B" symptom

For decisions on treatment, patients with non-Hodgkin's lymphomas are conveniently divided into two groups based on the stage of their disease.

Limited stage
• Stage I
• Stage II confined to <3 adjacent lymph node regions
• No B symptoms
• Nonbulky disease

Advanced stage
• Stage II with disease involving >3 adjacent lymph node regions
• Stage III or IV
• B symptoms
• Bulky disease

PROGNOSTIC FACTORS

There are five independent prognostic factors in non-Hodgkin's lymphoma: patient's age, performance status, stage of disease, extra-nodal involvement and LDH level. These form the basis for the International Prognostic Index (Table 14.6).

FOLLICULAR LYMPHOMA (INDOLENT OR LOW-GRADE)

CLINICAL FEATURES

Follicular lymphoma is the second most common adult lymphoma in North America and Europe, accounting for almost 25% of cases. It is typically a disease of older adults, and it affects men and women with equal frequency. The usual presentation is widespread nodal

Table 14.6 International Prognostic Index for non-Hodgkin's lymphoma

Factor	Score	
	0	1
Age (years)	≤60	>60
Performance status	0 or 1	2, 3 or 4
Stage	I or II	III or IV
Extra-nodal involvement	≤2 sites	>2 sites
LDH	normal	high

Category	Risk Category
Low	0 or 1
Low/intermediate	2
High/intermediate	3
High	4 or 5

enlargement, usually associated with involvement of the spleen and bone marrow. Occasionally, the peripheral blood and extra-nodal sites may be involved. The disease is indolent and runs a protracted course over years. Progression to diffuse large B-cell lymphomas occurs in about 45% of cases.

TREATMENT

Limited stage disease

About 15% of patients have limited stage disease at diagnosis. The main treatment is radiation therapy. About 80% of patients survive 10 years.

Advanced stage disease

Treatment is with single-agent chemotherapy (chlorambucil) or combination chemotherapy (CVP [cyclophosphamide-vincristine-prednisone] or CHOP [cyclophosphamide-doxorubicin-vincristine-prednisone]). Tumor responses last about 2 years, and <10% of patients remain in remission for more than 5 years. Rituximab, a monoclonal antibody directed to the CD20 antigen, is an effective treatment for B-cell lymphomas, either alone or combined with chemotherapy. Maintenance therapy with rituximab for 2 years prolongs the duration of disease remission.

DIFFUSE LARGE CELL LYMPHOMA (INTERMEDIATE OR AGGRESSIVE GRADE)

CLINICAL FEATURES

Diffuse large cell lymphoma makes up about 30% of adult non-Hodgkin's lymphomas. The median age of presentation is in the sixth decade, but it can occur at any age. In children, it constitutes about 5% of lymphomas. Patients often present with a painful, enlarging mass in nodal or extra-nodal sites. The most common extra-nodal site is the stomach, but the disease can affect the CNS, bone, kidney and testis.

TREATMENT

Limited stage disease

Patients with limited stage disease can be cured with combined modality therapy, consisting of CHOP chemotherapy, usually combined with rituximab, followed by radiation therapy. Five-year disease-free survival is 88%.

Advanced stage disease

Combination chemotherapy is the treatment of choice for patients with low or low/intermediate risk category lymphoma. A few active drugs are available, but the CHOP regimen is the standard. The addition of rituximab to CHOP significantly improves the results of treatment. The overall survival following chemotherapy is 33% at 6 years. For patients with worse prognostic features, conventional chemotherapy produces poor

results. High-dose chemotherapy with stem cell rescue is being studied in this group.

ANAPLASTIC LARGE CELL LYMPHOMA (CD30-POSITIVE)

CLINICAL FEATURES

Anaplastic large cell lymphoma represents 15% of lymphomas in children, and 3% in adults. The tumor cells express CD30 and are T-cell or NK cell types. Anaplastic large cell lymphoma presents as a systemic disease, involving lymph nodes or extra-nodal sites or as a cutaneous disease. Children with anaplastic large cell lymphoma have a better prognosis, and those with cutaneous lesions are more responsive to chemotherapy than those with nodal involvement. The disease may also arise as a high-grade transformation of an indolent extra-nodal lymphoma.

TREATMENT

Anaplastic large cell lymphomas respond to conventional chemotherapy, such as CHOP.

PERIPHERAL T-CELL LYMPHOMA (UNSPECIFIED)

CLINICAL FEATURES

Peripheral T-cell lymphoma makes up about 10% of lymphomas in North America and Europe, but it is more common in other parts of the world. It is morphologically heterogeneous, but has a mature T-cell immunophenotype. It affects mostly adults, who present with generalized disease associated with pruritis, eosinophilia or hemophagocytic syndromes. Lymph nodes, skin, liver, spleen or other viscera may be involved.

TREATMENT

In general, treatment has been less effective than in B-cell lymphomas. The anaplastic large T/null cell subtype has the best outcome of the peripheral T-cell lymphomas when treated with CHOP chemotherapy.

BURKITT'S LYMPHOMA/ LYMPHOBLASTIC LYMPHOMA

CLINICAL FEATURES

Burkitt's lymphoma is one of the most common childhood lymphomas in North America. The male:female ratio is 2-3:1. Two forms of the disease are seen. In African or endemic cases, the jaws or facial bones are most commonly involved, whereas in the non-African cases, the abdomen is frequently involved, especially the distal ileum, cecum or mesentery. The disease is highly aggressive with rapid tumor doubling times.

TREATMENT

Intensive multi-drug chemotherapy regimens are the mainstay of treatment. Induction therapy tends to follow the treatment protocols used for acute lymphoblastic leukemia with full CNS prophylaxis. The addition of rituximab to chemotherapy appears to improve the outcome. Particular management problems include tumor lysis syndrome and anatomical complications from large mediastinal masses. The prognosis is better in children than in adults. Despite its biological aggressiveness, the cure rate for low-stage disease is 85%, and for advanced stage about 40%

OUTCOME

The outcome of Non-Hodgkin's lymphomas, based on the International Prognostic Index risk category, is as follows:

Category	Risk Category	5-year survival(%)
Low	0 or 1	73
Low/intermediate	2	51
High/intermediate	3	43
High	4 or 5	26

HODGKIN'S LYMPHOMA

INCIDENCE

Hodgkin's lymphoma is an uncommon malignancy with an annual incidence of 3 in 100,000. The disease shows an unusual bimodal incidence pattern in western countries with peaks at age 15-40 years, and over 55 years. It is twice as common in men as it is in women. There has been a slight increase of Hodgkin's lymphoma in the elderly. The overall incidence is lower in underdeveloped countries, where the disease is more common in childhood.

RISK FACTORS

There is no known causative factor. The disease is more common among wood-workers, and the risk of developing Hodgkin's lymphoma is increased in persons who have had tonsillectomy or appendectomy. A familial association and linkage with certain HLA antigens are noted. Recently, the Epstein-Barr virus has been implicated as a causative agent in Hodgkin's lymphoma.

PATHOLOGY

The pathology of Hodgkin's lymphoma is unique and depends on identification of binucleate cells, called Reed-Sternberg cells, in an inflammatory background. A definite neoplastic cell has not been described. The variation in the morphology of the Reed-Sternberg cell and composition of the inflammatory background allow the description of four subtypes of Hodgkin's lymphoma (Table 14.7).

Table 14.7 REAL Classification of Hodgkin's lymphoma

Lymphocyte predominance	5-6%
Nodular sclerosis	60-80%
Mixed cellularity	15-30%
Lymphocyte depletion	1%

CLINICAL FEATURES

Hodgkin's lymphoma typically arises in lymph nodes, commonly in the neck or chest. The disease spreads to the contiguous nodes, e.g. from cervical nodes to supraclavicular nodes to mediastinal nodes before involving the subdiaphragmatic nodes. The lymph nodes may be painless, but can cause local discomfort as they enlarge. Typically, the enlarged nodes are present for many weeks or months.

Characteristic B symptoms may occur. In addition, patients may complain of itchiness. These symptoms are more common in the advanced stages of the disease. Some patients may note alcohol-induced pain in the enlarged nodes. Splenomegaly can cause upper abdominal pain or discomfort, and para-aortic nodes are responsible for back pain.

Examination reveals enlarged nodes, usually in the neck, which are firm or rubbery. The spleen may be enlarged and para-aortic nodes, if large, may be palpable. Mediastinal node involvement can lead to superior vena cava obstruction, and inguinal or iliac node involvement can cause leg edema. Extra-nodal spread of Hodgkin's disease is uncommon, and it usually occurs in the setting of extensive or bulky nodal disease.

DIAGNOSIS AND STAGING

An open node biopsy is required to establish the diagnosis and determine the histological subtype. The staging system for Hodgkin's lymphoma is the Ann Arbor system/ Cotwold Revision (Table 14.8).

Table 14.8 Staging system for Hodgkin's lymphoma

Stage	Involvement
I	Single lymph node region (I) or one extra-nodal site (IE)
II	Two or more lymph node regions, on the same side of the diaphragm (II) or local extra-nodal extension plus one or more lymph node regions on the same side of the diaphragm (IIE)
III	Lymph node regions on both sides of the diaphragm (III) which may be accompanied by local extra-lymphatic extension (IIIE)
	III_1 involvement limited to spleen, hilar portal or celiac nodes
	III_2 involvement of para-aortic, iliac or mesenteric nodes
IV	Diffuse involvement of one or more extra-lymphatic organs or sites

Bulk disease
Mediastinal/thoracic ratio <1:3 at T5-6 level; or mass >10 cm

INVESTIGATIONS

- Complete blood count may be normal or there may be mild anemia or leucocytosis
- Erythrocyte sedimentation rate is often elevated and is an indication of disease activity
- Biochemistry: serum creatinine, alkaline phosphatase, LDH, AST, bilirubin, calcium, albumin. LDH is a marker of disease activity

and a high LDH is a poor prognostic sign. Serum calcium may be elevated in few cases
- Hepatitis B surface antigen
- Imaging studies
  - Chest x-ray may indicate mediastinal node enlargement, pleural effusion or lung infiltrate

- CT scan of chest, abdomen and pelvis is important in assessing the abdominal viscera and nodes.
- PET scan may be used to assess response to treatment

Special tests

Condition	Test
B symptoms or WBC <4 x10^9/L or Hgb <120 g/L or platelets <125 x10^9/L	Bone marrow aspiration and biopsy
Stage IA or IIA disease without intrathoracic involvement on CXR or CT scan	Gallium scan or PET scan
Stage IA or IIA disease with upper cervical lymph node involvement	ENT examination

PROGNOSTIC FACTORS

Certain criteria identify patients with high-risk Hodgkin's lymphoma. Each of the following has an equivalent negative impact on survival.
- Age >45 years
- Male gender
- Stage IV disease
- Hemoglobin <105 g/L
- Serum albumin <40 g/L
- WBC >15 x 10^9/L
- Lymphocyte count <0.6 x 10^9 /L or <8% of WBC

The presence of 4 or more of these risk factors at diagnosis identifies patients at high risk.

TREATMENT

Treatment of Hodgkin's lymphoma depends on histological subtype, stage of the disease, and the age of the patient. The disease is both radio-sensitive and chemo-sensitive. Because most patients with Hodgkin's lymphoma are young and likely to be cured, the long-term toxicity of treatment is of clinical relevance. Treatment is, therefore, designed to offer the best chance of a cure while minimizing toxicity. The standard chemotherapy is the combination of doxorubicin, bleomycin, vincristine and dacarbazine (ABVD). The general approach to the management of Hodgkin's lymphoma is shown in Table 14.9. Radiation to the involved nodal regions follows a standard technique. A "mantle" field is used for disease above the diaphragm, and an "inverted-Y" field for disease below the diaphragm (Figure 14.1). The usual dose is 35-40 Gy over 4-5 weeks.

OUTCOME

The prognosis is good. Almost all patients with Stage I disease are cured. Even those with advanced stages (IIIB or IV) have an 80% cure rate with intensive chemotherapy.

Table 14.9 Treatment of Hodgkin's disease by stage and prognostic factors

Stage	Bulk	Risk factor	Treatment
IA IB IIA	low	0–3	ABVD chemotherapy x 2 cycles + radiation
IIB IIIA or B IVA or B	low	0–3	ABVD chemotherapy x 6-8 cycles
Any	high	0–3	ABVD chemotherapy x 6 cycles + radiation
Any	any	4–7	ABVD chemotherapy x 6 cycles + radiation

Figure 14.1 Radiation fields for Hodgkin's lymphoma

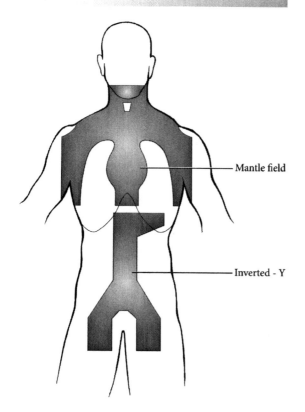

- Second cancers may occur infrequently. They include breast, lung and gastrointestinal cancers due to radiation; and leukemia due to chemotherapy
- Hypothyroidism can result from mantle radiation
- The risk of cardiovascular disease is increased by chest radiation

ACUTE LEUKEMIAS

Leukemia occurs as a result of a genetic event in a hematopoietic precursor cell that causes its progeny to proliferate and differentiate abnormally. The leukemias are classified on the basis of their cell lineage (myeloid vs. lymphoid) and their clinical course (acute vs. chronic). Four common leukemias are:

- Acute lymphoblastic leukemia (ALL) – 11%
- Acute myeloid leukemia (AML) – 40%
- Chronic lymphocytic leukemia (CLL) – 29%
- Chronic myelogenous leukemia (CML) – 14%

Acute leukemias arise from early precursor cells. The leukemic cells continue to proliferate, but do not differentiate beyond the blast stage. As a result, immature cells accumulate in the bone marrow, displacing the normal cells and leading to reduced production of red cells, white cells and platelets. The leukemic cells escape into the blood stream, and later infiltrate lymph nodes, spleen and other vital organs. The course

FOLLOW-UP

Follow-up of patients with Hodgkin's lymphomas is aimed to detect the long-term complications of treatment. These include the following:

is rapid, and untreated patients die within months of diagnosis.

In chronic leukemias, the neoplastic cells are more differentiated, and there is overproduction of relatively mature cells that resemble their normal counterparts: neutrophils in CML, and lymphocytes in CLL. They tend to run a more indolent course, and patients can live for several years after diagnosis. Over time, however, as more genetic mutations occur, the leukemic cells become more aggressive, and may eventually progress to a state more like acute leukemia.

ACUTE LYMPHOBLASTIC LEUKEMIA

INCIDENCE

Acute lymphoblastic leukemia (ALL) is relatively rare, but it is an important cause of death in children and young adults. The median age of diagnosis is 10 years. The incidence of ALL is 1.3 per 100,000, and it is twice as common in Caucasians compared with African-Americans.

RISK FACTORS

A few risk factors have been recognized, but the majority of cases are not associated with any known risk factors.
- Genetic factors
  - An increased risk is associated with certain genetic syndromes, e.g. Down's syndrome, Fanconi's anemia, Bloom's syndrome, infantile X-linked agammaglobulinemia and ataxia telangiectasia
  - There is a high concordance for the disease between identical twins
- Environmental factors
Risk factors of proven significance
  - Exposure to atomic bomb radiation
  - Previous radiation therapy for cancer or ankylosing spondylosis

Risk factors of uncertain or unproven significance
  - Occupational low-dose radiation
  - Exposure to electromagnetic fields
  - Infection by RNA retrovirus

CLASSIFICATION

The most important distinction to be made in acute leukemias is the cell lineage: myeloid versus lymphoid. There are two classification systems in general use: the French-American-British (FAB) (1994) and World Health Organization (WHO) (2001). Both of these systems are based on the cellular morphology and histochemical staining characteristics, but the WHO classification also takes into account immunotyping and cytogenetic abnormalities of the leukemic cells. The WHO classification for acute lymphoid leukemias is shown in Table 14.10.

Table 14.10 WHO classification of acute lymphoblastic leukemias

Precursor B-cell acute lymphoblastic leukemia

Cytogenetic subgroups
t(9:22)(a34;q11); bcr/abl
t(v;11q23); MLL rearranged
t(1:19)(q23;p13) E2A/PBX1
t(12;21)(p12;q22) ETV/CBF-alpha

Precursor T-cell acute lymphoblastic leukemia
Burkitt-cell leukemia

CLINICAL FEATURES

The symptoms and signs of acute leukemias are not specific and reflect the disturbance in the hematologic cell lines.

Symptoms

From anemia: fatigue, malaise and dyspnea.
From low platelets: epistaxis, easy bruising, hematuria, hemoptysis and GI bleed.

From bone marrow crowding: bone pain.
General: weight loss, abdominal pain, night sweats and fever.

Signs

From anemia: pallor. Anemia is present in most patients at diagnosis.
From low platelets: petechiae, ecchymoses, hemorrhage, fundal hemorrhage. Thrombocytopenia is present in about 25% of patients at presentation.
From granulocytopenia: infection, sepsis and perirectal abscess. About one-third of patients have significant infections at initial diagnosis. Although the granulocyte count is reduced, the total white cell count may be normal or high. Blasts may be present in the peripheral blood and the bone marrow is hypercellular.
From visceral infiltration: Peripheral lymphadenopathy, mediastinal mass, hepatosplenomegaly and renal enlargement. Testicular infiltration may occur with enlargement of the testes. Meningeal infiltration leads to neurological signs, and this may occasionally be the presenting feature of ALL.

PROGNOSTIC FACTORS

Feature	Favorable	Unfavorable
Age	≤50 year	>50 years
Gender	Female	Male
Mediastinal mass	Absent	Present
WBC count at diagnosis	Low (≤50x10⁹/L)	High (>50x10⁹/L)
Time to achieve remission	Early (≤4 weeks)	Late (>4 weeks)
Cell lineage	T-cell	Mature B-cell
Cytogenetic abnormalities	Hyperdiploidy t(9;22)	Philadelphia chromosome t(8;14); t(1;19); t(4:11)

DIAGNOSIS

The diagnosis of ALL is straightforward on examination of the peripheral blood or bone marrow. The differential diagnosis that must be considered is infectious mononucleosis or other viral illnesses, which may sometimes resemble ALL with a large number of lymphocytes in the peripheral blood. The concomitant complications of hemolytic anemia or immune thrombocytopenia can be misleading. Immunological and cytogenetic studies confirm the diagnosis.

INVESTIGATIONS

- Complete blood count and differential frequently shows pancytopenia with blast cells present in the peripheral blood smear
- Coagulation studies: INR, PTT and fibrinogen
- Biochemistry: electrolytes, creatinine, LDH, uric acid, calcium, phosphorus
- Examination of bone marrow aspirate and biopsy is the important diagnostic test. Cytogenetic analysis, molecular testing and immunotyping of the leukemic cells are necessary
- Chest x-ray may show a mediastinal mass or leukemic infiltrates in the lungs
- CT scan of chest or abdomen (in patients with mature B-cell ALL)
- Cytological examination of CSF
- HLA typing in younger high-risk patients

TREATMENT

The aim of treatment of the acute leukemia is to eradicate the leukemic cells and restore normal hematopoiesis. This can be achieved with chemotherapy. However, significant myelosuppression or even transient aplasia is a consequence, and patients require intensive hematological support during the period of bone marrow suppression. ALL treatment is given in three phases.

Induction therapy

This is an 8-week treatment, consisting of 4 or 5 drugs, using an anthracycline like daunorubicin, cyclophosphamide, vincristine, L-asparaginase and prednisone. Multidrug regimens induce a clinical complete remission in 80% of patients.

Intensive consolidation therapy

This is given after attainment of a clinical remission when no leukemic cells are present in the peripheral blood or bone marrow. Consolidation therapy consists of Ara-C combined with an anthracycline or etoposide. Prophylactic treatment to the CNS is also given as described below.

Protracted maintenance

Standard maintenance therapy typically uses 6-mercaptopurine and methotrexate with four-weekly pulses of vincristine and prednisone for 1-3 years.

Special considerations

CNS treatment and prophylaxis
Because of the high frequency of meningeal involvement, diagnostic CSF cytology is done as soon as blast cells are cleared from the peripheral blood. If the CSF is involved with leukemic cells, intrathecal or intraventricular (via an Ommaya reservoir) treatment with Ara-C or methotrexate should be given until cytological clearing is achieved. If the CSF is not involved, prophylactic intrathecal chemotherapy is given with each cycle of systemic chemotherapy for a total of six doses. Cranial radiation is also recommended in either circumstance.

Bone marrow transplantation
Poor-risk patients (adults, Philadelphia positive chromosome) who achieve a complete clinical remission are candidates for bone marrow transplantation. This intensive treatment requires high-dose chemotherapy and whole-body radiation. This causes ablation of the bone marrow, which has to be replaced. During this period of marrow aplasia, intensive support of the patient is required with red cell and platelet transfusions, and antimicrobial prophylaxis against bacterial, viral and fungal infections.

Allogeneic transplantation is the only therapy with curative potential for patients with ALL who do not attain an initial complete remission or who relapse with chemo-resistant disease. The cure rate is in the order of 10-20%.

Philadelphia chromosome positive ALL
Philadelphia chromosome positive ALL is one of the high-risk adult ALL variants with a poor prognosis. Treatment has been improved by the use of the tyrosine kinase inhibitor imatinib, either alone or in combination with chemotherapy, for both previously untreated as well as those with relapsed or chemotherapy-resistant disease. (See also acute myeloid leukemia below.)

Complications of therapy

- Sepsis and hemorrhage due to profound myelosuppression
- Tumor lysis syndrome

- Leucostasis due to sludging of leukocytes in the microcirculation, causing intracerebral or pulmonary hemorrhage and death
- Metabolic disturbances: increase in serum uric acid and potassium
- Bleeding diathesis or disseminated intravascular coagulation (DIC)
- Graft versus host disease. This is a complication of bone marrow transplantation in which the graft tissues react to the host tissues. Generally, this begins with gastrointestinal symptoms, skin rash and liver dysfunction. Management includes immunosuppressive drugs, like methotrexate or azathioprine, or measures to remove the T-lymphocytes, which mediate this reaction, from the donor marrow

OUTCOME

In children, complete remission can be attained in 90% of children with a cure rate of 70%. In adults, the complete remission rate is about 75%, with a 3-year disease-free survival of 35%.

ACUTE MYELOID LEUKEMIA

INCIDENCE

The incidence of acute myeloid leukemia (AML) is 2.5 per 100,000. There has been no significant change in the incidence over the past 20 years, and there is a uniform worldwide incidence. It affects Caucasians and African-Americans equally. The median age of diagnosis of AML is 65 years.

RISK FACTORS

AML shares similar risk factors to ALL. Chemical exposure to benzene and benzene-containing solvents, such as kerosene, increases the risk for AML. In addition, secondary AML can be induced by some cancer chemotherapeutic drugs, e.g. alkylating agents or podophyllotoxins.

CLASSIFICATION

Both the FAB and WHO classifications are used with the important difference between the two systems is that the FAB requires a minimum of 30% blasts in the marrow, while the WHO system requires only 20% blasts to make the diagnosis. Table 14.11 shows the WHO classification of acute myeloid leukemias.

Table 14.11 WHO Classification of Acute Myeloid Leukemias (AML)

AMLs with recurrent cytogenetic translocations
    AML with t(8:21)(q22;q22), AML1 (CBF- alpha)/ETO
    Acute promyelocytic leukemia
    AML with abnormal bone marrow eosinophils
    AML with 11q23 abnormalities
AMLs with multilineage dysplasia
    With prior myelodysplastic syndrome
    Without prior myelodysplastic syndrome
AMLs and myelodysplastic syndromes, therapy-related
    Alkylating agent-related
    Podophyllotoxin-related
    Other types
AML not otherwise specified

CLINICAL FEATURES

The clinical features are similar to ALL.

Symptoms

From anemia: fatigue, malaise and dyspnea.
From low platelets: easy bruising and bleeding gums.
From bone marrow crowding: bone pain.
General: weight loss, abdominal pain, skin rash, sweats and fever.

Signs

From anemia: pallor. Anemia is present in most patients at diagnosis.
From low platelets: petechiae, ecchymoses, hemorrhage and fundal hemorrhage.
From granulocytopenia: infection, sepsis and perirectal abscess.
From visceral infiltration: extramedullary leukemic mass (chloroma) sometimes occurs; they are rubbery and fast growing. Infiltration of gums or skin is more common than in ALL. Hepatosplenomegaly may be present due to leukemic infiltration of these organs.

Some patients with a variant of AML, acute promyelocytic leukemia (APML), may present with life-threatening bleeding due to release of thromboplastin from the leukemic cells. Almost always there is a chromosomal translocation t(15:17) that results in the fusion of the retinoic acid receptor gene alpha (RAR alpha) with a transcriptional factor gene called PML.

PROGNOSTIC FACTORS

Feature	Favorable	Unfavorable
Age	≤40 years	>40 years
Previous myelodysplastic disease	Absent	Present
WBC at diagnosis	≤100 x10^9/L	>100x 10^9/L
DIC	Absent	Present
Multidrug resistant gene-1	Negative	Positive
Cytogenetic abnormalities	t(8;21)	t(9;11)
	inv (16)	trisomy 13
	t(15;17)	chromosome 5, 7 abnormalities

DIAGNOSIS

The diagnosis of AML is generally made on examination of the peripheral blood or bone marrow. The differential diagnoses that must be considered are as follows:

- Small round cell neoplasms, e.g. Ewing's sarcoma. Immunological and cytogenetic markers allow the distinction between these
- Leukemoid reactions to certain benign conditions, such as tuberculosis, but the young myeloid cells rarely reach 20% in benign diseases

INVESTIGATIONS

These are similar to those for ALL.

TREATMENT
Induction chemotherapy

The most frequently used regimen consists of daunorubicin and Ara-C. A few alterations have been made to this with the addition of agents such as vincristine, thioguanine or etoposide. In general, most patients achieve a clinical remission after 1 or 2 cycles of treatment.

Consolidation therapy

This is not as well established as for ALL, but it is general practice to give additional therapy to prolong the period of remission or, possibly, produce a cure. Several cycles of chemotherapy, using the same drugs as in the induction phase, are given. More prolonged low-dose maintenance is usually not given.

Bone marrow transplantation

High-dose chemotherapy, with or without total body irradiation, followed by bone marrow transplantation is increasingly being used in the treatment of AML. In patients less than 50 years of age, who fail to achieve a complete remission with induction chemotherapy, allogeneic marrow transplantation offers a 20% chance of a cure. For patients who relapse after primary treatment, bone marrow transplantation is the only therapy with curative potential.

Complications

Complications of therapy are as outlined for ALL. DIC may occur with any type of AML, but it is most frequent with acute promyelocytic leukemia. This requires prompt blood component support, including platelets and frozen plasma. All-trans retinoic acid can control DIC.

OUTCOME

Induction chemotherapy produces a complete remission in 60-80% of patients. After achieving complete remission, consolidation chemotherapy with Ara-C can lead to a 5-year disease-free survival of 40%.

CHRONIC LYMPHOCYTIC LEUKEMIA

INCIDENCE

Chronic lymphocytic leukemia (CLL) is the most common leukemia with an annual incidence of 3 per 100,000. It is less common in Asians and Japanese compared with Caucasians. CLL is a disease of older persons, most being over 60 years of age at diagnosis. Men are affected twice as often as women.

RISK FACTORS

No specific risk factor is known for the common form of CLL in North America. Familial clustering of CLL has been reported. In Japan and the Caribbean, a rare T-cell variant is associated with human T-cell lymphotrophic virus Type 1 (HTLV-1).

PATHOLOGY

CLL is a monoclonal disorder involving B-cell (95%) or T-cell (5%) lineage. CLL cells express CD5 antigen, which is normally present in T-cells and fetal lymphoid cells. Trisomy of chromosome 12 or abnormality of chromosome 14 is present in about one-half of patients with CLL. A related condition is prolymphocytic leukemia, in which the leukemic cells are larger than the more mature cells of CLL. It occurs in elderly men, who have very high white cell counts and splenomegaly.

CLINICAL FEATURES

In the early stages of the disease, patients are asymptomatic, and the diagnosis comes to light because of an increased lymphocyte count when a blood count is done for unrelated reasons. Enlargement of the peripheral lymph nodes, especially cervical nodes, is the presenting complaint in some patients. In the late stages of the disease, there are recurrent infections, fever, sweats and weight loss.

INVESTIGATIONS

• Complete blood count
The hallmark of CLL is peripheral lymphocytosis in the range of 40-150 x 10^9/L. A total lymphocyte count of >5 x 10^9/L is required to make the diagnosis. The lymphocytes are similar to normal small B-lymphocytes, but on immunotyping, they express CD5. Anemia is present in 20% of cases, but it is usually mild. Some patients have Coombs-positive hemolytic

anemia. Thrombocytopenia occurs in about 10% of patients at presentation.

- Serum biochemistry: creatinine, bilirubin, LDH, SGOT, alkaline phosphatase
- Serum protein electrophoresis: at diagnosis, 25% of patients have hypogammaglobulin-emia, and in later stages of the disease, this rises to 70%
- Chest x-ray
- Bone marrow examination shows a lympho-cytic infiltrate of >40% of the total cell population. Three patterns of marrow involvement are seen: interstitial, nodular and diffuse

DIAGNOSIS

The diagnosis of CLL is usually straightfor-ward. The differential diagnoses include in-fectious mononucleosis, cytomegalovirus in-fection, pertussis or tuberculosis. In most of these, there is evidence of infection. Other lymphoproliferative conditions can resemble CLL, but immunophenotyping and histo-pathology are reliable in making the distinction between these and CLL.

STAGING

The Rai staging system is widely used.

Stage	Risk	Clinical findings
0	Low	Lymphocytes >5 x 10^9/L in blood or >40% in bone marrow
I	Intermediate	Lymphocytosis + lymphadenopathy
II	Intermediate	As in Stage I + splenomegaly and/or hepatomegaly
III	High	Lymphocytosis + anemia (Hgb <110g/L)
IV	High	Lymphocytosis + thrombocy-topenia (platelets <100x10^9/L)

TREATMENT

CLL is an indolent condition and patients with early stages of the disease require no immediate treatment and active surveillance may be appropriate. Indications for treatment include:

- Anemia or thrombocytopenia
- Massive lymphadenopathy
- Massive hepatomegaly or splenomegaly
- Evidence of progressive enlargement of lymph nodes, liver or spleen
- A doubling time of peripheral lymphocytes of less than 6 months

Chemotherapy

Fludarabine, a purine analogue, is the standard chemotherapy. Chlorambucil is also a useful drug that has been extensively used in the past for CLL. Either drug produces a tumor response in the majority of patients. The addition of rituximab, an anti-CD20 antibody, has im-proved the results of treatment of CLL.

Other treatments

- Radiation

Low-dose radiation (20-30 Gy over 2-3 weeks) can produce significant reduction in peripheral nodes or enlarged spleen.

- Splenectomy

Occasional patients may benefit from removal of the spleen. This is most helpful when there is symptomatic splenomegaly or hemolytic anemia not controlled by chemotherapy.

- Treatment of infections

A major complication of CLL is opportunistic infections. High-dose intravenous immuno-globulin therapy decreases the frequency of bacterial infections. Treatment with fludarabine also increases the risk of *Pneumocystis carnii*, and prophylaxis with trimethoprim-sulfamethoxa-zole and fluconazole may be considered.

- Bone marrow transplantation

Non-myeloablative bone marrow transplantation may be indicated in selected cases refractory to chemotherapy.

OUTCOME

There is a good correlation between the Rai stages and median survival of patients. In a small proportion of patients, CLL transforms into a more aggressive lymphoma (diffuse large cell lymphoma), termed Richter's syndrome. The median survival in this situation is poor, usually 4 months.

Stage	Median survival (months)
0	140
I	100
II	70
III	20
IV	20

CHRONIC MYELOGENOUS LEUKEMIA

INCIDENCE

Chronic myelogenous leukemia (CML) is an uncommon disease with an incidence of 1-2 per 100,000. It typically affects adults with the median age of diagnosis being 50 years. It is more common in men, with a male to female ratio of 1.4-2:1.

RISK FACTORS

Exposure to ionizing radiation is the only known risk factor.

PATHOLOGY

CML results from the overproduction and accumulation of cells of the myeloid lineage. The cells are relatively mature and retain most of their normal functions. A common feature is the Philadelphia chromosome or Ph chromosome, which is found in over 90% of cases. This is the result of translocation between the long arms of chromosomes 9 and 22, causing the abl oncogene on chromosome 9 to become contiguous with bcr on chromosome 22. In patients without Ph chromosome, molecular abl/bcr translocation occurs. The translocation results in the production of an oncogenic hybrid protein, called p210.

CLINICAL FEATURES

There are three phases of CML: chronic, accelerated and blast crisis. More than 90% of patients are diagnosed during the chronic phase, and 25% of these come to attention because of an elevation of the granulocyte count on a routine blood test. Other common presenting symptoms are fatigue, weight loss and night sweats. Because the granulocytes retain their normal function, infections are uncommon. Left upper quadrant abdominal discomfort may occur due to enlargement of the spleen. An uncommon complication is leucostasis when the granulocyte count is over 400×10^9/L. This is characterized by dyspnea, drowsiness, confusion and decreased visual acuity due to sludging of the white cells in the capillaries.

Examination reveals clinical signs of anemia, and purpura is often present. Peripheral lymph nodes are not usually prominent. The most common sign is splenomegaly, which can be massive. Hepatomegaly may also be present. During the blast crisis, the clinical features are similar to acute leukemia.

CML follows a chronic course, but two-thirds transform into an accelerated phase, heralded by an increase in blasts to >15% or basophils to >20% in blood or marrow. One-third of patients develop blast crisis rapidly.

INVESTIGATIONS

- Complete blood count shows elevation of the white blood cell count, ranging from 10-1,000 x 10^9/L. The majority are neutrophils, although basophilia is common. There is mild anemia, and platelets may be increased
- Biochemistry: electrolytes, creatinine, liver enzymes. Vitamin B12 levels are elevated. LDH is increased
- Bone marrow shows marked myeloid hyperplasia, but blasts are usually <5%. Ph chromosome is present. During the blast crisis, blast cells make up >30% of the myeloid cell population

DIAGNOSIS

The diagnosis is usually evident on examination of the peripheral blood and bone marrow in conjunction with splenomegaly. The presence of the Ph chromosome or bcr/abl rearrangement confirms the diagnosis.

TREATMENT

During the chronic phase, the goal of treatment is to reduce the peripheral white cell counts to under 15 x 10^9/L, and to relieve the symptoms of splenomegaly. A number of different chemotherapeutic agents have been used in the past, the most common being hydroxyurea and busulfan. The majority of patients will have a hematologic remission and reduction of splenomegaly. However, treatment with either drug is not curative, does not prolong overall survival, and only rarely results in attainment of a cytogenetic response. Interferon is usually given as maintenance therapy.

Hematopoietic cell transplantation and the oral tyrosine kinase inhibitors have supplanted chemotherapeutic agents and/or interferon therapy, although they can be of benefit to patients who are not transplantation candidates and who are intolerant or refractory to treatment with tyrosine kinase inhibitors.

With an understanding of the molecular defect in CML, drugs have been developed which are highly effective in the treatment of this disease. The first and second generation oral tyrosine kinase inhibitors (e.g. imatinib, dasatinib, nilotinib) have become the initial treatment of choice for almost all newly diagnosed patients with CML. Imatinib, a tyrosine kinase inhibitor which is targeted against the abl/bcr hybrid protein induces cytogenetic remission in more than 80% of patients.

Allogeneic hematopoietic cell transplantation is a curative treatment option, which may be considered in younger patients with stable disease who have a suitable donor. About 15% of patients in blast crisis who receive an HLA-matched sibling transplant can be cured. Higher cure rates can be achieved if bone marrow transplantation is done during the accelerated phase (40%) or chronic phase (65%).

Splenic radiation may be helpful in alleviating the symptoms due to a large spleen. When hyperviscosity of the blood is present, leucophoresis can bring about a rapid reduction in the white cell count. In the acute phase, treatment of the blast crisis follows that of acute leukemia.

OUTCOME

The median survival of patients with chronic phase CML is about 4 years, but this is improving with the use of imatinib. The onset of the acute blast crisis is an ominous development with a short survival time, but an increasing number of patients are being treated with high-dose chemotherapy and bone marrow transplantation, some of whom achieve durable remissions.

MULTIPLE MYELOMA

INCIDENCE

Multiple myeloma is an uncommon condition that affects men and women equally. Over the past several decades, it has been diagnosed with increasing frequency, which may reflect improved diagnostic procedures.

RISK FACTORS

There is no recognized risk factor. Exposure to radiation, benzene and other organic solvents, herbicides and insecticides may play a role, but are not conclusively proven as risk factors.

PATHOLOGY

Multiple myeloma is a neoplasm of plasma cells and it is part of the spectrum that spans benign monoclonal gammopathy to solitary plasmacytoma to multiple myeloma. One-fifth of those with monoclonal gammopathy and two-thirds of those with plasmacytoma eventually develop multiple myeloma. The bone marrow shows infiltration with plasma cells, with >10% plasma cells being diagnostic of multiple myeloma. Bone destruction is a common feature, and this is due to osteoclast activating factors, such as interleukins, tumor necrosis factor and macrophage colony-stimulating factor.

CLINICAL FEATURES

Local infiltration of the bone marrow by plasma cells leads to anemia. Thrombocytopenia is mild at presentation. Bone pain is common due to bone destruction. There may be nerve root compression or spinal cord compression secondary to bone destruction.

Generalized symptoms include the following:

- nausea/vomiting, thirst, polyuria, constipation and confusion due to hypercalcemia
- nausea/vomiting, malaise, fluid retention and pruritis due to renal failure from deposition of paraprotein or secondary amyloidosis of the kidneys
- headaches and confusion due to hyperviscosity from high levels of paraproteins

Examination reveals signs of anemia and bone tenderness, usually in the ribs and spine. Pathological fractures may be present. Weakness of the legs, sphincter dysfunction and neurological signs may uncommonly be present at diagnosis.

DIAGNOSIS

The diagnosis requires the presence of any two of the following:

- Presence of monoclonal immunoglobulin (M protein) in blood or urine
- Lytic bone lesions
- More than 10% plasma cells in the bone marrow

The following additional features are helpful supportive evidence when present:

- Depression of the levels of uninvolved immunoglobulins
- Hypercalcemia
- Amyloid deposit in biopsied tissues

Differential diagnosis

The main differential diagnosis is from bone metastases from other common cancers, primarily those of the breast, lung, prostate, kidney or thyroid. The presence of an M protein usually suggests the diagnosis. Occasionally, a patient may present with a solitary plasmacytoma. A biopsy is advised in these cases to confirm the diagnosis and rule out a metastatic deposit from another cancer. Patients with Waldenström's macroglobulinemia have IgM paraproteinemia, but none of the features of multiple myeloma.

INVESTIGATIONS

- Complete blood count: anemia is present. Peripheral blood smear shows rouleaux formation
- Erythrocyte sedimentation rate is elevated
- Biochemistry: total protein is raised. Hypercalcemia may be present and creatinine may be elevated
- Serum protein electrophoresis shows a band containing the paraprotein: IgG (50%), IgA (20%), IgM (10%), light chain only (10%), IgD (2%), heavy chain (1%). Rarely, two different M proteins may be present
- Bence-Jones protein may be present in the urine
- Serum β_2-microglobulin is raised and it is a useful marker of disease activity
- Chest x-ray and skeletal survey (skull, spine, humeri, pelvis, femurs and ribs). Typically, multiple lytic lesions are present. (Isotope bone scan may be falsely negative, since the lesions are primarily lytic with little osteoclastic reaction)
- Bone marrow examination with cytogenetic study for del 13q

TREATMENT

Most patients require treatment at diagnosis. Chemotherapy is the treatment of choice. Even though a cure is not possible, chemotherapy often offers satisfactory palliation. The standard regimen for younger patients (below 65-70 years of age) is high dose chemotherapy and autologous hematopoietic stem cell transplant. For older patients, melphalan and prednisone are used.

Rarely, multiple myeloma runs an indolent course, either progressing slowly or remaining static for long periods. Hence, therapy may be initially withheld in patients who fulfill all of the following criteria:

- No symptoms
- Satisfactory peripheral blood counts
- No paraprotein in the urine
- Normal serum calcium
- Stable serum paraprotein level
- No non-irradiated lytic bone lesions
- No renal or neurological disease due to myeloma
- No more than one lytic bone lesion
  Secondary treatments for recurrent myeloma include the following:
- Bortezomib, a proteasome inhibitor
- Thalidomide, which can inhibit angiogenesis and also may directly inhibit the growth and survival of myeloma cells, is used in patients with relapsed or resistant myeloma
  Other measures include:
- Radiation therapy to relieve pain due to bone lesions. It is also indicated for pathological fractures, and in cases of spinal cord compression
- Red cell transfusion for anemia
- Management of hypercalcemia (hydration and diuresis with bisphosphonates)
- Management of renal failure
- Bisphosphonates are effective in preventing some of the skeletal destruction caused by myeloma, and they improve patient survival

OUTCOME

The typical course of multiple myeloma lasts 3-4 years. There is, however, a wide variation in survival, ranging from a few months to >10 years in 5% of patients. In the presence of renal failure or elevated β_2-microglobulin, the median survival is <1 year.

IMMUNIZATIONS FOR PATIENTS WITH LYMPHOID MALIGNANCIES

Patients with malignant lymphomas, Hodgkin's lymphoma, chronic lymphocytic leukemia and multiple myeloma do not have a normal immune system. They are, therefore, at increased risk for infections and certain immunizations are recommended. In patients who are receiving chemotherapy or radiation therapy, immunizations, except influenza vaccine, should be delayed until completion of treatment.

Type of immunization	Frequency
Influenza vaccine	Yearly in the autumn
Pneumococcal vaccine	At diagnosis and then every 6 years
Tetanus/diphtheria/pertussis/polio	Every 10 years
Meningococcal types A, C	Once only, if the spleen is removed or radiated

Chapter 15

ENDOCRINE TUMORS

THYROID CANCER

INCIDENCE

Thyroid cancers are infrequent and account for only about 1% of all cancers, but the incidence is increasing. Thyroid nodules are commonly found in asymptomatic persons, but the probability of finding an underlying cancer is 5-10%. Cancers of the thyroid affect women more frequently than men (4:1 ratio). The median age of diagnosis of well-differentiated thyroid cancer is the early 40s, whereas anaplastic cancers are seen in the elderly. Thyroid cancers are a diverse group of neoplasms with distinct epidemiology and natural history. Table 15.1 lists the common thyroid cancers and their relative distribution.

Table 15.1 Classification of thyroid cancers

Type	Percentage of total
Well-differentiated	70
Papillary (20)	
Follicular (50)	
Medullary	4
Anaplastic	25
Lymphoma	1-3
Sarcoma and others	<1

WELL-DIFFERENTIATED THYROID CARCINOMA

RISK FACTORS

Radiation exposure is the only clear-cut risk factor. This exposure can be from external sources (nuclear plant accidents, atomic blasts, medically administered radiotherapy), or internal by ingestion of radioactive iodine which concentrates in the thyroid gland. The lag time from radiation exposure to the diagnosis is 5-40 years with a peak around 15 years. Follicular thyroid cancer is more common in endemic goitre areas of the world, while papillary cancer occurs with higher frequency in areas where there is an excess of iodine in the diet.

Well-differentiated thyroid cancer is occasionally associated with multiple endocrine neoplasms type I (MEN-I), while medullary thyroid cancer is associated with MEN-II. Other rare associations include Pendred's syndrome (goitre and nerve deafness), Gardner's syndrome (colon polyposis, osteomas and sebaceous cysts) and Cowden's disease (multiple hamartomas).

PATHOLOGY

Macroscopic

Thyroid cancers form minute sub-capsular white scars to large tumors (>5 cm in diameter). They are well-circumscribed with a pseudocapsule due to compressed thyroid tissue at the site of the primary.

Microscopic

Most cancers of the thyroid arise from the epithelial cells of the thyroid follicles (papillary and follicular) and are well-differentiated. Medullary carcinoma arises from parafollicular C cells. Anaplastic carcinomas are poorly differentiated with no identifiable follicular elements.

Spread

Local invasion leads to spread of the cancer to the contralateral lobe via the isthmus. Capsular invasion leads to involvement of the surrounding structures, such as strap muscles, trachea, larynx and recurrent laryngeal nerve.

Lymphatic invasion is common, leading to multiple microscopic lesions within the thyroid, and metastasis to the neck nodes is present in 40% of cases at the time of diagnosis.

Blood-borne spread occurs infrequently. The lung is the most common site of metastasis, followed by bone, liver, skin, brain and kidney.

CLINICAL FEATURES

The usual presentation is an asymptomatic thyroid nodule, but infrequently there may be hoarseness (recurrent laryngeal nerve) or dysphagia (extrinsic compression of the pharynx or upper esophagus).

Examination reveals a firm mass in the thyroid. Recurrent laryngeal nerve involvement can cause stridor. Enlarged lymph nodes may be palpable in the neck or supraclavicular areas.

DIAGNOSIS

Thyroid nodules are present in as many as 50% of adults, increasing in prevalence with age. Many of these are small and clinically inapparent, and they are due to many different pathological processes, including cancer. Because of the possibility of a malignancy, thyroid nodules should be systematically evaluated, especially if they are new or measure more than 1 cm in diameter. The important distinction to be made is whether the nodule is cystic or solid. This may be confirmed by ultrasonography or by fine needle aspiration biopsy (FNA). FNA provides material for cytological analysis and it is, therefore, preferred to ultrasound.

When a malignancy is confirmed, surgery is recommended. If the cytology is suspicious, but not confirmatory for cancer, a repeat FNA can be done; if the diagnosis is still uncertain,

further investigations are required. A radioisotope scan of the thyroid determines if the nodule is "hot" (functional) or "cold." A hot nodule likely represents a solitary autonomous nodule, and follow-up is appropriate with periodic clinical examination, with or without thyroid suppressive therapy. A nodule that increases in size during follow-up is suspicious for cancer, and repeat FNA or surgery is advised. If the nodule is cold on thyroid scan, surgical intervention is recommended.

INVESTIGATIONS

- Serum markers
  - thyroglobulin is a useful marker for well-differentiated thyroid cancer
  - calcitonin is elevated in medullary cancer (suspected in those with a family history of thyroid cancer at a young age or associated diarrhea)
  - CEA is occasionally elevated in medullary thyroid cancer
- Chest x-ray can demonstrate lung metastasis
- Isotope thyroid scan with technetium-99 or iodine-131 will show a cold spot in the presence of a cancer
- CT scan is useful to define the extent of the thyroid mass and the presence of neck nodes

TREATMENT

Patients with thyroid cancer require some form of thyroid ablation therapy, followed by thyroid hormone replacement to prevent hypothyroidism. The dose of thyroid hormone replacement should be titrated to suppress the TSH level to reduce the risk of stimulating any residual TSH-dependent cancer.

Surgery

Surgery is the mainstay of therapy; this may require a lobectomy, subtotal thyroidectomy or total thyroidectomy. Complications of total thyroidectomy include recurrent laryngeal nerve injury, and hypocalcemia due to removal of the parathyroid glands. Metastases to the neck nodes are managed by neck dissection.

Radioiodine therapy

Radioiodine concentrates in any thyroid remnant or cancer persisting after surgery. Radioiodine therapy is recommended for patients who have a well-differentiated cancer and are at risk for recurrence. It emits β-particles which ablate the thyroid or cancer. (It also emits γ-photons which are a radiation hazard.) Radioiodine therapy is indicated when there is risk for recurrent disease based on the following features:

- Tumor size >2.5 cm
- Multifocal disease
- Follicular histology
- Capsular invasion by the tumor
- Metastatic nodal disease
- Patients older than 40 years

Ablation of the thyroid is usually accomplished by 30-200 millicuries. Following thyroidectomy, thyroid hormone replacement is withheld, and radioiodine is given when the serum TSH is >50 UIU/ml. Following radioiodine ablation, thyroxine is started at doses to keep levels of T3 and T4 in the upper limit of the normal range, while keeping serum TSH level suppressed to <1 UIU/ml.

Another indication for radioiodine is the treatment of metastatic or recurrent well-differentiated thyroid cancer which takes up radioiodine. A larger dose (100-200 millicuries) is usually used.

OUTCOME

Well-differentiated thyroid cancers have a favorable survival rate. The 10-year survival rate for papillary tumors is 90% and for follicular tumors 80%. In contrast, anaplastic tumors have a poor prognosis, and most patients die within 6 months.

MEDULLARY THYROID CANCER

Medullary thyroid carcinoma (MTC) is a neuroendocrine tumor of the parafollicular or C cells of the thyroid gland, and accounts for approximately 4% of thyroid cancers. A characteristic feature of this tumor is the production of calcitonin. About 80% of medullary thyroid cancers are sporadic. The typical age of presentation is in the fifth or sixth decade, and there is a slight female preponderance. In most patients, metastasis is evident at the time of diagnosis: 50% of patients have clinically detectable cervical lymph node; 15% have dysphagia or hoarseness due to involvement of the upper aero-digestive tract; and 5% have distant disease. Systemic symptoms may occur due to hormonal secretion. Calcitonin or other substances can cause diarrhea or facial flushing; occasional tumors secrete corticotropin (ACTH), causing Cushing's syndrome.

MTC is also familial and occurs as part of the multiple endocrine neoplasia type II (MEN-II, see below) syndrome, in which there is multicentric hyperplasia of the parafollicular C cells. Genetic screening for the RET proto-oncogene permits the precise identification of those at risk for MTC.

OUTCOME

Patient's age at diagnosis is an important prognostic factor; the 5-year disease-free survival (DFS) rates are higher in patients <40 years compared with patients >40 years (95 vs. 65%); the respective 10-year DFS rates are 75 vs. 50%.

Other factors that predict a poor prognosis

include cellular heterogeneity, low immuno-staining for calcitonin, high immunostaining for galectin-3, or immunostaining for CEA associated with scant staining for calcitonin. Patients with high preoperative serum CEA, and persistent hypercalcitoninemia after thyroidectomy fare less well.

GASTROENTEROPANCREATIC NEUROENDOCRINE TUMORS

There are two groups of gastroenteropancreatic neuroendocrine tumors: carcinoid tumors and pancreatic neuroendocrine tumors.

CARCINOID TUMOR

INCIDENCE

Carcinoid tumors are rare, with an incidence of 2.5-4.5 per 100,000. The incidence has increased in the past two decades. The average age of diagnosis is 50 years, and men and women are affected equally. The tumor occurs most commonly in the small bowel, but it may be found anywhere in the GI tract, and occasionally in other sites, such as lung, ovary, testis, thyroid, bile duct and bladder. Carcinoid tumors may be associated with MEN-I, neurofibromatosis type 1 and familial adenomatous polyposis syndrome. A familial carcinoid tumor syndrome is also recognized.

PATHOLOGY

Macroscopic

Carcinoid tumor appears as a yellow plaque with intact overlying mucosa that later ulcerates. The tumor encircles the bowel, leading to obstruction. Frequently, it invokes a fibrotic response in adjacent tissues.

Microscopic

The tumor arises from cells that make up the diffuse endocrine system. The cells tend to be uniform and small.

Special test

Ki67, a nuclear protein expressed by cycling cells, is a useful prognostic marker; tumors with Ki67 index <2% behave in an indolent manner while those with an index >20% are more aggressive tumors.

CLINICAL FEATURES

Carcinoid tumors are often found incidentally at surgery, particularly at appendectomy. They are slow growing and seldom metastasize unless they are >2 cm. They can spread to the regional nodes and liver. When the tumor metastasizes to the liver, the carcinoid syndrome occurs as a result of the secretion of vasoactive substances produced by the tumor into the systemic circulation; these tumors are referred to as functioning tumors. The carcinoid syndrome comprises flushing, diarrhea and bronchospasm. Carcinoid flushing and diarrhea may be precipitated by alcohol, caffeine, stress, or certain foods (e.g. bananas, avocado, eggplant, pineapple or plums). Carcinoid heart disease develops in up to 40% of patients with long-standing carcinoid syndrome. This involves the endocardium of the right side of the heart and its valves, leading most commonly to tricuspid insufficiency or pulmonic stenosis. Right heart failure eventually results.

SPECIAL INVESTIGATIONS

- Urinary 5HIAA (5-hydroxyindoleacetic acid), a metabolite of 5-hydroxytryptamine is elevated in functioning carcinoid tumors
- Serum chromogranin A is a good marker for

both functioning and non-functioning carcinoid tumors
- Somatostatin receptor imaging with Indium-111-labelled octreotide (OctreoScan) is a useful staging scan, especially for patients undergoing surgery

TREATMENT

Resection of localized tumor can be curative. Because of the generally indolent nature of the disease, patients with liver metastases can live for years, and resection of the liver metastases, when possible, can therefore be useful. Hepatic artery embolization also leads to control of the metastatic liver disease for long periods.

Carcinoid syndrome responds well to treatment with somatostatin analogues, such as octreotide or lanreotide, with marked improvement of diarrhea and flushing. Interferon therapy may also provide good control of the symptoms. The risk of valvular heart damage may be reduced by treatment with somatostatin analogues, presumably by suppressing the serum levels of serotonin, which is believed to be the underlying cause of the valvular heart disease.

Chemotherapy has a limited role. Streptozotocin with 5FU or doxorubicin, or temozolomide with capecitabine can bring about partial tumor responses in a small proportion of patients. Targeted therapies with anti-angiogenesis drugs or mTOR inhibitors, like everolimus, show some activity.

Radio-targeted therapy, with lutetium-177 or yttrium-90 tagged to octreotide, or iodine-131-mIBG (meta-iodobenzyl guanidine) may be a useful palliative measure in patients with tumors that show avid uptake of octreotide or mIBG, respectively.

Patients with functioning carcinoid tumors require treatment with octreotide before any invasive procedures, such as surgery, to avert a carcinoid crisis (flushing, extreme changes in blood pressure, bronchoconstriction, arrhythmias and confusion).

OUTCOME

Patients with localized or regional nodal disease may be cured by surgical resection. Because carcinoid tumors are generally slow-growing, some patients with liver metastases can live for several years. The overall 5-year survival is 67%.

PANCREATIC NEUROENDOCRINE TUMORS

These are rare tumors with an annual incidence of 0.4 per 100,000. Although exocrine pancreatic cancers (adenocarcinoma) are far more common, in young individuals under 40 years, endocrine tumors make up 50% of all pancreatic tumors. Men and women are affected equally. Pancreatic neuroendocrine tumors are associated with MEN-1, von Hippel-Landau syndrome and neurofibromatosis type 1.

Several distinct clinical syndromes are recognized, but up to one-half are non-functioning and secrete no detectable hormones. These remain clinically silent and are found incidentally or come to attention due to their mass effect. They are a heterogeneous group that can be subdivided into the following types:
- Functioning tumors
  - insulinoma (25%)
  - gastrinoma (15%)
  - VIPoma
  - glucogonoma
  - somatostatinoma
  - rare tumors (GFRoma, ACTHoma, PTHoma)
- Non-functioning tumors

Surgical excision is recommended for localized tumors and can be curative. Even in the presence of metastases, the prognosis is good as they are generally slow-growing tumors. Somatostain analogues, such as octreotide or lanreotide, can suppress secretion of the hormones and improve symptoms. Chemotherapy with streptozotocin plus 5FU or doxorubicin, or temozolomide plus capecitabine can bring about partial responses in up to 40% of patients. Targeted drugs, including anti-angiogenesis agents and mTOR inhibitors (everolimus), show some activity. Radio-targeted therapy, with lutetium-177 or yttrium-90 tagged to octreotide, is also a useful therapeutic modality.

MULTIPLE ENDOCRINE NEOPLASIA (MEN)

MEN Type I

Multiple endocrine neoplasia type I (MEN-I) is an autosomal dominant predisposition to tumors of the parathyroid glands, anterior pituitary and pancreatic islet cells, referred to as the "3 Ps." Additionally, a few other tumors can occur, including duodenal gastrinomoma, carcinoid tumor, thyroid and adrenal adenomas, and lipomas.

MEN Type II

Multiple endocrine neoplasia type II (MEN-II) is subdivided into three distinct syndromes: MEN-IIA, MEN-IIB, and familial medullary thyroid cancer (FMTC).

- MEN-IIA is inherited as an autosomal dominant disease. The syndrome comprises medullary thyroid cancer (MTC), pheochromocytoma, and primary parathyroid hyperplasia. Men and women are equally affected. MTC occurs in almost all patients, whereas the development of the other tumors is more variable

- MEN-IIB is an autosomal dominant disorder consisting of MTC and pheochromocytoma, but not hyperparathyroidism. As with MEN-IIA, MTC is evident in almost all patients, and it develops at an earlier age and is more aggressive than in MEN-IIA. Other manifestations of the syndrome are mucosal neuromas, usually involving the lips and tongue, and intestinal ganglioneuromas. Patients with MEN-IIB also have altered body habitus (decreased upper/lower body ratio), skeletal deformities (kyphoscoliosis or lordosis), joint laxity, Marfanoid features, and myelinated corneal nerves. Patients may also have chronic constipation and megacolon

- FMTC is a variant of MEN in which there is a strong predisposition to MTC, but not the other clinical manifestations

PHEOCHROMOCYTOMA

Pheochromocytomas are rare tumors arising from chromaffin cells that migrate from the neural crest to the adrenal gland during fetal development. The vast majority of these tumors arises in the adrenal medulla, but about 10% are extra-adrenal, involving the aortic bifurcation, sympathetic chain, bladder, paravertebral region and carotid arch. Most are benign, but malignant pheochromocytomas can spread locally and invade the kidney and retroperitoneum. Lymphatic spread is uncommon, but blood-borne spread can occur to lung, bone and liver.

Pheochromocytomas can affect individuals of any age with the peak age of incidence being 35-55 years. Common symptoms are headaches, postural dizziness, pallor, sweating, tremor, palpitations, chest pain and feelings of fear.

Investigations include urinary VMA and

catecholamines. CT scan can define the tumor. Diagnostic mIBG scan is usually positive.

Treatment is surgical excision by adrenalectomy. Therapeutic mIBG may be used to treat metastatic disease if the tumor uptake of mIBG is good. Chemotherapy is not useful. Radiation therapy may be used to palliate local symptoms, such as bone pain from metastasis. Even with metastatic disease, patients may live for several years, and usually succumb to car-diovascular complications, such as myocardial infarction or cerebrovascular accident.

Chapter 16

SARCOMA AND BONE ONCOLOGY

Sarcomas are malignant tumors that arise from the skeletal and extra-skeletal connective tissues, including the peripheral nervous system. They may arise almost anywhere in the body and are conveniently subdivided into two groups: soft tissue sarcomas and bone sarcomas.

SOFT TISSUE SARCOMAS

Classification

Tissue type	Benign	Malignant
Fibrous tissue	Fibroma Nodular fasciitis Desmoid tumors	Fibrosarcoma
?Fibroblastic	Fibrous histiocytoma	Malignant fibrous histiocytoma
Fat	Lipoma Angiomyolipoma	Liposarcoma
Smooth muscle	Leiomyoma	Leiomyosarcoma
Skeletal muscle	Rhabdomyoma	Rhabdomyosarcoma
Blood and lymph vessel	Hemangioma	Angiosarcoma Kaposi's sarcoma Lymphangiosarcoma
?(unknown)	–	Synovial sarcoma
Peripheral nerve tissue	Neurofibroma Schawnnoma	Malignant peripheral nerve sheath tumor (neurogenic sarcoma)

INCIDENCE

Soft tissue sarcomas are rare cancers, which account for 1% of adult malignancies and 15% of childhood malignancies. Men and women are affected equally. In adults, the cancer can occur at any age, but it is more common between 50-70 years.

RISK FACTORS

There is no clear etiology for the majority of cases, but a number of predisposing factors have been identified.

• Genetic factors
Soft tissue sarcomas occur with increased frequency in several hereditary conditions, including Li-Fraumeni syndrome, neurofibromatosis type 1 (von Recklinghausen's disease), Gardner's syndrome, retinoblastoma, Werner's syndrome, Gorlin's syndrome, multiple neuro-endocrine neoplasia, Carney's triad and tuberous sclerosis.
• Chronic lymphedema from a variety of causes, such as chronic congenital lymphedema, infections (e.g. filariasis), post-surgical or post-radiation therapy
• Exposure to ionizing radiation and radioactive contrast agent (Thorotrast)
• Chemical exposure to vinyl chloride, arsenic, chlorophenols, and herbicides
• Androgenic steroids (hepatic angiosarcoma)
• Immunosuppressive therapy for renal trans-

plant and other conditions

PATHOLOGY

Macroscopic

Soft tissue sarcomas are distributed throughout the body with about half occurring in the extremities while the remainder are in the retroperitoneum, viscera (bladder, bowel and uterus), trunk and head/neck area. The tumor appears as a large, fleshy mass with central areas of necrosis. Invasion of the adjacent structures may be evident.

Microscopic

Histologically, soft tissue sarcomas form a diverse group of tumors, and they are categorized according to the normal tissue they resemble. For several sarcomas, the cell of origin is unknown, and they may arise from mesenchymal cells distributed throughout the skeleton and somatic soft tissues.

Tumor grade

Tumor grade is an important parameter in assessing sarcomas. The biological aggressiveness of the tumor can be determined by its grade, and this is a good predictor of metastasis and patient survival. The assignment of tumor grade takes into account cellularity, tumor differentiation, amount of necrosis, degree of nuclear pleomorphism and number of mitoses. Two grades are recognized: low and high grades.

Biology

Unlike epithelial cancers which develop by a multi-step process, such as the adenoma-carcinoma sequence in colorectal cancer, sarcomas do not arise in the setting of a pre-existing benign mesenchymal lesion. However, some low grade sarcomas can transform into high grade malignancies, a process referred to as "dedifferentiation."

CLINICAL FEATURES

Local symptoms predominate at initial presentation of sarcomas.
• Extremity sarcoma
Most patients with extremity sarcomas usually present with a painless mass. Because the disease is uncommon, diagnosis is often delayed; it may be misdiagnosed as "pulled muscle," intramuscular hematoma, sebaceous cyst or benign lipoma. As the tumor grows, it presses on nearby structures, causing pain or numbness. Any mass >5 cm arising deep to fascia with rapid growth should be suspect.
Examination reveals a large mass on the limb or trunk. When it is close to a joint, movement may be impaired.
• Intra-abdominal or retroperitoneal sarcoma
Patients with intra-abdominal or retroperitoneal sarcoma often present late, since the tumors can reach a large size before they cause symptoms. Patients may complain of vague abdominal discomfort. Occasionally, the tumor can cause gastrointestinal bleeding or incomplete bowel obstruction. A large retroperitoneal mass may be palpable on abdominal examination. Pressure or invasion of the nerve plexus in the retroperitoneum leads to neurological symptoms.

The differential diagnosis is from other types of retroperitoneal malignancies: lymphoma or germ cell tumor or metastasis from another primary carcinoma.

Gastrointestinal stromal tumors (GIST)

These rare tumors are among the most common mesenchymal gastrointestinal malignancy. They can cause acute GI bleed and perforation. The malignant cells show over-expression of the cell receptor protein c-kit. This has been the basis for a dramatic change in the treatment of GIST. Imatinib, which inhibits the intracellular tyrosine kinase domain of mutated c-kit, brings about a partial remission in up to 80% of patients with advanced GIST with significant improvement in patients quality of life and survival. Imatinib improves the disease-free survival after resection for GIST and is often used as postoperative adjuvant treatment for high-risk tumors.

Rhabdomyosarcoma

There are three main histological subtypes: pleomorphic and alveolar rhabdomyosacromas in adults; and embryonal rhabdomyosarcoma in children. (Embryonal rhabdomyosarcoma is discussed in Chapter 19.)

In adults, pleomorphic rhabdomyosarcoma is the most common form of rhabdomyosarcoma. It is a high-grade malignancy. Alveolar rhabdomyosarcoma commonly arises in the extremities in adolescents and young adults. The tumor cells form ill-defined aggregates of poorly differentiated round or oval cells, which are less cohesive centrally, giving rise to irregular "alveolar" spaces. Most have a specific translocation t(2,13) (q37;q14), involving the PAX3 gene on chromosome 2 and the FKHR gene on chromosome 13. Translocation between chromosome 1 and chromosome 13 t(1:13)(p36;q14) may also be present. The prognosis for pleomorphic and alveolar rhabdomyosarcoma is poor.

Kaposi's sarcoma

Kaposi sarcoma is an uncommon vascular sarcoma. There are four varieties, which have different clinical features and different natural history despite their similar histological appearances.

- Classical Kaposi's sarcoma occurs in elderly men of Jewish or Mediterranean origin. It appears as a single or multiple, purple-red nodules, usually around the ankles. Its course is indolent, but metastases eventually develop. There is an increased risk for non-Hodgkin's lymphomas
- A second form is seen in Bantu men in Africa. Its course is variable and it can run an aggressive course
- Kaposi's sarcoma may also occur in patients who have had an organ transplant and are on immunosuppressive therapy
- Epidemic Kaposi's sarcoma runs a more aggressive course. There are multiple lesions involving the skin, oral mucosa, lymph nodes and visceral organs. The disease is observed in homosexual and bisexual men with HIV infection, and there is a strong association with human herpesvirus 8. Homosexual men without HIV infection are also at increased risk of Kaposi's sarcoma, but it is more indolent and affects the genitalia and extremities. Interestingly, heterosexual men and intravenous drug users with HIV have a lower risk of Kaposi's sarcoma than homosexual men with HIV. Kaposi's sarcoma associated with AIDS is controlled with anti-viral therapy for the HIV infection. However, the disease can be fulminant when drug resistance develops in the late stages of AIDS or in patients with untreated AIDS. When the disease involves the oral mucosa or visceral organs, low-dose liposomal doxorubicin can be effective

Notes on other soft tissue tumors

- Lipoma

Lipoma is the most common benign tumor and is found in about 1% of the population, usually in adults 40-60 years of age, but may occur in children. It can arise in any site of the body where fat is located. Superficial lipomas are soft, mobile and painless; most occur on the trunk, thighs and forearms. Microscopically, it is well-encapsulated and composed of fat cells.

• Liposarcoma

Liposarcoma is the second most common sarcoma in adults, with peak incidence in the age group 50-65. Although it can occur anywhere, it is most common on the thigh and in the retroperitoneum.

• Smooth muscle tumors

Benign smooth muscle tumors or leiomyomas are common in the uterus and gastrointestinal tract. Its malignant counterpart, leiomyosarcoma, occurs commonly in the retroperitoneum or intra-abdominal site, often growing to a large size.

• Malignant fibrous histiocytoma

This is the most common extremity sarcoma in adults. It usually occurs in the seventh decade of life, although younger adults can develop it. It presents as an enlarging, painless mass, usually in the lower extremity, followed by the upper extremity and the retroperitoneum.

• Angiosarcoma

Angiosarcoma may arise in either blood or lymphatic vessels. Hemangiosarcoma is usually located in the skin or superficial soft tissue. Angiosarcoma may occur in irradiated tissues, particularly the pelvis of women who had radiation therapy for gynecological cancers. Angiosarcoma of the breast is an uncommon condition with a tendency for local recurrences; it may metastasize to the lung. A cutaneous form of lymphoangiosarcoma, known as Stewart-Treves syndrome, can occur in the setting of chronic lymphedema of the arm following radical surgery and radiation for breast cancer.

DIAGNOSIS AND INVESTIGATIONS

The distinction between a benign and malignant soft tissue tumor is important, and this requires careful histological evaluation. In general, any soft tissue mass in an adult that is >5 cm or persists for more than 4-6 weeks requires a biopsy. A core biopsy is often satisfactory to allow a precise histological diagnosis and tumor grading, whereas a fine needle aspiration provides inadequate tissue for accurate assessment. When a biopsy is done, it must be planned so that subsequent surgery removes the site of the biopsy *en bloc* with the tumor. Careful attention to this detail reduces or eliminates the risk of tumor contamination of the nearby tissue planes.

Imaging studies for soft tissue sarcomas depend on the site of the lesion. MRI is best for evaluation of the primary tumor and involvement of local structures. Appropriate imaging studies are also required to rule out metastases. Patients with sarcomas of the extremities tend to develop lung metastases, while patients with retroperitoneal or visceral tumors are more likely to have liver metastases.

STAGING

The UICC/AJCC staging system is widely used. This includes the grade of the tumor, size of the lesion (≤5 cm or >5 cm), and presence of lymph node metastasis or distant metastasis.

T1	Tumor <5 cm
	T1a - superficial tumor
	T1b - deep tumor
T2	Tumor >5cm
	T2a - superficial tumor
	T2b - deep tumor
N0	No node involved
N1	Regional nodes involved
M0	No distant metastasis
M1	Distant metastasis present

Stage grouping

Stage	T N M	Grade
I	T1a, 1b, 2a, 2b N0 M0	Low
II	T1a, 1b, 2a N0 M0	High
III	T2b N0 M0	High
IV	Any N1 M0	High or Low
	Any N0 M1	High or Low

Note: The presence of lymph node metastasis is regarded as evidence of advanced disease.

TREATMENT

The complexity of management and the relative rarity of sarcomas make it desirable for treatment to be carried out in a major referral centre with a multidisciplinary team.

Surgery

Wide *en bloc* resection is the cornerstone of treatment for soft tissue sarcomas of the extremities or trunk. Sarcomas arising at other sites, such as the retroperitoneum, head and neck region or breast, require special consideration. The principle of surgery is adequate resection followed by radiation, if necessary.

Selected patients with limited lung metastases may benefit from surgical resection of these. The 5-year survival following pulmonary metastatectomy is about 30%.

Radiation therapy

Because of the risk of recurrence for large (>5cm) or high-grade sarcomas, postoperative adjuvant radiation is often recommended. Postoperative radiation is added for small or low-grade tumors if there is concern about the margins of excision. This situation arises in sarcomas of the head/neck or hands, where wide excision is often difficult to obtain. Radiation may also be used for unresectable lesions or in medically inoperable patients, but the results are not as good as surgical resection.

Chemotherapy

Because almost half of patients with sarcomas develop metastases, the use of adjuvant chemotherapy has been examined in many clinical trials. This may delay disease relapse, but it does not improve overall patient survival. Chemotherapy for advanced or metastatic sarcomas is palliative. The most commonly used drugs are doxorubicin and ifosfamide. A newer drug is trabectedin. For asymptomatic patients with slowly growing tumors, active surveillance and deferred treatment may be appropriate.

OUTCOME

The average 5-year survival is 60% after surgery. The prognosis for extremity sarcomas is better than that for sarcomas of the retroperitoneum, trunk or visceral organs. Generally, the prognosis is worse with:

- Tumor size >5 cm
- High-grade tumors
- Age >60 years
- Spread to lymph nodes or distant sites

SARCOMAS OF BONE

CLASSIFICATION

The classification of bone tumors is based on the cell type. Bone consists of cartilaginous, osteoid and fibrous tissues, and bone marrow elements. Tumors, both benign and malignant, can arise from all of these.

Classification

Type of tissue	Benign	Malignant
Cartilaginous	Osteochondroma Endochondroma	Chondrosarcoma
Osteoid	Osteoid osteoma Osteoblastoma	Osteosarcoma
Fibrous	Desmoplastic fibroma*	Fibrosarcoma
? Unknown	–	Ewing's sarcoma

may be locally aggressive, but does not metastasize

OSTEOSARCOMA

INCIDENCE

Osteosarcoma is rare, but it is the third most frequent malignancy in young adults after leukemia and lymphoma. Men are affected slightly more commonly. The disease usually involves the long bones, and the axial skeleton is rarely affected. It coincides with growth spurts in adolescents when the long bones show increased growth rates. The most common sites are bones of the knee joint (distal femur or proximal tibia) and proximal humerus. A second peak of incidence occurs later in life in those over 60 years, related to Paget's disease of the bone, where bone turnover rates are high.

RISK FACTORS

- Genetic factors
  - Li-Fraumeni syndrome, a germ-line mutation of the p53 gene. Other cancers that are part of this syndrome are those of the breast, brain, adrenal cortex and leukemia
  - Hereditary retinoblastoma
- Other factors
  - Chronic bone diseases, such as Paget's disease, benign bone tumors, fibrous dysplasia, chronic osteomyelitis, and sites of bone infarcts or implants
  - Previous treatment with radiation and alkylating drugs

PATHOLOGY

Macroscopic

Osteosarcoma forms a solid lesion that grows centrifugally. A pseudo-capsule may form, comprised of compressed tumor cells and fibrovascular tissue.

Microscopic

Osteosarcoma is a high-grade, spindle cell malignancy. The detection of osteoid or reactive bone in the background of sarcomatous cells confirms the diagnosis.

Molecular genetics

The genetics of osteosarcoma parallels that of retinoblastoma, and patients with hereditary retinoblastoma have a relative risk of 500 for developing osteosarcoma. In both, there is loss of the rb gene. In addition, loss of p53 has been detected in 25% of patients with osteosarcomas, and amplification of the MDM-2 gene, which is speculated to inactivate p53, has been described in about 20% of patients.

Growth pattern and spread

Osteosarcoma has a distinct pattern of growth. Initially, the surrounding normal tissues are compressed and bone is resorbed by osteoclasts. Later, the tumor invades and destroys adjacent tissues. Because bone lacks any lymphatic supply, metastasis is almost exclusively blood-borne. The lung is the most common site of metastasis, followed by other parts of the skeleton. High-grade sarcoma embolizes within the marrow sinusoids to form "skip" metastases. A skip metastasis shows up as a tumor nodule located within the same bone as the primary tumor, but not in continuity with it. This is infrequent and occurs in <1% of cases. Bone sarcoma may occasionally extend through an adjacent articular cartilage.

CLINICAL FEATURES

Local pain is the usual presenting symptom; this is frequently present for a few months and occurs at night.

Systemic symptoms are uncommon at presentation; lung metastases, when present, seldom cause respiratory symptoms.

Examination reveals a firm mass, fixed to the underlying bone. Swelling and deformity of the bone are present. The mass may be hot and red. There is usually no effusion in the adjacent joint, and range of movement of the joint is full. Pathological fracture is infrequent.

DIAGNOSIS

The technique used to obtain a biopsy must be carefully considered. A trephine or core biopsy is recommended, and it must be properly placed to allow subsequent excision of the biopsy site at surgery. A poorly placed biopsy can be a deciding factor whether an amputation or limb salvage surgery is needed. Because of this, it is preferred that the biopsy of a suspicious skeletal lesion be performed by the surgeon who will carry out the definitive surgical procedure.

INVESTIGATIONS

- Complete blood count: this may be normal or there may be an increase in the white cell count
- Biochemistry: serum alkaline phosphatase is elevated about 50% of cases. (Adolescents can have an elevated alkaline phosphatase during bone growth.) LDH may also be elevated
- Imaging studies
  - Plain films of the primary shows local destruction of bone with marked periosteal reaction with lifting of the cortex (Codman's triangle), and calcification in adjacent soft tissue ("sunburst"). A pathological fracture may be present
  - Bone scan is useful to rule out polyostotic involvement, metastatic disease and intra-osseous extension of the cancer
  - CT scan of the bone is useful to assess bone involvement
  - MRI is a good technique for assessing medullary marrow and extra-osseous extension and it is the investigation of choice
  - CT scan of the chest is useful for identifying lung metastases

STAGING

The commonly used staging system is the Surgical Staging System, which evaluates three parameters:
- Tumor grade
  - G1 – low grade vs. G2 – high grade
- Surgical site

This is designated intra-compartmental (T1) or extra-compartmental (T2), depending on whether the tumor is contained within an anatomic compartment bounded by the natural barriers to tumor extension.

- Presence of metastasis

Lymph node metastasis or distant metastasis (lymphatic spread is a sign of wide dissemination); this is designated as M1.

Stage	Grade	T stage	Metastasis
IA	G1	T1	M0
IB	G1	T2	M0
IIA	G2	T1	M0
IIB	G2	T2	M0
III	any	any	M1

TREATMENT

Surgery

Surgery is the main modality of treatment. Limb-sparing techniques are now practiced more widely for selected cases. Patients with lung metastases may benefit from surgical resection of these whenever possible.

Chemotherapy

About 85% of patients with osteosarcoma develop metastases if treated by surgery alone. With the addition of postoperative adjuvant chemotherapy, 70% of patients with osteosarcoma survive without recurrent disease. Most regimens now include doxorubicin and cisplatin with or without ifosfamide or methotrexate. Although there is no survival benefit for preoperative compared with postoperative chemotherapy, preoperative administration may permit a greater number of patients with extremity tumors to undergo limb-sparing procedures. Response to preoperative chemotherapy is a major prognostic factor. Five-year survival rates for patients with an extremity sarcoma and a "good" response to chemotherapy (>90 percent necrosis in the surgical specimen) are significantly higher than for those with a lesser response.

Radiation therapy

Radiation has a limited role, since the cancer is not radio-sensitive. However, for unresectable disease, high-dose radiation (60 Gy in 6 weeks), followed by chemotherapy, may be used. In certain sites, such as the spine, it is not possible to give high doses of radiation, since this dose exceeds the tolerance of the spinal cord.

Treatment of recurrent disease

Patients with lung metastases are candidates for surgical metastatectomy, especially if there are unilateral, few (<5) in number, and occur after a long disease-free interval. Surgery is followed by further chemotherapy. Those with bone metastases have a poorer prognosis.

OUTCOME

The average 5-year survival for non-metastatic extremity osteosarcoma is 65%. Patients with lung metastases have a 20% long-term survival following resection of the metastases. When osteosarcoma occurs in the setting of Paget's disease, the prognosis is poor with a 5-year survival of <10%.

EWING'S SARCOMA

Ewing's sarcoma is primarily a childhood disease. It is discussed in Chapter 19.

Chapter 17

HEAD AND NECK ONCOLOGY

Head and neck cancers include a wide variety of malignancies that arise from the mucosal lining of the upper aero-digestive tract. They comprise 5% of all new cancers. Most are squamous cell carcinomas, but cancers may also arise from other tissues including connective tissues (sarcomas) or lymphoid tissues (lymphomas).

LARYNGEAL CANCER

INCIDENCE AND RISK FACTORS

Cancer of the larynx affects middle-aged or older persons, mostly men, who have smoked tobacco and drank alcohol. The effects of these two factors are syngeristic. In addition to cigarette smoking and alcohol, other factors implicated in laryngeal cancer include voice abuse, chronic laryngitis, chronic gastric reflux, dietary deficiencies of some vitamins (A, C and E), fruits and vegetables, exposure to wood dust, asbestos and ionizing radiation. Human papillomavirus has been identified in laryngeal cancers, but a direct causal relationship is not confirmed.

PATHOLOGY

Macroscopic

The tumor forms an ulcer or grows as an exophytic lesion.

Microscopic

More than 95% of laryngeal cancers are squamous cell carcinomas. Other uncommon subtypes comprise sarcoma, adenocarcinoma and neuroendocrine tumor.

Spread

The site of the primary determines its pattern of spread.

• Glottis or vocal cord cancer

Lesions arising from the glottis or true cord, the most common site of origin of laryngeal cancer, usually infiltrate locally. The sparse lymphatic supply makes metastasis of early lesions unlikely.

• Supraglottic cancer

Supraglottic lesions also spread locally, but spread to the ipsilateral and contralateral cervical lymph nodes is common due to the rich lymphatic drainage.

• Subglottic cancer

Lesions arising in the subglottis are uncommon, but metastases to the cervical nodes occur in 30% of cases.

CLINICAL FEATURES

The presenting symptoms depend on the location of the cancer. Cancer of the glottis causes symptoms early as a result of distortion of the vocal cord. Hoarseness or a change in voice is an early symptom. Persons with a hoarse voice for more than four weeks should be examined for the possibility of an underlying cancer.

Supraglottic cancer may cause subtle symptoms, such as pain in the throat or referred pain to the ear. A scratchy sensation on swallowing or an intolerance to hot or cold foods may also be present. Hoarseness occurs in the more advanced stage of the disease when the large primary cancer directly invades the glottis.

Subglottic cancer is usually silent until the disease is at an advanced stage. Cervical lymphadenopathy may be the presenting complaint.

DIAGNOSIS

Routine laryngeal inspection confirms the diagnosis. Flexible laryngoscope permits a full examination of the entire larynx.

TREATMENT

• Glottis

Because cancer of the glottis causes symptoms early, diagnosis is made at an early stage of the disease. Carcinoma *in situ* is highly curable by micro-excision, laser vaporization or radiation therapy. For early stage invasive carcinoma, excellent local control is achieved by radiation or partial laryngectomy. Patients with more advanced local disease are managed by a combination of total laryngectomy and radiation with or without chemotherapy.

• Supraglottis

Early-stage cancer is curable by partial laryngectomy or by radiation therapy. For a more advanced lesion, total laryngectomy and radiation are required; the addition of chemotherapy may be considered. Because of the high probability of cervical nodal metastasis, radical neck dissection is generally recommended.

• Subglottis

Total laryngectomy and neck dissection, including thyroidectomy, followed by postoperative radiation are usually recommended. The cure rates are, however, low.

CARCINOMA OF NASOPHARYNX

INCIDENCE AND RISK FACTORS

Nasopharyngeal cancer is endemic in southern China and northern Africa and in Greenland Inuit. A common risk factor in these regions is the consumption of salt-cured food. Infection with Epstein-Barr virus is implicated in the development of nasopharyngeal cancer. Unlike other head/neck cancers, there is no clear association with alcohol or smoking. Persons with certain HLA loci (H2 locus, BW46 antigen or B17 antigen) are more susceptible to the disease. Nasopharyngeal carcinoma is more common in men than women (2:1 ratio) in the fifth or sixth decade of life. However, in endemic areas, the disease occurs at an earlier age, 15-25 years.

PATHOLOGY

Three types are recognized:
• keratinizing squamous cell carcinoma, type 1 – more common in Caucasians
• non-keratinizing carcinoma, type 2
• undifferentiated carcinoma, type 3 – most common in Asians and in endemic populations

Spread

Local spread of nasopharyngeal cancer has dire consequences. The infiltration may be mainly sub-mucosal, producing little evident mucosal change even though there is deep extension outside the nasopharynx. Extension can occur to the parapharyngeal space through the sinus of Morgagni; into the paranasopharyngeal space with involvement of the pterygoid muscle, leading to trismus; along the base of the skull with lower cranial nerve involvement; through the cavernous sinus with involvement of the cranial nerves III, IV and VI; and along the fascial planes surrounding the jugular vein and artery. Growth into the posterior orbit may also take place.

Lymphatic spread occurs to the posterior neck nodes (60-90%) or to bilateral neck nodes (50%). Another common pattern of spread is to the nodes in the retropharyngeal space.

Blood-borne spread occurs late, but is evident in

10% of patients at presentation. Bone is the most common site, followed by lungs, liver and extra-regional nodes.

CLINICAL FEATURES

Nasopharyngeal cancer often presents as a neck mass due to metastasis to cervical nodes. It may also cause tinnitus, reduced hearing due to blockage of the Eustachian tube, nasal obstruction, epistaxis and trismus. Lower cranial nerve palsies may be evident from extension of the disease to the base of the skull. Palsies of cranial nerves III, IV and VI signify further extension to the cavernous sinus.

Distant metastasis is uncommon at initial diagnosis. However, the majority of patients will develop distant metastases during the course of their disease, and this is the primary cause of death.

INVESTIGATIONS

Because of the propensity for deep spread, CT scan or MRI is important to define the local extent of the disease. PET scan may be helpful to assess involvement of nodes.

TREATMENT

Radiation therapy directed to the nasopharynx and both sides of the neck is the standard treatment. The role of surgery is limited as adequate margins cannot be attained. Palliative chemotherapy with a cisplatin-based regimen is indicated for fit patients with metastatic disease.

CARCINOMA OF TONGUE

INCIDENCE AND RISK FACTORS

Carcinoma of the tongue is one of the most common cancers of the head and neck region. It afflicts men more than women (3:1 ratio), and the median age of diagnosis is 60 years. It is increasing in young men, possibly due to marijuana use. In common with other head/neck cancers, inhalation of tobacco smoke from cigarette, cigars or pipes is a major risk factor. Heavy alcohol consumption acts synergistically with tobacco to promote development of these cancers. In addition, alcoholics have poor nutrition with deficiency of vitamins A and C, which could increase their cancer risk. Chronic irritation from poor dentition may lead to cancer at the site of trauma, usually on the lateral borders of the tongue.

PATHOLOGY

Macroscopic

Cancer of the tongue grows as an exophytic lesion or it may be infiltrative.

Microscopic

The histology is squamous cell carcinoma. Ulceration may be present.

Spread

Local invasion occurs into the deeper muscles or to adjacent structures.
Lymphatic spread is common to the jugulodigastric nodes. Bilateral nodal involvement occurs in 25% of cases.
Blood-borne spread is uncommon at diagnosis, but may occur in the later stages of the disease. Common sites of metastases are lungs and bone.

CLINICAL FEATURES

The main symptom at diagnosis is pain, although the lesion may be painless. A history of preceding leucoplakia may be obtained, especially in young women. Difficulty in speech or swallowing is occasionally present.

INVESTIGATIONS

- Examination of the ear, nose and throat (ENT) as well as indirect laryngoscopy
- X-rays to rule out invasion of the jaw bones
- Chest x-ray
- CT scan or MRI of the oral cavity and neck is useful to define the local extent of the cancer
- PET scan may be helpful to assess involvement of nodes
- Fine needle aspirate of any enlarged neck nodes can confirm metastasis

TREATMENT

- Anterior two-thirds of tongue

Small cancers can be treated by wide excision, brachytherapy or external beam radiation. Locally advanced lesions are managed by combined modality treatment, including radical surgery and radiation therapy with or without chemotherapy.

- Base of tongue

Small cancers can be resected, but larger lesions are managed by radiation therapy with or without chemotherapy.

- Lymph node metastasis at presentation

Two options are available:

- Surgical resection of the primary and the regional nodes
- Treatment of the primary by brachytherapy and surgical dissection of the neck nodes
- Unresectable or metastatic disease

This is an incurable situation. Palliative radiation and chemotherapy may be used to control symptoms.

CANCER OF TONSIL AND SOFT PALATE

RISK FACTORS

Cancers of the tonsil and soft palate share similar risk factors to other head/neck cancers.

PATHOLOGY

Most are squamous cell carcinomas. The oropharynx contains lymphoid tissues and lymphomas may occasionally develop at this site.

CLINICAL FEATURES

Tonsillar fossa cancer usually presents in the advanced stage of the disease. It often involves the base of tongue and lateral pharyngeal wall. The common symptoms are pain, dysphagia and a neck mass. Involvement of the pterygoid muscle causes trismus.

Soft palate cancer tends to be more indolent, and it is diagnosed at an earlier stage than tonsillar fossa cancer.

TREATMENT

Early stage disease

Surgical resection or radiation therapy is recommended.

Advanced disease

Advanced stage cancers require combined modality treatment with surgery and postoperative radiation therapy.

OUTCOME OF HEAD/NECK CANCERS

The cure rates for head/neck cancers are related to the site and stage of the disease. In the absence of lymph node metastasis, patients with early stage disease have 5-year survival of 70-95%, whereas for those with more locally advanced disease, the 5-year survival is only

20-30%. Metastasis to the regional lymph nodes reduces the probability of cure by more than half, but some patients may still be cured of their disease. Patients with distant metastases are seldom cured.

FOLLOW-UP OF HEAD/NECK CANCERS

With the exception of nasopharyngeal cancer, most recurrences of head/neck cancers occur within the first year. Prompt detection of recurrent disease may permit salvage therapy, such as surgery or radiation therapy. Cervical lymph node metastases may also be treated with curative intent.

In addition to disease recurrence, patients with head/neck cancers are at risk for developing a second primary cancer of the upper aero-digestive tract.

Overall assessment by clinical examination with attention to symptoms of pain, dysphagia and hoarseness, and examination of the primary site and regional nodes are recommended monthly for the first year, 3-monthly in the second and third years, 6-monthly in the fourth year, then yearly. Annual chest x-ray is recommended, and other investigations (e.g. CT scans or other x-ray studies) are done as required by clinical symptoms or signs. Patients with nasopharyngeal, base of tongue or laryngeal cancer should have fibre-optic endoscopy on each follow-up visit.

Chapter 18

CENTRAL NERVOUS SYSTEM ONCOLOGY

CLASSIFICATION OF BRAIN MASS

Non-neoplastic lesions

- Cerebral abscess
- Resolving cerebral infarct
- Giant aneurysm
- Arteriovenous malformation
- Cerebral contusion
- Radiation necrosis

Neoplastic lesions

Primary
- Intracranial neoplasm
- Spinal neoplasm

Secondary

The common sites from which brain metastases arise are lung, breast, kidney and skin melanoma.

PRIMARY CENTRAL NERVOUS SYSTEM TUMORS

INCIDENCE

Primary tumors of the central nervous system are uncommon, accounting for about 2% of cancer deaths. There is a bimodal distribution with an early peak from birth to age 4 years, and a steady increase in incidence after age 15 years, reaching a plateau by age 70 years. Central nervous system tumors are the most prevalent solid neoplasms of childhood, and the second leading cause of death in children younger than 15 years. Nonetheless, most intracranial tumors occur after age 45 years. The incidence is higher in men and in individuals in upper social classes. African-Americans have a higher incidence compared with Caucasians, but the international variation is not very striking.

RISK FACTORS

There are a few recognized risk factors, but for the majority of patients, none is present.
- Genetic factors

About 15% of patients with brain tumors have a positive family history, suggesting a hereditary predisposition. Brain tumors may also occur as part of other defined genetic syndromes, such as tuberous sclerosis, neurofibromatosis, Li-Fraumeni syndrome, Turcot's syndrome, Gorlin's syndrome, Sturge-Weber disease and von Hippel-Landau syndrome.
- Environmental factors

Proven risk factors
- Exposure to high-dose ionizing radiation
- Industrial exposure to vinyl chloride or benzene

Suspected but unproven risk factors
- N-nitroso compounds in tobacco smoke, cured meats and cosmetics
- Exposure to low-dose electromagnetic radiation (e.g. high current power lines) or radiofrequency radiation (e.g. mobile phones)
- Infective process

In patients with human immunodeficiency virus (HIV), primary CNS lymphoma is associated with Epstein-Barr virus.

PATHOLOGY

Primary brain tumors are diverse with over 50 different subtypes, most of which arise from the glial cells (astrocytes, oligodendrocytes and ependymal cells). Astrocytomas account for the majority of primary brain tumors and can be subdivided into three groups:

- low grade astrocytomas (Grades 1 and 2)
- anaplastic astrocytomas (Grade 3)
- glioblastomas (previously called glioblastoma multiforme or GBM) are grade 4 astrocytomas with high mitotic activity

Eighty percent of brain tumors occur intracranially, and 20% are spinal. In children, CNS tumors are predominantly located in the cerebellum, whereas in adults they are in the cerebral hemispheres.

The most common types are listed in Table 18.1.

Table 18.1 Frequency of primary central nervous tumors

Gliomas	66%
◆ Astrocytoma (58%)	
◆ Oligodendroglioma (5%)	
◆ Ependymoma (3%)	
Meningioma	9%
Pituitary adenoma	7%
Medulloblastoma	4%
Vascular tumors	2%
Others	12%

CLINICAL FEATURES

Intracranial tumors

Primary brain tumors tend to remain localized to the CNS. Symptoms are often nonspecific, and a distinguishing feature of brain tumors is that symptoms develop slowly, unlike vascular lesions such as bleeding or ischemia, which are acute in onset and rapid in progression. Even so, about 25% of patients with brain tumors present with seizure activity. A brain tumor should be considered in all patients with new onset seizure activity, particularly focal epilepsy. In general, the symptoms of an intracranial neoplasm are due to increased intracranial pressure or infiltration of normal brain tissue.

Increased intracranial pressure
The mass effect from the tumor itself or surrounding edema within the rigid boundaries of the skull results in increased intracranial pressure. The common presenting complaint is headache, which is due to stretching of the nerve endings in the dura mater. The headaches can vary in severity and quality, and occur in the early morning or on awakening. Some patients may complain of a discomfort in the head. Vomiting is also common, especially in children. Impaired consciousness follows with drowsiness, stupor and, finally, coma. Increased intracranial pressure leads to papilledema due to compression of some part of the ventricular system. An expanding tumor in one hemisphere causes a horizontal shift of the midline structures to the contralateral side. If left untreated, the brain stem is compressed. As this occurs, there is pressure on the third or sixth cranial nerves leading to palsy; this may be misleading as to where the lesion is actually located. Herniation of the brain stem follows with ptosis and ipsilateral enlargement of the pupil due to third nerve palsy. Later, the pupils become fixed. Extension spasm of the arms and legs occurs, and there is hyperventilation. Eventually, the corneal and pupillary reflexes are lost, the pupils become pinpoint, flaccid paralysis sets in and there is hypoventilation, followed by death.

Infiltration of normal brain tissue
Direct infiltration of the brain is the main mode of spread of brain tumors, and this is responsible for death in most patients. Neural tissues lack a lymphatic system and spread through the lym-

phatic system is, therefore, not observed. Distant metastases are very rare, but may occur with aggressive tumors that breach the dural veins. The location of the tumor determines what the symptoms and signs are (Table 18.2). Right-sided tumors in the non-dominant lobe of the brain generally present later than left-sided tumors.

Table 18.2 Common symptoms and signs of brain tumors

Supratentorial tumors

Frontal lobe	Changes in personality, such as apathy, occasional outbursts of aggression, lack of sense of responsibility in personal affairs, vulgarity in speech, slovenliness in personal habits
Temporal lobe	Hemianopia and aphasia
Parietal lobe	Contralateral motor and sensory abnormalities
Occipital lobe	Hemianopia and visual agnosia

Infratentorial tumors

Cerebellum	Ataxia, dysarthria, signs of increased intracranial pressure due to obstructive hydrocephalus and direct compression of brain stem
Brain stem	Focal cranial nerve signs, e.g. Bell's palsy, bilateral pyramidal weakness of extremities, hemi-sensory syndromes, gait disturbances, hiccups
Mid-brain	Cranial nerve signs (VI, VII, IX, X), dysarthria, head tilt and personality changes

Spinal tumors

Spinal tumors can be classified according to their origin in relation to the spinal cord anatomy. There are three categories: extradural, intradural-extramedullary and intradural-intramedullary.

• Extradural tumors

Extradural tumors include metastatic cancer (commonly lung, breast and prostate cancers, and lymphoma) or primary bone tumors (osteoma, sarcoma, plasmacytoma/multiple myeloma). Patients may present with localized spinal pain, which progresses to neurological deficits.

• Intradural-extramedullary tumors

Intradural-extramedullary tumors arise outside the spinal cord. Meningioma and nerve sheath tumors account for the majority of these lesions. Occasionally, seeding of the spinal or subarachnoid space may occur from a primary central neoplasm, e.g. medulloblastoma, ependymoma or lymphoma.

• Intradural-intramedullary tumors

Intradural-intramedullary tumors arise within the spinal cord, and they represent true spinal cord tumors. Most are astrocytomas or ependymomas.

From a clinical standpoint, there are two chief modes of presentation.

Spinal cord compression

When the tumor is located between the foramen magnum and the lower end of the spinal cord (at the level of L1-L2 vertebral bodies), it leads to cord compression with upper motor neuron deficits. Involvement of the long tracts within the cord causes weakness of the limbs with a sensory level corresponding to the location of the tumor, and bladder and bowel sphincter disturbance.

Cauda equina syndrome

When the tumor lies below the end of the spinal cord, the nerve roots are impinged, leading to lower motor neuron deficits. This presents as leg weakness, dermatome sensory loss and sphincter dysfunction.

DIAGNOSIS AND INVESTIGATIONS

Imaging studies

Once a brain tumor is suspected by clinical symptoms or signs, the diagnosis can be supported by imaging studies. Considerable progress has been made in imaging of the brain.

- CT scan can provide reliable information about cerebral tumors (Figure 18.1)
- MRI is more sensitive than CT, especially for lesions in the posterior fossa, spinal cord or leptomeninges. It has the advantage of imaging the sagittal and coronal planes and it is the investigation of choice (Figure 18.2)
- Angiography is useful for delineating the arterial blood supply to the tumor as a prerequisite to surgical management
- Positive Emission Tomography (PET) can provide useful information to complement CT scan or MRI

Biopsy

Definitive management of CNS tumors requires histological confirmation. For intracranial tumors, this is achieved by biopsy or concomitant with an open procedure for resection. If the tumor is unresectable because of its location in an eloquent area, such as the motor cortex, a stereotactic needle biopsy is indicated. Spinal cord tumors require open procedures for tissue diagnosis. Tumors of the skeletal spine can be biopsied by percutaneous needle techniques under image guidance.

Lumbar puncture for CSF cytology

Lumbar puncture may be useful when there is leptomeningeal invasion by providing CSF for cytological studies. (This must only be done when increased intracranial pressure is ruled out by fundoscopy and CT or MRI of the brain, since there is a high risk of coning – compression and herniation of the brain stem through the foramen magnum – if the intracranial pressure is high.)

Figure 18.1 CT scan of head. Right frontal lobe astrocytoma showing typical features of primary brain tumors: local mass effect, midline shift and hydrocephalus (top). There is minimal enhancement of the lesion with contrast dye (bottom)

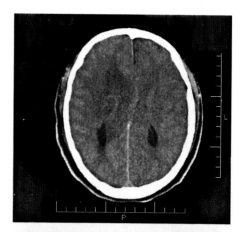

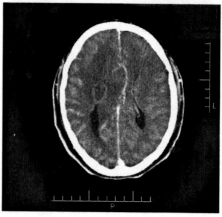

Figure 18.2 MRI of head demonstrating left cerebellar astrocytoma. T2 weighted axial image showing left cerebellar high-signal mass with local compression of brainstem (left). Post-Gadolinium T1 weighted image showing enhancement of lesion in left cerebellum and relationship to midline and cerebral hemispheres. Note hydrocephalus secondary to compression of the fourth ventricle (right)

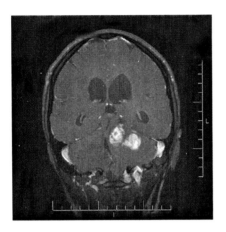 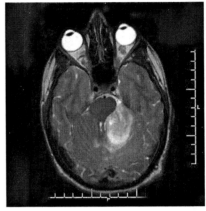

TREATMENT

Surgery

Surgical resection is the primary mode of treatment. While the goal is complete removal of the tumor, this may not be achieved, since the surgery must be planned to ensure the maintenance of adequate neural function. The poor regenerative potential of CNS tissues limits the amount of tissue that can be resected. When complete resection cannot be accomplished, tumor bulk reduction may be carried out, since this can delay the onset of compressive symptoms.

Radiation therapy

Most primary brain tumors are unifocal and, therefore, treatable by radiation therapy. Its major limitation is the tolerance of the surrounding normal tissue to radiation due to the risk of permanent neurological impairment. Recent advances in treatment planning and delivery have improved the results of radiation therapy. Conformal radiation uses multiple beams to conform to the tumor volume. This allows high doses to be given over several weeks without significant risk of late complications. An alternative to surgery is stereotactic radio-surgery. This is a specialized form of radiation that uses a focused beam of radiation to treat small lesions in a single treatment with sparing of the surrounding normal brain tissues.

Patients who undergo a gross total resection of high-grade gliomas have a high recurrence rate because of the infiltrative nature of the tumors. Postoperative radiation treatment extends the median survival from 5 to 11 months compared with surgery alone.

Chemotherapy

The nitrosoureas and temozolomide are the common drug used for brain tumors, but their role is limited. Temozolomide, an oral alkylating agent, is now favored for initial treatment of patients with malignant gliomas.

Chemotherapy and radiation provide an improved survival benefit for Grades 3 and 4 astrocytomas, compared with radiation alone. For Grade 4 astrocytoma, radiation with concurrent temozolomide, followed by 6 months of temozolomide gives a small 3-month survival benefit compared with radiation alone; the 2-year survival improves from 10% to 27%.

Other drug therapies

• Corticosteroids

Corticosteroids, especially dexamethasone, are often helpful in the alleviation of symptoms caused by edema that results from the tumor as well as surgery or radiation therapy. These drugs counteract the vasogenic brain edema and reduce the rate of trans-capillary water and albumin flow into the peritumoral tissue. The effect is usually apparent within 24-48 hours with improvement of neurological symptoms.

• Mannitol

In patients with acutely raised intracranial pressure, mannitol can reduce the pressure.

• Anticonvulsants

Seizures are common in patients with brain tumors, and those with a history of seizures should be treated with an anticonvulsant, such as phenytoin or carbamazepine. Other choices are phenobarbital and valproic acid. Because of the frequent presence of residual tumor, scarring from surgery or radiation, most patients require lifelong anticonvulsant therapy.

PROGNOSIS

Adverse prognostic factors for survival of patients with malignant astrocytomas are:
• neurological deficit at diagnosis
• older age (>50 years)
• KPS performance status <70
• high tumor grade (Grade IV)

The median survival for younger patients with a good performance status is 59 months for grade III tumors, and 18 months for grade IV tumors. The median survival for older patients with a good performance status is 37 months for grade III tumors, and 11 months for grade IV tumors. In contrast, the median survival for patients over 50 years with a poor performance status is only 18 months for grade III tumors, and 5 months for grade IV tumors.

BRAIN METASTASES

Brain metastases develop in more than 20% of all cancer patients, and they are far more common than primary brain tumors. Lung cancer (especially small cell lung cancer) and melanoma are the two most common cancers that metastasize to the brain. Other cancers that give rise to brain metastases include breast, kidney and testis. Cancers of the stomach and colorectum can give rise to brain metastases, but not commonly. Cancers of the prostate, bladder and ovary rarely metastasize to the brain.

In about one-third of cases, the brain metastasis is solitary, whereas in the other two-thirds there are multiple brain lesions. Surgery may be required to establish a tissue diagnosis if a solitary brain lesion is detected in a patient without a known history of cancer. Even in patients with known cancer, a craniotomy for resection of a single brain metastasis, followed by cranial radiation, may be advised if the anticipated life expectancy is over 6 months. While this may not be curative, such an approach can preserve the quality of life in these patients. Patients with a single brain metastasis have a 1-year survival rate of 40%, and a 2-year survival of 20%. Patients with multiple brain metastases have a poorer prognosis and, in general, the median survival is 3-4 months.

LEPTOMENINGEAL METASTASES

Spread of a cancer to the leptomeninges leads to diffuse involvement of the meninges around the brain and spinal cord. Leptomeningeal metastasis is more common with leukemia and lymphoma, but it is also a complication of other cancers, particularly breast cancer, small cell lung cancer and melanoma. It may present with headaches, vomiting, lethargy, confusion and radicular or back pain. Focal deficits due to cranial nerve or nerve root involvement are common. The diagnosis is confirmed by MRI and CSF cytology. Intrathecal or intraventricular injections of chemotherapy with methotrexate or Ara-C can clear the CSF of malignant cells in the chemo-sensitive cancers, such as lymphoma or leukemia. Leptomeningeal metastasis from breast cancer may also be treated in a similar fashion, but the results are not as good. Radiation therapy has a limited role, and is used to slow the progression of disease and relieve symptoms. The prognosis of patients with leptomeningeal metastases is poor with a median survival of <6 months.

SPINAL CORD COMPRESSION FROM VERTEBRAL METASTASES

Spinal cord compression can result from metastasis to the vertebral body. The common cancers that spread to the spine are those of the prostate, breast and lung. The onset of back pain is one of the first symptoms, and this complaint in a cancer patient should be taken seriously. The back pain is usually accompanied by a radiculopathy, and this is followed by epidural compression of the spinal cord. The course can be rapid or it may progress slowly over days or weeks. Occasionally, a complete transverse lesion of the spinal cord occurs due to occlusion of the artery. In this situation, the course is rapid with painless weakness of the legs. The diagnosis is confirmed by an MRI of the spinal cord. Treatment consists of high-dose dexamethasone. Radiation therapy to the involved spine is standard treatment. Vertebrectomy is considered in certain situations: disease limited to single level, spinal instability, progressive neurological deficit despite radiation, or if a histological diagnosis is needed.

Chapter 19

PEDIATRIC ONCOLOGY

Cancers are rare in children, with an annual incidence of 1.4 per 100,000 children under age 15 years. However, they are a major cause of mortality in this age group. The most common cancers in children are acute lymphoid leukemia and cancers of the central nervous system. Table 19.1 lists the common childhood cancers. The leukemias are discussed in Chapter 14, and brain tumors in Chapter 18.

Some childhood cancers have a well-defined genetic association, but the cause of most is unknown. The cancers are unique in their responsiveness to chemotherapy and high cure rates can be achieved. Management of cancers in this group must take into account the effects of treatment on growth and development of the child.

Table 19.1 Types of cancer in children in order of their frequency of occurrence

Cancer	Frequency
Acute leukemias	28%
Central nervous system tumors	20%
Bone and soft tissue sarcomas	15%
Neuroblastoma	7%
Non-Hodgkin's lymphoma	7%
Wilms' tumor	6%
Hodgkin's lymphoma	5%
Ewing's sarcoma	2%
Others	10%

NEUROBLASTOMA

INCIDENCE

Neuroblastoma is the most common intra-abdominal malignancy in children. It is more common in boys with the median age of diagnosis being 2 years.

PATHOLOGY

Macroscopic

Neuroblastoma arises from primitive sympathetic ganglion cells. The neuroectodermal cells that comprise these tumors originate from the neural crest during fetal development, and are destined for the adrenal medulla and sympathetic nervous system. The most common site is within the abdomen, and the adrenal gland accounts for almost 40% of cases. The tumor is an encapsulated, soft mass with areas of hemorrhage, necrosis, cystic degeneration and calcification.

Microscopic

Histologically, there are nests of neoplastic cells separated by fibrovascular septa. The tumor cells are uniform and round with hyperchromatic nuclei. An interesting feature is spontaneous maturation or regression of the tumor. Neuron specific enolase (NSE) stain is positive, but PAS is negative.

Neuroblastoma is one of the "small, blue, round cell" tumors of childhood. The other members of this group include lymphoma, Ewing's sarcoma, germ cell tumors, rhabdomyosarcoma and primitive neuroectodermal tumors (PNETs).

Spread

Local infiltration of surrounding structures is the common mode of spread.
Lymphatic spread to regional nodes may occur.
Blood-borne metastases are common to bone and liver. Lung metastasis is uncommon.

Genetics

Cytogenetic rearrangements observed include amplification of the N-myc oncogene, gain of the long arm of chromosome 17, and deletion affecting chromosome 1.

Prognostic factors

- Age

Children under the age of 1 year have a better prognosis than those above 1 year of age.
- Tumor marker levels

Patients with advanced stage disease who have a low VMA/HVA ratio of <1.5, NSE >100 ng/mL, and LDH >1000 IU have a lower survival rate.
- N-myc

Increased number of N-myc copies in the tumor cells is associated with poor prognosis.
- Tumor diploidy

Tumor diploidy is a poor prognostic sign, whereas hyperploidy carries a good prognosis.
- Serum ferritin

A high level (>142 ng/mL) at diagnosis is associated with a poor prognosis.
- Expression of nerve growth factors

High expression of nerve growth factors TRK-A is associated with an improved survival. (TRKs are tyrosine kinase receptor genes.)

CLINICAL FEATURES

Local growth leads to abdominal swelling or mass, which is the most common reason children come to medical attention. There may be bowel or urinary obstruction. Cancers arising in the head/neck region present as a painless mass. Neurological symptoms due to involvement of paravertebral sympathetic ganglia may occur.

Blood-borne metastases are present in two-thirds of children at diagnosis. These lead to bone pain or liver dysfunction.

Generalized symptoms are common. Fever is present in about 25% of patients at diagnosis. Anorexia, malaise and weight loss may occur. Normal sympathetic tissues secrete catecholamines, and most patients with neuroblastomas have elevated levels of catecholamines – vanillylmandelic acid (VMA), homovanillylic acid (HVA), norepinephrine, dihydroxyphenylalanine (DOPA), and dopamine. Excessive production of catecholamines causes flushing, palpitations, diarrhea and headaches.

Examination reveals an abdominal or neck mass. Tumors in the thorax can lead to venous obstruction with dilated neck veins and edema. Acute cerebellar signs may rarely be present. Spinal cord compression may occur due to extension of the tumor through the intervertebral foramina.

INVESTIGATIONS

- Complete blood count: this is usually normal, but extensive bone metastases can lead to pancytopenia
- Urinalysis
- Blood urea and creatinine
- Serum ferritin
- Urinary catecholamines
- Abdominal x-rays
- CT scan or MRI of abdomen
- Bone scan
- Bilateral trephine bone marrow biopsies and aspirates are important due to the high incidence of bone metastases
- MIBG scan (Meta-iodobenzyl guanidine is used as a precursor in catecholamine synthesis and when it is labelled with radioactive iodine, it can serve as a tracer in scanning)

STAGING

Evans or Children Cancer Group classification

Stage I   Tumor confined to site of origin

Stage II   Tumor extending beyond site of origin, but not crossing midline, including lymph nodes

Stage III   Tumor extending beyond site of origin across midline, including lymph nodes

Stage IV   Distant metastasis

Stage IVS   Infants (<2 years) with local tumor not crossing midline, but with liver, skin or bone marrow involvement

TREATMENT

Surgery

For limited stage disease, surgery alone can be curative. Postoperative radiation is given to older children (>1 year) or those with poor prognostic factors. For more advanced stage disease, surgical resection is followed by chemotherapy.

Radiation therapy

Neuroblastoma is sensitive to radiation, and it is used to reduce the frequency of local recurrence as well as eradicate microscopic and macroscopic metastases.

Chemotherapy

The drugs most commonly used are cisplatin, etoposide, cyclophosphamide, doxorubicin and vincristine. Response rates to chemotherapy are low and efforts to improve the results now examine the use of autologous bone marrow transplant (ABMT). Patients with N-myc amplification or high-stage disease have a substantial risk of recurrence and should be considered for ABMT.

Other therapy

Biological therapy with agents such as retinoids is also used when there is minimal disease left after surgery to promote differentiation of the malignant tumor to a benign tumor. MIBG can be used to deliver radioactive iodine directly to the tumor cells in patients with recurrent disease.

OUTCOME

The prognosis for localized disease is good with high cure rates. Almost all children with Stage I disease and 80% of those with Stage II disease are cured. Those with Stage IVS also have a good prognosis with an 80% cure rate. For older patients with metastatic disease, however, the prognosis is poor with cure rates of 10-40%.

WILMS' TUMOR

INCIDENCE

Wilms' tumor (nephroblastoma) is a rare renal cancer in children under 15 years of age. It is slightly more frequent in girls. The mean age of diagnosis is about 45 months for those with unilateral tumors, and 30 months for those with bilateral tumors.

RISK FACTORS

• Genetic factors

A familial association is seen in 2% of cases.

• Associated congenital conditions

Wilms' tumor is associated with other congenital conditions, such as Bloom's syndrome, aniridia, hemi-hypertrophy, cryptorchidism, hypospadias, and Beckwith-Weidemann syndrome.

PATHOLOGY

Macroscopic

The tumor forms a mass in the kidney. Five percent are bilateral. It can be lobular and it is surrounded by a pseudo-capsule. There are areas of necrosis, hemorrhage and cysts within the tumor.

Microscopic

There is marked cellular diversity with varying amounts of three cell types: blastemal, stromal and epithelial. Monomorphic epithelial variants have a better prognosis, whereas tumors with anaplastic areas, especially if these are diffuse rather than focal, are associated with a worse prognosis.

Wilms' tumor must be distinguished from clear cell sarcoma and rhabdoid tumor of the kidney, both of which follow a more aggressive course.

Spread

Local invasion from the renal parenchyma to the renal pelvis and renal vein is the common mode of spread.
Lymphatic spread is infrequent.
Blood-borne metastases occur commonly to the lung.

Genetics

Several chromosomal abnormalities are associated with Wilms' tumor. They include trisomy 8, and deletions on chromosomes 1, 11 and 16.

CLINICAL FEATURES

Local growth leads to abdominal swelling or mass, accompanied by abdominal pain. Gross hematuria occurs in 20% of cases. A tumor thrombus in the inferior vena cava or renal vein may cause a varicocele.
Blood-borne metastases to the lung rarely cause symptoms.
Generalized symptom: Fever may be present.
Examination reveals an abdominal mass. Hypertension, due to increased levels of renin, occurs in about 25% of patients.

STAGING

National Wilms' Tumor Study Group Staging system

Stage I   Tumor confined within the capsule of the kidney and completely resected
Stage II   Tumor extends beyond the capsule of the kidney, but completely resected
Stage III Residual tumor is present in abdomen after surgery
Stage IV   Blood-borne metastases present
Stage V   Bilateral kidney involvement

INVESTIGATIONS

- Complete blood count: anemia may be present
- Blood urea and creatinine
- Urinalysis: proteinuria and hematuria may be present
- Abdominal ultrasound
- Real-time ultrasonography to check the patency of the inferior vena cava
- Chest x-ray and chest CT scan to rule out lung metastases

TREATMENT

Surgery is the major treatment modality. Wilms' tumor is responsive to radiation therapy, and this is used in locally advanced cases when there is residual local tumor after surgery. The tumor is sensitive to several chemotherapeutic drugs, including actinomycin D, vincristine, doxorubicin, etoposide and cyclophosphamide.

Treatment is determined by the stage of the disease and histological grade of the tumor as follows:

Stage I favorable or anaplastic histology, or Stage II favorable histology
  Surgery followed by chemotherapy
Stage III favorable histology
  Chemotherapy and postoperative whole abdominal radiation
Stage IV favorable histology
  Chemotherapy; abdominal radiation if there is residual local tumor; those with lung metastases receive whole lung radiation
Stages II- IV anaplastic histology
  Chemotherapy; all patients receive abdominal radiation; patients with lung metastases receive whole lung radiation
Stage V
  Nephrectomy of the more involved kidney and partial nephrectomy of the smaller lesion in the remaining kidney. This is followed by chemotherapy and radiation

OUTCOME

Wilms' tumor is chemo-sensitive and radio-sensitive, and the prognosis is, therefore, good. For Stages I and II disease, the cure rate is 80-90%. In the presence of distant metastases, the cure rate is lower, about 40%.

MEDULLOBLASTOMA

INCIDENCE

Medulloblastoma is the most common intra-cranial tumor in children under the age of 15 years and they make up 25% of pediatric CNS tumors. The peak age is 3-5 years.

RISK FACTORS

There are no known risk factors. Medullo-blastoma may arise in association with Gorlin's syndrome.

PATHOLOGY

Medulloblastoma belongs to a family of tumors called primitive neuroectodermal tumors or PNETs. If present in the posterior fossa, they are designated medulloblastoma. In the supra-tentorial compartment, they are generally referred to as PNETs. (Ependymoblastoma and pineoblastoma are other tumors of the PNET group.)

Macroscopic

Medulloblastoma originates in the cerebellum or brainstem.

Microscopic

The cells arise from primitive neural tissues and form a characteristic rosette or circular pattern with varying degrees of differentiation. They stain positively with S-100.

Spread

Local spread through the cerebrospinal fluid (CSF) is common with blockage of the fourth ventricle or aqueduct. Tumor deposits occur in the meninges within the skull and spinal cord. *Blood-borne* metastasis to the bone occurs rarely.

CLINICAL FEATURES

With its location in the posterior fossa, symptoms are those of increased intracranial pressure (headaches), and those related to the cerebellar tracts (difficulty in walking). Not infrequently, the early symptoms are insidious, and irritability and failure to thrive are observed by parents. Spread through the CSF can lead to nerve root compression with weakness of the arms or legs.

Examination reveals cerebellar signs: ataxia, in-coordination and dysarthria. Meningeal deposits of the tumor can lead to cranial nerve palsy or weakness of the limbs. Obstruction of CSF flow causes hydrocephalus with signs of increased intracranial pressure.

INVESTIGATIONS

• CT scan or MRI of the head and spine
MRI is better than CT scan, especially for assessing the posterior fossa. Spinal MRI also demonstrates any spinal deposits.

STAGING

There is no standard staging, but two groups of children are recognized, based on prognostic factors.

Factor	Good risk	Poor risk
Age	>3 years	<3 years
Extent of disease	no spread	metastatic disease
Tumor excision	total or <1.5 cm³ residual tumor	subtotal or >1.5cm³ residual tumor

TREATMENT

Medulloblastoma is treated by surgical re-section. A temporary external ventricular drain is required until the CSF pathway is restored. Postoperative radiation is given to the cranium and spinal cord due to the propensity of the tumor to spread through the cranio-spinal axis. In good risk patients, a lower dose of radiation is used in combination with chemotherapy in an attempt to decrease the late complications of radiation. For poor risk patients, high-dose radiation and chemotherapy are required.

OUTCOME

The overall long-term survival is 50-70%.

EWING'S SARCOMA

Ewing's sarcoma was first described as an undifferentiated tumor of bone, but less commonly it arises in soft tissue. Both are part of a group of tumors called Ewing's sarcoma family of tumors or EFT. This family also includes the more differentiated peripheral primitive neuro-ectodermal tumor or PPNET. Both bone and soft tissue tumors share common chromosomal translocations.

INCIDENCE

Ewing's sarcoma is a rare tumor of children and young adults with a peak incidence in the second decade. It is more common in males and more prevalent in Caucasians.

RISK FACTORS

There is no recognizable risk factor.

PATHOLOGY

Macroscopic

Ewing's sarcoma may affect any bone and it involves the extremities and central axis equally. It arises within the medullary cavity of the diaphysis and grows subperiosteally.

Microscopic

Sheets of small, round, "blue" cells, rich in glycogen, are present.

Spread

Local extension occurs through the cortex of the bone into the soft tissues. A marked periosteal reaction occurs with successive layers being formed, giving rise to an "onion peel" appearance on x-rays.
Lymphatic spread is very uncommon.

Blood-borne metastasis can occur, most commonly to the lungs, but may also affect the bone marrow or bone (spine).

Genetics

Ninety percent of Ewing's tumors are associated with rearrangement of the EWS gene on chromosome 22, most commonly with the FLI-1 gene on chromosome 11. This leads to a fusion protein which promotes tumor growth. A similar effect occurs when a second translocation between chromosome 21 and chromosome 22 is present. CD99 surface marker is characteristic of Ewing's sarcoma.

CLINICAL FEATURES

Local growth frequently causes pain or a mass. A pathological fracture may be present in some patients.
Lymphatic spread is very rare.
Blood-borne spread is present in about 25% of patients at diagnosis, mainly to the lungs, bone marrow and bone. Liver metastasis is very uncommon.
Generalized effect: Fever is present in 20% of patients at diagnosis.
Examination reveals a tender mass which can be large.

DIAGNOSIS

A biopsy of the mass is required to confirm the diagnosis. This should be planned to allow subsequent excision of the biopsy site during definitive surgery.

INVESTIGATIONS

- Complete blood count: this may be normal or the white cell count may be raised
- Serum biochemistry: alkaline phosphatase is raised. LDH may also be elevated
- X-ray of bone shows a lytic lesion in the diaphysis and the typical onion peel appearance
- Radionuclide bone scan to evaluate the entire skeleton for multiple lesions
- Chest x-ray or CT scan of chest is required to rule out lung metastasis
- CT scan is useful to assess the primary and associated bone destruction
- MRI of the bone provides detailed information of the primary tumor and possible invasion of marrow
- Bone marrow biopsy to exclude widespread metastatic disease

TREATMENT

Ewing's sarcoma is a chemo-sensitive and radio-sensitive cancer, and it is usually treated by a multimodality approach. The standard chemotherapy is a combination of vincristine, doxorubicin and cyclophosphamide, alternating with ifosfamide and etoposide. After an induction course of chemotherapy, radiation is delivered at a dose of 50-60 Gy over 5-6 weeks. Surgery is an alternative to radiation when the involved bone (rib or fibula) is "expendable."

Treatment of patients with clinically detectable metastatic disease and those who relapse after initial therapy also require multimodality therapy. Up to 40 percent of patients with limited pulmonary metastatic disease who undergo intensive chemotherapy and pulmonary resection with or without radiation therapy may be long-term survivors. The prognosis for other subsets of patients with advanced disease is less favorable.

OUTCOME

The 5-year survival is 70-80% for non-metastatic disease. Favorable prognostic factors include sites in distal bones or ribs, tumor <100 mL, young age, normal LDH and good response to initial chemotherapy.

Long-term follow-up is needed because disease relapse, treatment-related complications and second malignancies are common beyond five years after treatment.

EMBRYONAL RHABDOMYOSARCOMA

INCIDENCE AND RISK FACTORS

Embryonal rhabdomyosarcoma is the commonest soft tissue sarcoma in children, with two-thirds of cases occurring under the age of 6 years. The tumor is part of Li-Fraumeni syndrome and it is also associated with Beckwith-Wiedemann syndrome.

PATHOLOGY

Macroscopic

Embryonal rhabdomyosarcoma arises commonly in the head and neck region, including the orbit, or genitourinary tract. The botryoid variety originates in the mucosa of the vagina or urinary bladder, and forms polypoid masses, likened to a bunch of grapes.

Microscopic

The tumor cells are embryonal, rich in glycogen. Myofibrils are evident within the tumor.

Genetics

The DNA content is variable, ranging from diploid to hyperploid, and there is a specific deletion at chromosome 11p15, which is distinct from other forms of rhabdomyosarcoma.

Spread

Local growth is rapid and the tumor spreads along the tissue planes.
Lymphatic spread can occur, especially in those tumors arising in the genitourinary tract.

Blood-borne metastases occur early and up to 20% of patients have bone marrow metastases at initial diagnosis.

CLINICAL FEATURES

Symptoms depend on the site of the primary. Usually there is a painless, enlarging mass. Visual disturbances may accompany those tumors arising in the orbit; nasal obstruction and epistaxis occur with tumors in the head/neck; hematuria with bladder tumors; and vaginal bleeding with those arising in the vagina or uterus.
Signs also depend on the site of the primary and a mass may be evident. A fleshy mass at the introitus may be seen with vaginal botryoid tumors.

DIAGNOSIS AND INVESTIGATIONS

- Imaging studies
  - Chest x-ray may show lung metastases
  - CT scan and MRI of the primary site define the local extent of the tumor
- Bone marrow examination
- Biopsy of the affected site is essential to confirm the diagnosis

TREATMENT

Embryonal rhabdomyosarcoma is managed by multimodality therapy. The tumor is chemosensitive and chemotherapy, consisting of vincristine, actinomycin D and cyclophosphamide (VAC), is given to all patients, followed by definitive surgery or radiation. Chemotherapy is then continued for up to 1 year.

OUTCOME

The prognosis is generally good with an overall cure rate of 80%. However, the prognosis is less favorable when there is distant metastasis with cure rates <20%. Patients with tumors arising in the orbit, paratesticular region or vagina have a better prognosis than those with tumors in the parameninges, prostate or perineum.

Chapter 20

CANCER OF UNKNOWN PRIMARY SITE

DEFINITION

Patients with a histologically confirmed meta-static cancer in whom the primary site is not evident after a careful history, full physical examination, tumor marker measurements, chest x-ray and an imaging study of the abdomen and pelvis belong to this category.

INCIDENCE

About 2.5% of all cancer patients have metastatic cancer of unknown primary site. The incidence increases with age, and it occurs with equal frequency in men and women. On post-mortem examination, the lung and pancreas are the most frequent sites of the primary, but in about one-half of patients a primary site is not identified.

CLINICAL CONSIDERATIONS

The common cancers – lung, breast, colorectal, prostate and pancreas – should always be considered as the condition may represent an uncommon presentation of a common cancer. The next step is to rule out curable cancers (e.g. germ cell tumors or lymphomas), or treatable cancers (e.g. breast, prostate, thyroid or ovary) for which therapy can provide good palliation. Particular attention should, therefore, be placed on the history to rule out the possibility of these malignancies. The presence of "B" symptoms may suggest a lymphoma or back pain in a young man may be a clue to a retroperitoneal mass due to lymph node metastases from a primary testicular cancer. A thorough and complete physical examination is essential, including an examination of the lymph node-bearing regions (cervical, Waldeyer's ring, epitrochlear, supraclavicular fossae, axillae and groins), prostate, testis, thyroid, breast and pelvic organs. In certain situations, regional nodal spread from head/neck cancer, skin melanoma, anal or vulvar cancer may represent a potentially curable disease.

INVESTIGATIONS

- Hematology/biochemistry: complete blood count, renal and liver function tests
- Tumor marker assays can be helpful in providing a clue to the possible primary site of the cancer. A reasonable panel includes CEA (GI cancers), CA19-9 (upper GI cancers), CA125 (ovarian cancer), CA15-3 (breast cancer), PSA (prostate cancer), and hCG or alpha-fetoprotein (germ cell tumors)
- Imaging studies
  - Chest x-ray
  - CT scan of the abdomen and pelvis (useful to assess pancreas and ovaries)
  - Mammograms should be done where a primary breast cancer is a possibility, although breast cancers seldom present in this manner
- Others
  - Fecal occult blood as a preliminary screen may be useful for patients with abdominal symptoms

The results of these tests may give a hint of the possible primary site and guide further investigation, but multiple tests are to be avoided, since the diagnostic yield is poor. However, a limited number of investigations are justified to rule out certain cancers, whose identification has therapeutic implications.

PATHOLOGY

A careful pathological assessment is mandatory to guide treatment. The histology can be useful in pointing to the possible primary site (Table 20.1).

Table 20.1 Possible sites of primary cancer based on histology

Histology	Possible sites of primary
Adenocarcinoma	Lung
	GI tract
	Ovary
	Breast
	Prostate
Squamous cell	Lung
	Head and neck
	Esophagus
Small cell	Lung
Poorly differentiated	Lymphoma
	Germ cell
	Neuroendocrine tumor
	(GI tract or pancreas)

An open biopsy or a core biopsy is often required, and fine needle aspiration biopsy may be insufficient. Accessible sites of disease, such as peripheral lymph nodes, are best for obtaining adequate tissue for diagnosis.

When the diagnosis is not clear from routine pathology examination, special immunohistochemistry can be helpful in establishing the likely diagnosis among the common epithelial cancers (Table 20.2). They can also suggest the diagnosis in up to 25% of patients with malignancies, such as germ cell tumors, lymphomas and neuroendocrine tumors. In addition, cytogenetic studies can be of value in some cancers, particularly those in children, where specific chromosomal abnormalities have been identified; these include Ewing's sarcoma (t11;22), non-Hodgkin's lymphoma ((t8;14) and rhabdomyosarcoma 9(t2;13).

Table 20.2 Immunohistochemistry in primary unknown cancer

IHC test	Possible sites of primary
Alpha-fetprotein	testicular, liver
Alpha-1 antitrypsin	liver
Calcitonin	medullary cancer of thyroid
CA125	ovary
CA19.9	pancreas, stomach
CA15.3	breast
CD117 (c-kit)	GI stromal tumors
CEA	GI (especially colorectal)
CK7/CK20 profile (cytokeratin 7/20)	colon
Chromogranin	neuroendocrine tumors
Desmin	leimyosarcoma, rhabdomyosacrcoma
Estrogen receptor	breast
GCDFP-15 (gross cystic disease fluid protein-15)	breast
HCG	testicular
Leucocyte common antigen	lymphoma
Melan A (melanoma antigen)	melanoma
Myoglobin	rhabdomyosarcoma
Neurone-specific enolase	neuroblastoma, primitive neuroectodermal tumors
Pancytokeratin/epithelial membrane antigen	squamous cell
PSA	prostate
S100	melanoma, small cell lung
TTF-1 (thyroid transcription factor-1)	lung
Thyroglobulin	follicular cancer of thyroid
Vimentin	sarcoma
WT-1 (Wilms' tumor-1)	ovary

SPECIAL SITUATIONS

There are certain clinical situations for which useful treatment is available and should, therefore, not be overlooked.

- Axillary nodes in a woman may be due to a breast cancer. If the disease is regional with no distant metastatic disease, potentially curative therapy can be offered. Hormone receptor assay can be helpful
- Lytic-blastic bone lesions in a woman with an adenocarcinoma are most likely due to a breast cancer. Chemotherapy or hormone therapy directed to breast cancer should be considered
- Metastatic adenocarcinoma in the lungs, liver or retroperitoneal nodes associated with blastic bone lesions in a man may be of prostatic origin. Serum PSA measurement may confirm the diagnosis
- Abdominopelvic adenocarcinoma or malignant ascites in a woman with elevation of CA125 is presumptive evidence of an ovarian cancer, and chemotherapy protocols for this type of cancer can produce meaningful clinical remissions
- In the presence of a midline tumor (mediastinal and retroperitoneal nodes) with a poorly differentiated histology, a germ cell tumor should be considered. The tumor specific markers (hCG and alphafetoprotein) may be negative. In such cases, immunohistochemical stains for lymphoma must be negative. Cisplatin-based chemotherapy is advised for these patients
- An uncommon syndrome of carcinoma of the retroperitoneum, mediastinum, lungs or lymph nodes with the histological findings of a poorly differentiated neuroendocrine tumor is responsive to chemotherapy with cisplatin and etoposide
- Squamous cell cancer of an inguinal node

may be from a perineal, anal or genital cancer. Careful examination of these sites for a primary tumor is required. Surgical excision followed by radiation therapy is recommended

- Squamous cell cancer of cervical nodes likely arises from a primary in the head/neck area. This requires a full ENT examination, including fibre-optic endoscopy. Even if a primary is not detected, radical radiation to include the pharynx is recommended. This may be followed by radical neck dissection in selected patients

These special subgroups represent only the minority of patients with a primary unknown cancer. More commonly, patients present with metastases to the lungs, liver or bone. When the lesion is solitary, a thorough search for other sites of disease is required. In some cases, these solitary lesions may, in fact, be an uncommon primary cancer, such as cholangiocarcinoma (liver) or plasmacytoma (bone). If no other site of cancer is found, aggressive local treatment by surgery or radiation is justified. However, the most common presentation of unknown primary cancer is multiple metastatic deposits in the lungs or liver. The histology is usually adenocarcinoma.

TREATMENT

Treatment for primary unknown cancer is generally unsatisfactory due to the widespread nature of the disease at presentation. Treatment must, therefore, be carefully selected to provide maximum benefit and avoid unnecessary toxicity. This takes into consideration the probable site of the primary cancer, based on the clinicopathological assessment, and the extent of the metastatic disease. A fit patient with squamous cell cancer confined to the cervical lymph nodes may be a candidate for radical surgery and radiation, whereas an elderly person with a poor performance status and widespread adenocarcinoma of the lungs or liver may well be considered for palliative measures to relieve symptoms.

Local complications, such as pain, obstruction or bleeding may be managed by radiation or palliative surgery. Patients with spinal cord compression require urgent assessment to ensure prompt treatment by radiation therapy or neurosurgical decompression to enhance the chance of neurological recovery.

Chemotherapy has a limited role and appropriate choice of drugs and careful selection of patients for treatment are important to avoid unnecessary toxicity. The decision about chemotherapy is guided by the patient's age, general condition, and site and extent of the metastatic disease (e.g. predominantly nodal vs. visceral). In the presence of widespread visceral metastases and a poor performance status, chemotherapy is unlikely to provide any meaningful benefit, and symptomatic measures are indicated. For those who are deemed fit for drug therapy, empiric chemotherapy with drugs that have a broad spectrum of activity, such as cisplatin-gemcitabine or carboplatin-paclitaxel, may be considered.

Hormone therapy may be offered to those with suspected cancers of the breast or prostate with the expectation of a favorable medium term outcome.

OUTCOME

The outcome is determined by certain adverse prognostic factors:
- male gender
- adenocarcinoma histology
- visceral organ involvement (vs. lymph node)
- involvement of liver
- increasing number of organs involved

For the majority of patients with metastatic adenocarcinoma of primary unknown site, the prognosis is not good with a median survival of about 6 months, and less than 25% of patients are alive at 1 year. A few with germ cell tumor or lymphomas can live for a long time and may be cured.

Chapter 21

ONCOLOGICAL EMERGENCIES

The morbidity experienced by cancer patients is usually the result of the disease process itself or the complications of treatment. There are several conditions that pose a threat to the patient's well being, and it is important that these are recognized promptly and managed appropriately.

INFECTIONS

Anticancer therapy often affects both cell-mediated and humoral immune systems, leaving patients at high risk for infections. A decrease in the granulocyte count below 1.0 x 10^9/L increases the risk of infections. Several cancer drugs also cause mucositis, permitting entry of potential pathogens into the blood. The concurrence of granulocytopenia and mucositis is, therefore, particularly worrying. Patients with a temperature above 38.5°C persisting over 2-6 hours must be assumed to have an infection until proven otherwise. In the face of granulocytopenia, a careful systematic assessment is necessary. This includes a full history and physical examination with attention to signs of inflammation that could be a clue to the site of infection. In particular, the mouth and perineal area must be inspected to rule out an incipient infection. Not uncommonly, however, patients with granulocytopenia may exhibit minimal signs of infection. Other causes of fever in this setting include drug fever, especially from drugs like bleomycin and Ara-C, or tumor fever due to tumor necrosis. Febrile reaction to blood products may also occur, but its temporal relationship to the onset of the fever is usually evident.

The evaluation of fever in a cancer patient should include blood counts and chemistry (electrolytes and creatinine), chest x-ray, urinalysis, cultures of blood and urine, and any other relevant source of an infection, such as indwelling venous catheters. If a source of infection is not readily apparent, a broad spectrum antibiotic should be prescribed if there is concomitant granulocytopenia. A fourth generation cephalosporin, e.g. cefepime, or a carbapenem, e.g. imipenem, is an appropriate choice. Granulocyte colony-stimulating factors (G-CSF) can accelerate hematopoietic recovery after chemotherapy, and they are indicated in patients with fever and granulocytopenia.

Patients with persistent fevers for more than seven days despite antibiotics require a reassessment to rule out a new infection or an unusual causative organism, such as fungus, parasite or virus. An antifungal agent, e.g. amphotericin B or fluconazole, may be started empirically in these situations.

Special situations

- Patients with Hodgkin's lymphoma are more susceptible to infection due to their compromised immune system even when in remission
- Patients with splenectomy are at risk for infections by encapsulated organisms, e.g. *Streptococcus pneumoniae, Hemophilus and Neisseria*. They should receive prompt antibiotic treatment if they develop fever or signs of infection. Immunization of these patients against these organisms is advised
- Anaerobic infection should be considered in patients with damage to the GI tract mucosa. Typhlitis or necrotizing colitis of the cecum is an uncommon but serious condition due to infiltration of the cecum by

anaerobic organisms, like *Clostridium septicum*, and gram negative organisms, mainly *Pseudomonas aeruginosa*. Patients present with right lower quadrant abdominal pain, which rapidly becomes generalized and is associated with fever and diarrhea. Prompt antibiotic coverage and surgery are required

- Immunocompromised patients are prone to viral infections (herpes zoster and cytomegalovirus), and an antiviral agent, like acyclovir, should be started if these organisms are identified or suspected
- Patients with acute leukemia or those on chronic steroid therapy are susceptible to *Pneumocystis carinii*. Prophylactic trimethoprim-sulfamethoxazole may be considered

HYPERCALCEMIA

Hypercalcemia is a potentially life-threatening condition caused by circulating humoral factors (parathyroid-like hormones, prostaglandins or osteoclast-activating factors) produced by cancers. These lead to increased osteoclastic activity with release of calcium from bone. A corrected plasma calcium concentration >2.6 mmol/L defines hypercalcemia. Hypercalcemia occurs particularly in lung, breast and prostate cancers and myeloma.

Patients present with anorexia, polydipsia, polyuria, nausea and vomiting, constipation, confusion, seizures and coma. Symptoms can be severe at first presentation depending on the rapidity of increase of the serum calcium levels. The first line of treatment is normal saline with furosemide diuresis. A bisphosphonate, such as pamidronate or etidronate, which stabilizes osteoclastic activity, can be helpful in controlling the serum calcium levels in most patients.

SYNDROME OF INAPPROPRIATE ANTI-DIURETIC HORMONE SECRETION

The syndrome of inappropriate anti-diuretic hormone secretion is most common in patients with small cell lung cancer, and it is caused by ectopic secretion of the anti-diuretic hormone (ADH) by the tumor. This leads to hyponatremia and water retention, resulting in serum hypo-osmolarity. In most cases, the process is chronic with slow disturbance of the water-electrolyte balance, and symptoms can be mild. Common symptoms are fatigue, nausea, irritability and confusion. If the process is rapid, patients can experience profound confusion, seizures and coma. For mild to moderate cases (serum Na^+ >120), fluid restriction to <1 L/day may correct the imbalance. If symptoms are more severe with serum Na^+ <120, intravenous normal saline with furosemide is required to promote free water excretion. Oral urea, which causes an osmotic diuresis and, therefore, removes free water, may be used in severe cases. Demeclocycline and lithium carbonate, which interfere with the renal action of ectopic ADH, are useful ancillary measures. Management of the underlying cause is important for the long-term control of the syndrome.

SUPERIOR VENA CAVA SYNDROME

Superior vena cava syndrome (SVCS) is caused by reduction of venous return to the right side of the heart due to obstruction of the superior vena cava by a pulmonary or mediastinal mass. The most common cancer responsible for SVCS is lung cancer, but it may also occur in patients with mediastinal lymphoma, esophageal cancer or metastases to the mediastinal lymph nodes from breast or testicular cancer. Infrequent causes of SVCS are thrombosis due to an indwelling venous catheter or benign diseases, such a retrosternal goiter. Patients often complain of a band-like tightness around the head, followed by the appearance of periorbital edema (usually worse in the morning), facial swelling, and shortness of breath. The presence of stridor indicates a serious situation. Examination reveals periorbital edema, engorged conjunctivae, dilated neck veins and dilated collateral veins over the chest and arms. Chest x-ray or CT scan demonstrates a thoracic mass. Treatment of the underlying malignancy is necessary for long-term control of SVCS, but oxygen and high-dose corticosteroids (e.g. dexamethasone) can bring about some relief of symptoms in the acute situation. Because the most common cause of SVCS is small cell lung cancer, which is a chemo-sensitive disease, chemotherapy (cisplatin and etoposide) can produce rapid tumor reduction and symptomatic improvement. Radiation therapy may also be considered in urgent situations. Unless there is severe respiratory compromise, it is preferable to obtain a tissue diagnosis before embarking on treatment with chemotherapy or radiation. In refractory cases, a vascular stent can be inserted.

SPINAL CORD COMPRESSION

Spinal cord compression is a medical emergency, which occurs in up to 3-5% of cancer patients. Prompt diagnosis and management are essential to prevent irreversible neurological damage. The most common cancers associated with spinal cord compression are those of the lung, breast and prostate; other tumors include renal cell cancer, melanoma and lymphoma.

The cause is frequently tumor involvement of the vertebral body, and less commonly involvement of the paravertebral or epidural spaces. Lesions above L1, the lower end of the spinal cord, causes upper motor neuron signs, while lesions below this level produce lower motor neuron signs and perianal numbness. The most common site of compression is the thoracic spine (60%), followed by lumbosacral spine (30%) and cervical (10%).

The usual early presenting symptom is pain localized to the involved vertebral body, which may be present for days to weeks. New onset of back pain, especially if it radiates around the chest like a band, should be a warning sign of a possible spinal cord complication. Neurological symptoms and signs follow, often with vague sensory symptoms, leg weakness and numbness in the legs. Sphincter motor dysfunction leading to urinary retention and constipation occurs later. The neurological deficits can progress rapidly to paraplegia. CT scan or MRI of the spine often confirms the diagnosis.

Treatment with high-dose corticosteroids should be initiated, followed by radiation therapy or surgery with decompression laminectomy. Radiation is indicated if the cancer is radio-sensitive or if there are several levels of compression. It is also advised when patients are unfit for surgery. Surgical decompression is recommended if the cancer is radio-resistant, the spine is unstable, the cervical cord is involved, the compression is severe or if there is a solitary vertebral metastasis. Surgery also offers the opportunity to obtain a biopsy and may be advised if the histology is uncertain.

TUMOR LYSIS SYNDROME

This is an uncommon complication precipitated by chemotherapy of bulky, chemo-sensitive tumors, such as leukemia, lymphoma and myeloproliferative disorders. The acute lysis of tumor cells results in severe metabolic disturbances with hyperuricemia, hyperkalemia, hyperphosphatemia and hypocalcemia. The syndrome leads to renal failure, and cardiac arrhythmias can occur due to electrolyte imbalance. Preventive measures are advised when treatment of these high-risk tumors is started.

Hydration and alkalinization of the urine to pH >7 by sodium bicarbonate as well as pretreatment with allopurinol are advised. In severe cases with rapid progression to renal failure, dialysis may be required. Close monitoring of the blood electrolytes, uric acid, phosphorus, calcium and creatinine permits early recognition of the syndrome.

Chapter 22

GENERAL APPROACH TO PAIN MANAGEMENT

Pain is one of the symptoms most feared by cancer patients and it is important to reassure them at the outset that there is effective treatment. About one-third of patients report pain at the time of diagnosis of their cancer, and the prevalence in advanced stages of the disease is about 75%. The impact of pain on patient's physical and psychological well-being and social functioning can be gauged by quality-of-life assessments that are now commonly used.

A number of patients may also express fears of drug addiction or tolerance, especially to the opioids like morphine. Proper education of patients and their families can be reassuring.

Several mechanisms can be responsible for pain in cancer patients:
• Infiltration or compression of nerve
• Involvement of soft tissue
• Treatment-related e.g. post-mastectomy pain or radiation-induced inflammation

Broadly, there are two types of pain. Pain due to stimulation of nerve receptors is nociceptive pain, while that due to damage of the nerves is neuropathic. Recognition of which type of pain a patient is experiencing is important in selecting the appropriate therapy.

CLINICAL ASSESSMENT OF PAIN

Cancer pain is chronic and distinct from acute pain of trauma or postoperative pain. The initial evaluation of cancer pain includes a detailed history of the location, nature and intensity of the pain; a physical examination, including a full neurological examination; psychological assessment; and appropriate diagnostic tests to elucidate its cause.

Evaluating pain intensity is a good first step in the assessment. An ordinal scale in which patients rate their pain from 0 (no pain) to 10 (worst pain) is helpful in communicating pain intensity and evaluating changes over time. When the character or intensity of pain changes, reassessment may disclose another cause. It is not infrequent that another disease process, such as infection or gallstones, may be responsible, and this possibility should not be overlooked.

The ABCDE system, developed by the Agency for Health Care Policy and Research, is a good tool.

A   Ask about pain regularly. Assess pain systematically
B   Believe the patient and family in their reports of pain and what relieves it
C   Choose pain control options appropriate for the patient, family and setting
D   Deliver intervention in a timely, logical and coordinated fashion
E   Empower patients and their families. Enable them to control their course to the greatest extent possible

TREATMENT

Pharmacologic management

Three pharmacologic classes of drugs are used in the management of pain: nonsteroidal anti-inflammatory agents, opioids and adjuvant treatment. An important consideration in the management of cancer pain is the prescription of analgesics around the clock and not "as required," since the aim is the prevention of pain.

Acetaminophen and nonsteroidal anti-inflammatory drugs or NSAIDs

These are suitable for mild to moderate pain and may also be used in conjunction with opioids.

- Acetaminophen 500 mg every 4 hours orally. The combination of acetaminophen and codeine is particularly useful in mild to moderate pain. This does not irritate the gastric mucosa or cause platelet dysfunction
- Ibuprofen 600-800 mg every 6-8 hours orally. This, however, may not be suitable for patients with GI ulcer disease or renal insufficiency
- Because of their anti-platelet properties, aspirin and NSAIDs are often avoided in cancer patients who are also receiving chemotherapy

Opioid analgesics

Opioids are indicated for moderate to severe pain. Patients whose pain is not controlled by a nonopioid analgesic should be switched to an opioid analgesic without delay. Morphine is the usual first choice for treatment of cancer pain, but other commonly used drugs include hydromorphone, fentanyl and oxycodone. Methadone may be indicated when pain control is not optimal with these drugs. Table 22.1 shows the usual doses and analgesic equivalence for commonly used opioids. All opioids can cause constipation, although fentanyl and methadone less so, and stool softeners and other measures are required.

- Morphine comes as a short-acting analgesic whose dose is titrated to achieve pain control. A usual starting dose is 10-20 mg orally every 4 hours, but this dose can be escalated to ensure adequate pain control. Preparations that extend analgesia for 8-12 hours are available, and patients may be switched to the long-acting formulations when their daily analgesic requirement is determined. For chronic cancer pain, long-acting opioids may be appropriate for initial treatment. To deal with occasion break-through pain, patients on long-acting morphine should be prescribed short-acting morphine, usually 10-15% of their daily dose equivalent, on a 2-hourly basis. Morphine sometimes causes confusion, especially in the elderly. If this occurs, oxycodone or fentanyl is a better choice
- Hydromorphone is a good alternative to morphine and is recommended for patients who are unable to tolerate morphine. A long-acting formulation is available
- Fentanyl is a potent opioid analgesic available as a trans-dermal patch, which is applied for 48-72 hours duration
- Oxycodone is often combined with other drugs, e.g. acetaminophen and aspirin, for analgesia. It is also available alone in short-acting and long-acting preparations Oxycodone may be a good choice for patients who are reluctant to take morphine
- Methadone can provide good analgesia. Its long half-life can lead to its accumulation, which can be a problem in elderly patients.
- Meperidine, which is a common analgesic for surgical patients, is not recommended for treatment of cancer pain. Its active metabolite can accumulate and lead to adverse side effects, including seizures, in patients who receive it for more than a few days

Adjuvant drugs

Adjuvant drugs are used in conjunction with standard analgesics to enhance their therapeutic efficacy as well as provide some analgesic action on their own. There are several types of drugs that are useful adjuvants.

- Corticosteroids exert a number of beneficial effects: mood elevation, stimulation of appetite, reduction of nausea/vomiting. They also are useful for the acute pain due to pathological fractures
- Tricyclic antidepressants, such as amitriptyline, can help in the control of neuropathic pain by potentiating the effects of opioids
- Anticonvulsants may reduce neuropathic pain, especially those that are burning or lancinating. Gabapentin is commonly used for this
- Neuroleptics, e.g. methotrimeprazine, have been used as an adjuvant in chronic pain

- Local anesthetics can be effective in controlling neuropathic pain

Non-pharmacologic management

Certain measures not requiring drugs may be of value in pain management in selected patients.
- TENS: trans-cutaneous electrical nerve stimulation can be helpful in neuropathic pain
- Specific nerve blocks
- Neurosurgical procedures, such as cordotomy, rhizotomy or thalamotomy
- Massage therapy with use of heat and cold to tender areas

Table 22.1 Approximate analgesic equivalents for opioids

	Approximate equivalent dose compared with morphine 10 mg IM		Usual starting dose for moderate to severe pain	
	Oral	Parenteral	Oral	Parenteral
Morphine	20-30	10	15-30 mg q3-4h	10 mg q3-4h
Hydromorphone	4-6	2	2-4 mg q4h	1-2 mg q2-4h
Oxycodone	15-20	na	10 mg 3-4h	na
Codeine	200	100	60 mg q3-4h	60 mg q2h
Fentanyl	na	0.07-0.1*	na	25µ/hr
Methadone	2-4	na	2-5 mg q8h	na

* trans-dermal patch of fentanyl that delivers 25µ/hr is roughly equianalgesic to 90 mg of morphine given orally in a 24-hour period

INDEX